WHAT TO EXPECT®
BEFORE YOU'RE EXPECTING

By Heidi Murkoff
and Sharon Mazel

Foreword by Charles J. Lockwood, MD,

Chair, Department of Obstetrics, Gynecology, and Reproductive Sciences, Yale University School of Medicine

SIMON & SCHUSTER

London · New York · Sydney · Toronto

A CBS COMPANY

To Emma and Wyatt, my greatest expectations
To Erik, my everything
To Arlene, with so much love, always and forever
To all the mums and dads, and babies everywhere

First published in 2009 by Simon & Schuster UK Ltd
A CBS COMPANY

1 3 5 7 9 10 8 6 4 2

Simon & Schuster UK Ltd
1st Floor
222 Gray's Inn Road
London
WC1X 8HB

www.simonandschuster.co.uk

Simon & Schuster Australia
Sydney

Book design: Janet Parker
Interior illustrations: Karen Kuchar

A CIP catalogue copy for this book is available
from the British Library.

ISBN: 978-1-84737-705-0

Printed and bound in Finland by
WS Bookwell

Contents

Part 1: Getting Ready to Make a Baby

Part 2: Making a Baby

Part 3: Bumps on the Road to Baby

Part 4: Keeping Track

Thanks Again

So, here I am again – about to deliver yet another book. Or should I say . . . another baby. As I'm pretty sure I've pointed out before (about a hundred and seventy-two times), gestating a book is very much like gestating a baby (and I know this because I've gestated both more than once). And not just for the obvious reasons – both take a lot of work, both keep you up at night and get you up way too early in the morning, both can bring you joy one mument and stress the next – but also because you can't (strictly speaking) create them by yourself.

My human babies, Emma and Wyatt, were created with the most wonderful man in the world – my husband, best friend, soul mate, and partner in all things, Erik. My book babies, well, that's a team effort with a much bigger team – and this new baby is no exception. Some members are new to the What to Expect team, but many have been by my side since book one.

More than I can say, thanks to Arlene Eisenberg, my first partner in What to Expect and my most important one. Your legacy of caring, compassion, and integrity lives on forever; you'll always be loved and always be remembered.

For all your valuable contributions, I thank:

Suzanne Rafer, my long hopefully-not-suffering-too-much editor, for talking me down, pumping me up, and letting me play with my words . . . a lot. And more than that, for your friendship and xo, Suz.

Peter Workman, for giving What to Expect the very best publishing home, Workman Publishing (not to be confused with a publishing house – like they say, a house is not a home without some love, and no one loves publishing books like Peter). And Walter Weintz, for everything you – and the whole sales team – do for What to Expect, which is a lot – books don't sell themselves, after all!

All of the rest of the What to Expect team (many more than I can name), including David Matt, for always getting "it" – and somehow, always getting "it" on paper. You manage to make my artistic vision come to life, even before I've figured out what it looks like. And for bringing us Tim O'Brien – creator of cover mums so radiant and babies so adorable that they almost make me want to run out and get pregnant again . . . thanks, Tim.

Karen Kuchar, for clearly and beautifully illustrating the art and science of conception (and for making reproductive parts look so pretty!). Janet Parker, for thinking outside the design box, and to Barbara Peragine for fitting in all those boxes. Peggy Gannon for your flow mojo – and for understanding (I hope) that I can never leave well enough alone. Julie Primavera and Monica McCready for your phenomenal production values (on time, on time, and – did I mention? – on time). And my many wonderful friends at Workman, some old, some new, all treasured: Suzie Bolotin, David Schiller, Jenny Mandel, Page Edmunds, Emily Krasner, Kristin Matthews, Erin Klabunde, Pat Upton, Andrea Fleck-Nisbet, Melissa Possick, and Melissa Broder.

Sharon Mazel, for being the only person in the world (besides Erik) who can finish my sentences (which really comes in handy sometimes) and read my mind (which we both know is a scary thought, in more ways than one). You light up my life, and my AOL (a day without e-mail from you is a day without sunshine – fortunately, those days are few and far between). You're my partner in pun crime, my BFF, and my mini-me – and I love you. Jay Mazel, as always, for filling in medical blanks – and sharing more than half of your better half with me. Daniella, Arianne, Kira, and Sophia, for raising yourselves when your mum and I have a deadline – which, let's face it, is most of the time. How is it I've watched you grow up, but never met you?

Dr. Charles Lockwood, our amazing medical adviser, for knowing it all (somehow, even before anyone else does), keeping us honest and accurate, and caring about pregnant women (and not-yet-pregnant women) as much as we do. Thanks for your insight, your wisdom, your eagle eye-for-medical detail – and for all your invaluable contributions to team What to Expect.

Steven Petrow (my beloved MG), Vince Errico (dimples), Mike Keriakos (TBD), Ben Wolin (ditto), Jim Curtis (CSOB), the amazing (how do you do it all?) Sarah Hutter, Nancy Cross Schimmel, and all my other incredibly awesome friends at Waterfront Media, for making virtual miracles happen every day. I love you all! And to the remarkable community of mums and dads (especially our den mums and dads) that makes WhatToExpect.com my very favourite home away from home – thanks for being part of the What to Expect family.

Marc Chamlin, for always being there for me, always protecting me, always caring for me, and always knowing when I need a little L&S (if you know what I mean, Marc), and Alan Nevins, for managing the unmanageable (is there anything you can't put on a spreadsheet?), putting out fires, cleaning up messes, and picking up pieces – in short, for being the best agent a girl could ever have.

Molly Lyons and Fran Kritz for getting us just the facts, ma'am. All the doctors who have lent their preconception know-how, including Jeremy Groll, MD, Frederick Licciardi, MD, and Shahin Ghadir, MD. And Dr. Howie Mandel, for always having time to talk obstetrics during my annuals (even though I'm not pregnant). The marvellous Lisa Bernstein, who long ago shared my dream of healthy pregnancies and babies for all – a dream that the What to Expect Foundation is making a reality for more and more mums (with the help of Energizer Bunny/mum of Bluebell, Ruth Turoff). And how could I forget Zoe, Oh-That-Teddy, and Dan Dubno?

Erik, the love of my life (in fact, I can't remember having a life before you, and couldn't imagine one without you), for taking care of business and taking care of me. One day, I promise: you, me, and a two-week holiday. Emma and Wyatt, for making me one very happy mama (how did I get so lucky twice?). I love you both so much.

My fabulous family – father Howard Eisenberg, sister Sandee Hathaway (and Tim, Rachel, Ethan, and Liz), brother Evan Eisenberg (and Freda and Sara-Xing), Victor Shargai (and always, John Aniello), Abby and Norman Murkoff (the best MIL and FIL), and Deborah and Bob Wall – for your love and support.

ACOG, the CDC, the March of Dimes, and all the other health-care organizations that have recognized the importance of preconception prep – and have committed to helping women and their partners have healthier pregnancies and healthier babies before they even start trying to become pregnant. As always, thanks, too, to all the doctors, midwives, and nurses who care for mums – and wannabe mums. And speaking of which, here's to all mums and all dads – present and future!

Foreword

By Charles J. Lockwood, MD

THE ANITA O'KEEFE YOUNG PROFESSOR OF WOMEN'S HEALTH
AND CHAIR, DEPARTMENT OF OBSTETRICS, GYNECOLOGY, AND REPRODUCTIVE SCIENCES,
YALE UNIVERSITY SCHOOL OF MEDICINE

As an obstetrician practising in the twenty-first century, I have plenty of sophisticated procedures and high-tech equipment at my disposal to help me help mothers-to-be have healthier pregnancies and healthier babies. Ultrasound allows me to visualize a pregnancy's progress and a baby's development. Doppler helps me locate and amplify the tiniest of heartbeats. Fetal heart rate monitors enable me to assess a baby's health inside the uterus. And I can order a lab-full of tests to screen for birth defects and identify risk factors to help minimize the risks they pose.

But, do you know what I've always wished I had on hand? A piece of equipment – not currently available in even the most high-tech medical catalogues – that might prove an OB's most effective tool in optimizing pregnancy outcome. One that can prevent many complications. One that can help every pregnancy get off to the best potential start, even before sperm and egg met up.

I wish I had a time machine.

With a time machine, I could turn back the clock on the many women who show up at my office door *after* they're expecting, or after they've started trying to expect. Women who've come into their pregnancies with a less than ideal lifestyle, less than perfect control of medical problems, or less than model nutritional status, all of which can lead to less than perfect pregnancies. Most of these issues could have been minimized or even completely avoided with a few preconception modifications – stop smoking or drinking alcohol; a change in treatment plan for a chronic illness, such as diabetes, depression, or high blood pressure; a change in diet; increased exercise and a decrease in weight. Women who've waited a little too long to begin their families, or those who have waited too long before seeking help with their fertility issues could benefit from time travel as well.

Well, I've finally got my time machine, and now so do you: *What to Expect Before You're Expecting*. It's the book to read *before* the journey of pregnancy begins – not only before sperm meets egg, but before you've stopped your birth control and begun trying to conceive. It's a complete, medically sound preconception programme designed to prepare both your bodies for a healthy conception, and mum's body for a healthy gestation and a healthy baby.

It's all here, everything that I'd tell you if you showed up at my practice door before you started trying to conceive. The book reviews everything that doctors and major medical associations emphatically concur couples should address in the preconception phase. It emphasizes all the guidelines for a healthy preconception protocol such as the habits that should be kicked now and the ones that should be jump-started, the prepregnancy value of good nutrition and the right amount of exercise, and the importance for both prospective parents of achieving your optimal body mass index, or BMI (women who are overweight or too thin are more likely to have trouble conceiving and, if they do conceive, are more likely to experience pregnancy and childbirth complications) – and how to best achieve it. The book highlights the significance of lifestyle: why you and your partner should quit smoking now; how too much caffeine can impact your ability to get and stay pregnant; which precautions you should take at the workplace; which vitamins to take and which to avoid; which preconception tests you might need and which you can skip; which medications are safe to take while you're trying to conceive and which will have to be tweaked; when to see your doctor; when to turn to a reproductive specialist; which gynaecological and medical conditions can interfere with fertility; and which treatments may help you conceive.

The chapters on getting pregnant are a complete how-to of conception, packed with practical advice, fascinating trivia, and a lot of empathy and humour. Did you know sperm can retain their fertilizing potential for up to 6 days in a woman's genital tract, while if a newly released egg isn't fertilized within 12 to 24 hours pregnancy may not happen? Or that it takes less than an hour for a sperm to reach the egg and fertilize it? Or that more boys are conceived in October? Or that a woman smells more appealing to her mate when she's ovulating? The book will help you pinpoint ovulation, facilitate conception, and test for pregnancy, while debunking many common conception myths. The emotional side and relationship issues couples often encounter while trying to conceive, as well as ways of overcoming the stress that can occur when conception takes longer than expected, are also covered throughout.

Dads are included, too. Since their role in conception is vital, and not only in the obvious way, each chapter contains many helpful hints on how men can best contribute to a healthy pregnancy and a healthy baby, including how a prospective father's diet, exercise, lifestyle, and medical issues can sometimes significantly impact conception and a healthy pregnancy.

Comprehensive, medically up-to-the-minute and accurate, reassuring, and reader-friendly, *What to Expect Before You're Expecting* is the one resource that will fully prepare you and your partner for one of life's most miraculous experiences, at the time when preparation will benefit your future baby most: before you're expecting.

So my advice? Put time on your side before you conceive. Use this book to give your pregnancy the healthiest head start possible.

What Can You Expect Before You're Expecting
(And why does it matter, anyway?)

Pregnancy, as you probably know, is nine months long (or thirty-eight weeks from conception, if you're really serious about keeping count). And if you've ever been pregnant before, you probably think that's plenty long enough. Maybe even a little too long, especially once your belly's the size of a prize-winning watermelon and your breasts have worked their way through the cup alphabet . . . twice.

But is nine months really long enough? Does that time-honoured baby-making timetable really stand up to the latest obstetrical science?

According to more and more research – and more and more experts – the answer is, maybe not. From the Centers for Disease Control and Prevention (CDC) to a growing body of health professionals – including the American College of Obstetricians and Gynecologists, the March of Dimes, American College of Nurse Midwives, the American Academy of Pediatrics, and the American Academy of Family Physicians – that traditional nine-month figure is being challenged by a surprising new suggestion: It's time to add more months to pregnancy.

That's right, more months. At least three more months, in fact, for a full year (or even more) of baby making. But before you panic (three extra months of not seeing my feet? Of passing on the sushi? Of waiting to hold that bundle of joy?), here's what you need to know: Those extra months aren't meant to be spent being pregnant, they're meant to be spent *getting ready* to be pregnant.

The truth is, a healthy pregnancy begins before sperm and egg meet up. Before the home pregnancy test announces the good news. Before the queasies kick in and your waistline checks out. Even before you ditch your diaphragm or peel off your patch. A healthy pregnancy begins before you're expecting – which is why, if you're planning to get pregnant, you might want to start planning (and prepping) ahead.

And here's how. *What to Expect Before You're Expecting* – a complete, start-to-cuddly-finish preconception plan – is everything you need to know, and everything medical experts recommend you do, to get your body and your partner's body into the best baby-making shape possible before you start baby making. What baby-friendly foods to order up often, and which fertility-busting foods – and drinks – to keep off the menu. (Hint: Get your sushi while you can, but can the tuna.) How to get your weight where it needs to be for maximum fertility and optimum pregnancy health (packing on too many pounds – or too few – can compromise conception and complicate pregnancy). Which medications need to be shelved (including some surprises, like antihistamines), when to toss your birth control, why your partner should put hot tubs (and spinning classes) on ice, why kicking your smoking habit now can give fertility a boost (while protecting your future baby's health). How healthier mums and healthier dads can create healthier pregnancies and healthier babies.

Once you've prepped for pregnancy, it's baby-making time. Sounds like the easy (and fun) part – and sometimes it is. But a little conception know-how can help you fast-track your fertility and make those baby dreams come true sooner. You'll find out how to pinpoint ovulation, when to schedule in sex, how sex toys and lubes fit in, why wet isn't wild when it comes to baby-making sex, how to keep on-demand sex spicy – plus the lowdown on sex positions and conception. Have you heard a few conception tales already, or read them on the Internet? Fertility fiction and fact are sorted out here, too.

What if you encounter a bump on the way to baby? Fertility challenges – and how to overcome them – are covered, as well as the latest in fertility treatments, from the low tech (nutritional therapies) to the high tech (IVF and more). You'll also find out when to let nature take its course, and when to seek help.

Whether you've begun your conception campaign already, or you're just starting to think about getting pregnant, it's never too late – or too early – to start optimizing your preconception profile, giving the baby of your dreams the healthiest possible start in life. So put time on your side, and add a few months to your baby-making calendar. More pregnancy, it turns out, is more.

May all your greatest expectations come true!

heidi

PART 1

Getting Ready to Make a Baby

Prepping Before You're Expecting

A RE YOU GEARING UP FOR A PREG- nancy? Preparing for baby mak- ing isn't only about tossing your birth control (though you'll need to do that), charting your ovulation (you'll probably want to do that), and head- ing to bed (you'll be happy to do that). It's also about getting your body – and your spouse's body – into tip-top baby- making shape. From the drinks you and your partner-in-procreation sip to the medications you take, from the habits you're best off kicking to the vitamins you're best off popping – tak- ing charge of your preconception prep will start you off on the right foot, mak- ing conception easier (hopefully) and pregnancy safer and more comfortable (ditto). So before you dive into bed to make that baby, dive into this chapter to find out what steps you should consider taking first.

Talk the Talk

A re you TTC? You probably are, if you're reading this book – yet you may not have the slightest idea of what "TTC" means (it's short for "trying to conceive"). Lots of fertility acronyms have become part of preconception- speak (check out any fertility website or message board and you'll get an eyeful), and they pop up frequently throughout this book, too. Feel a little out of the preconception lingo loop? You'll find a full glossary of preconception acronyms in the fertility planner section (see page 254), but to get you started, here are the most commonly used ones:

TTC: trying to conceive

AF: Aunt Flo(w) – in other words, your period

BD: baby dance – aka, sex

O (or the Big O): ovulation

Your Health Prep

It stands to reason that your overall health has a lot to do with your overall fertility. After all, it takes a healthy body (make that two healthy bodies) to make a healthy baby. Which means there's no better time than now – when that baby-to-be is just a gleam in your hopeful eyes – to make sure that you and your partner are healthy overall. Just about every aspect of your health – from the medications you take, to the immunizations you should have, to the chronic conditions that need controlling and the dental work that needs doing – can have an impact on your fertility and on your healthy pregnancy to come. So check it all out, starting with those checkups.

Preconception Checkups

"I'm young, in good health, and my periods are regular. Do I really need to see a doctor before I start trying to get pregnant?"

The best prenatal care starts long before conception (and doesn't stop at your reproductive parts), so now's a great time to schedule that full-body tune-up. Even if you've never had a sick day, it's easier to tackle health issues before baby's on board than to play catch-up after your body is already baby building (and this preconception prep is more essential still if you're living with a chronic condition). To make sure all systems are go, make an appointment with your GP – and believe it or not, with your dentist, too – for complete preprenatal checkups.

General health checkup. First up, a trip to the doctor who tends to your general health. On the agenda:

For Dads Only

Making a baby is always a two-person production (one from column Mum, one from column Dad). But as is often the case with pregnancy, preconception can be pretty female-centric. It shouldn't be. Both partners in conception have their work cut out for them before sperm meets egg. Though this entire book will be enlightening for prospective parents of both sexes, the shaded boxes throughout provide tips, advice, and information specifically geared to wannabe dads. So if you're looking to become a father, look for these just-for-you boxes. You'll find a full listing of dad-centric topics under "male" in the Index.

▢ A weight check. Because your prepregnancy weight has a lot more to do with your fertility and pregnancy health than you probably think, you'll be stepping right up to the scale for a baseline weight check. If that bottom line isn't where it should be (close to the ideal weight for your size and body type), your doctor will help you set some goals to get your weight conception-ready. See Chapter 2 for more on your weight and fertility.

▢ A thorough physical. All the top-to-bottom basics will be covered, so get ready to open up wide, take those deep breaths, and stick out your arm for a blood pressure reading.

▢ A medication overview. Whether it's over-the-counter or prescription, discuss all the drugs (as well as vitamin and herbal supplements) you take. Depending on the medication (some are safe during pregnancy, others may not be), a change may be in the cards.

- A blood test. Nobody's favourite part of the checkup, but your practitioner may want to draw blood to check for the following. You'll likely need many of these tests once you get pregnant anyway, so you might as well get a head start on them now – they may not need to be repeated if you conceive within a few months of this workup.

  - Haemoglobin or haematocrit to use as a baseline during pregnancy and to test for anaemia (many women have lower iron stores than they think, thanks to that monthly flow)

  - Rh factor, to see if you are positive or negative. If you are negative, your partner should be tested to see if he is positive.

  - Rubella titre, to check for immunity to rubella (German measles)

  - Varicella titre, to check for immunity to varicella (chicken pox)

  - Urine, to screen for urinary tract infection and kidney disease

  - Tuberculosis (if you're in a high-risk group)

  - Hepatitis B (if you're in a high-risk category, such as being a health care worker, and have not been immunized)

  - Cytomegalovirus antibody titres, to determine whether you are immune to CMV (this test isn't commonly offered). If you have been diagnosed with a recent CMV infection, it's generally recommended you wait 6 months – when antibodies appear in the blood – before trying to conceive.

  - Toxoplasmosis titre, if you have a cat, regularly eat raw or rare meat, or garden without gloves. If you turn out to be immune, you don't have to worry about infecting your fetus with toxoplasmosis.

  - Thyroid function. Because thyroid function can affect pregnancy – and fertility – it's a good idea for everyone to be screened before conception. This is especially important if you have ever had thyroid problems in the past or have them now, or if you have a family history of thyroid disease (check with your mum and other females in the family).

  - Sexually transmitted disease (STD). You may be tested for STDs at your general checkup, or you can be tested at a GUM clinic.

The exam will also pick up any medical problems that need to be corrected beforehand or will need to be monitored during pregnancy. If any test does turn up a condition that requires treatment, now's the best time to take care of it. Also consider getting around to minor elective surgery and anything else medical – major or minor – that you've been putting off.

If you were a PKU baby (ask your parents if you aren't sure, or check your medical records), begin a phenylalanine-free diet 3 months before you conceive, and continue it throughout pregnancy. If you need allergy shots, take care of them now – if you start allergy desensitization now, you will probably be able to continue once you conceive. Because depression can interfere with conception (and with a happy, healthy pregnancy), it should also be treated before you begin your big adventure (see page 9

Preconception Prep and Chronic Conditions

If you have a chronic health condition (such as diabetes, asthma, a heart condition, epilepsy, renal disease, high blood pressure), deciding to start trying to conceive (TTC) isn't always as easy as stopping the Pill and starting getting busy. It's likely your preconception prep will be a little more involved, and your pregnancy care a little more involved, too. But there's lots of good news – especially since you're planning ahead.

Though it's true that there are risks for a pregnancy (and baby) if a mum's chronic condition isn't well controlled, those risks can be minimized or even eliminated entirely by bringing the condition under control, preferably before sperm meets egg. With the right care and precautions, most chronic conditions are perfectly compatible with getting pregnant and having a healthy pregnancy.

But first things first. And your first step on the road to pregnancy should be at your specialist's office for a preconception appointment. He or she will evaluate how you're managing your condition and determine whether you're ready to TTC or need to make some changes in your treatment plan or your lifestyle before you get going. Maybe you'll need to tweak your diet, lose or gain some weight, or finesse your fitness. Maybe you'll need to be weaned off certain medications you no longer need or switched to others that are fertility and pregnancy safe (or alternative therapies may be integrated into your care, such as acupuncture or meditation for the relief of stress). Maybe you'll be referred to a high-risk pregnancy practitioner, or maybe you'll find that your usual GP will be able to offer up all the care you need, in a team effort with your specialist.

for information on the use of antidepressants when trying to conceive).

Gynaecological health checkup. Your preconception checkup will include a Pap and all the standards of your annual visit. In addition to that Pap smear, your practitioner will perform a pelvic, breast, and abdominal exam, ask for a urine sample, and check for any gynaecological conditions that might interfere with fertility or pregnancy, including:

- Polycystic ovarian syndrome (PCOS), if you have a history of irregular periods, excess hair growth, acne, and obesity

- Uterine fibroids, cysts, or benign tumours

- Endometriosis (when the cells that ordinarily line the uterus spread elsewhere in the body)

- Pelvic inflammatory disease (PID)

- Irregular periods

- Recurrent urinary tract infections

- An STD (if you weren't already tested). All pregnant women are routinely tested for STDs, including chlamydia, syphilis, gonorrhoea, and HIV. Having these tests before conception (and getting any necessary treatment) is better still. Even if you're sure you couldn't have an STD, testing now is a good idea, just to be on the safe side.

Now – before you get started on baby making – is the time to get any gynaeco-

Your Family Health Tree

Time to call your folks. Not to tell them you're expecting (you'll make *that* call soon enough), but to get the scoop on the health history on both sides of the family tree – yours and your partner's. Dig as deeply as you can, and write down everything you unearth (you can do this on page 208), so you'll be ready to answer the family history questions you'll be getting from your practitioner. It's especially important to find out if there's a history of any medical issues (such as diabetes, high blood pressure, or thyroid disease) and genetic or chromosomal disorders (such as Down's syndrome, Tay-Sachs disease, sickle-cell anaemia, thalassaemia, haemophilia, cystic fibrosis, muscular dystrophy, Huntington's disease, or fragile X syndrome) in your immediate family.

Your family health tree may also clue you in on how your future pregnancy might play out. Are there twins in your future? Multiples (especially fraternal twins) can run in families, so look for trends on your side of the tree (and your partner's, too, since some evidence indicates that identical twins can be genetically influenced by both mum and dad). Also running in families are some pregnancy complications. Ask your mum and your partner's mum if she (or her mother) ever had preeclampsia – a

complication that can cause a pregnant woman's blood pressure to skyrocket. Research shows that sons and daughters born from preeclamptic pregnancies may carry genes related to the condition. Ask about gestational diabetes, depression (postpartum or general), and other complications, too – and have this information at the ready when your practitioner asks for it.

It'll also help to find out more about your mum's pregnancies with you and your siblings. That's because the apple often doesn't fall far from the mama tree when it comes to gynaecological and obstetrical history, which means that a look at your mum's pregnancy history may give you a peek into your pregnancy future. Keeping in mind that every pregnancy is different (even for the same woman, two pregnancies may be very different), mums may predispose their daughters to any number of pregnancy or delivery scenarios – both good (no stretch marks) and not so good (lots of varicose veins). So ask your mother anything you might be wondering about, remembering that her pregnancy story may or may not foreshadow yours: How long did it take you to get pregnant? Did you have morning sickness? How long were you in labour?

logical condition diagnosed and treated because certain ones may prevent you from getting pregnant in the first place and others can complicate pregnancy. You can also take this opportunity to ask your practitioner any questions you might have – from when to stop your birth control (he or she will let you know how long you should ideally wait, if at all, before you can start trying for that baby of yours)

to how to make sense of your cycle and figure out when you're most fertile.

Dental health checkup. Here's something to smile about – you're about to make a baby. But before that positive home pregnancy test (HPT) has you beaming ear to ear, make sure your teeth and gums are ready for baby making, too, by scheduling a checkup and teeth cleaning with your dentist. This may sound random and unrelated (after all, what do teeth have to do with making a baby?), but the fact is that gum disease is associated with pregnancy complications such as preterm labour, preeclampsia, and gestational diabetes. What's more, if you have gum disease before pregnancy, it's likely to worsen once you're officially expecting. The pregnancy hormones you'll hopefully soon be producing (most notably progesterone) cause tissue in your mouth to soften, swell, and become stretchier, making teeth prone to loosening and gums prone to bleeding. Also, indulging in too many sweets, so commonly craved during pregnancy, can also make gums and teeth more vulnerable. This is a recipe for gingivitis, gum infection, and even eventual tooth loss – unless you're careful. The good news is that dental treatment is free in pregnancy, and up until your baby's first birthday. Meanwhile, take care of that preconception smile. Don't forget to brush and floss regularly, and see your dentist for advice on how to keep your oral health in tip-top condition – while you're TTC, once you're expecting, and beyond.

Immunizations

"Do I need to get any vaccines before I become pregnant?"

That depends on which ones you've already had, and when. The blood tests you take at your preconception checkup will reveal if the relevant immunizations are already up to date. If they are, you're probably all set vaccine-wise. If they aren't up to date or you have some immunization holes that need filling in, now – before your TTC campaign begins – is the time to roll up your sleeve for all necessary vaccinations – not only for your safety, but also to protect your baby-to-be, who won't be fully immunized against these diseases until at least 6 months of age (and should you contract an illness, your new baby may catch it, too – and that would not be a good thing). Vaccines that might be on the preconception agenda include:

- Tetanus-diphtheria (Td or Tdap). Even if you had your full set of vaccinations as a child, some vaccines require boosters to keep immunities going strong. If you haven't had a tetanus-diphtheria booster in the past 10 years, you'll likely be advised to have one now.

- Measles, mumps, rubella (MMR). If you know you've never had rubella, mumps, and measles or been immunized against this trio of serious childhood diseases, or if testing showed you are not fully immune (sometimes immunity wears off), get vaccinated now with the MMR vaccine and then wait 1 month before you start trying to conceive (but don't worry if you accidentally conceive earlier – any risk is purely theoretical).

- Chicken pox (varicella). If testing shows you've never had chicken pox (and most women of childbearing age have either had it or have been vaccinated), it's recommended that you be immunized against it prepregnancy, at least 3 months before conception (but again, don't worry if you get pregnant before the waiting period is up). Your immunity to chicken pox is actually really important for your baby-to-be, who won't be able to be immunized against the disease until age 1.

- Hepatitis B. If you're at high risk for hepatitis B, immunization for this disease is also recommended now. The Hep B shots come in a series of three, and if you don't finish up the series before you conceive, it's safe to continue it while you're expecting.

Action Plan

Before you start TTC in earnest, call for appointments with your GP and your dentist to schedule thorough preconception checkups. Another item on your medical to-do list: Start looking into the maternity care facilities available in your local area. There might be a team of community midwives at your GP's practice or your care might take place at a clinic in your local hospital. This way you'll know what to expect for that first prenatal visit as soon as the home pregnancy test gives you the good news. Alternatively, if your finances allow it, you might want to look into the option of private maternity care – but there are very few private maternity units in the UK, and these are primarily in the London area (most private health companies view pregnancy as a routine event, so they don't cover it). Check out *What to Expect When You're Expecting* for the lowdown on the different kinds of maternity care available.

◌ HPV (human papilloma virus). If you're younger than 26, you might consider getting vaccinated against HPV, but you'll need to finish the full series of three before trying to conceive. If you become pregnant before completing the full series, you'll have to resume the shots postpartum.

Whether or not you have to bare your arm for any vaccines now, keep in mind that you'll be advised to line up for your flu shot if you end up expecting during flu season.

Medications

"Will I have to stop using all medications once I'm trying to conceive, or can I wait until I get pregnant?"

It's time to take stock of your medicine cabinet, but not necessarily to empty it. As you've already figured out, it won't be medications as usual once you're expecting. During pregnancy, some of the drugs you occasionally or regularly reach for may be off limits, some may be limited, still others may be yours for the taking, as needed. But what about the medications you take before you're expecting? Should you start thinking before you keep popping?

That'll depend on what you normally pop. Most over-the-counter and many prescription meds are considered safe while you're trying to conceive. Still, it's smart to get the green light on any medications or supplements (including vitamins and herbals) before you take them during the preconception period. That's because some (including herbal products specifically touted for fertility) may not only affect your future pregnancy, but also your chances of getting pregnant. Even something as basic (and seemingly random) as antihistamines may compromise fertility, and for a very unexpected reason: They could dry out your cervical mucus along with your nasal mucus.

Ask your doctor, gynaecologist, or midwife (if you have one) for help figuring out what's safe to take, what should be dropped while you're TTC and while you're pregnant (and thinking way ahead, while you're breastfeeding), and what's fine while you're TTC but should be dropped or limited once you're officially expecting.

If you depend on prescription drugs to treat a chronic condition (like asthma, diabetes, depression, migraines, or any other), discuss your TTC and pregnancy medication options with the doctor overseeing your care and with your GP. Together, you can come up with a plan that'll help keep you healthy, fertile, and ready to welcome a pregnancy (and it may or may not include the drugs you typically take, at the same or different doses). You might have to drop some drugs for as long as 6 months prior to conceiving (and, of course, while you're pregnant and while you're breastfeeding), but there are almost always safer alternatives you can switch to during your reproductive break.

For more information on vitamin supplements while you're trying to conceive, see page 60. For information on herbal medications, see page 118.

Antidepressants

"I've been taking antidepressants for the past five years, and the meds have kept my depression under control. I worry about going off them, but I wonder if they're safe to keep taking while I'm TTC and beyond."

Avoid a Repeat

If you've had a previous pregnancy with any complications, or one that ended with a premature delivery or late pregnancy loss, or if you've had multiple miscarriages, talk to your practitioner about any measures that can be taken now – before you start trying again – to head off a repeat. For example, research shows that taking folic acid supplements for a year or longer before conception may reduce the risk of premature delivery. For information on preventing repeat miscarriages, see page 181.

When it comes to life changes, there's probably no bigger one than having a baby – or even deciding to take the baby plunge. But if you suffer from depression or anxiety, you may not only be wondering how your baby plans might change your life, but how they'll affect your ability to handle life – especially if trying to become pregnant might mean giving up your antidepressants or anti-anxiety meds.

Happily, many safe options (including medication options) are available for expectant mums with depression, anxiety, and other mental health conditions, though your current treatment plan may be modified or changed entirely now that you're planning a pregnancy. In fact, stopping antidepressants or other meds that you really need – and slipping back into depression – can actually do you (and the baby you're hoping for) more harm than good. Being clinically depressed or extremely anxious during pregnancy (and while you're trying to conceive) can make you less likely to eat well, sleep well, or otherwise live a baby-friendly lifestyle. Studies show that women who suffer from untreated depression during pregnancy may have a greater chance of pre-term delivery and are also at higher risk for postpartum depression, which can make it difficult for them to take care of and enjoy their babies after they're born.

So before you consider tossing your meds, talk to both your prescribing doctor and your GP (or gynaecologist). Together, you can weigh the benefits of continuing medication with the potential risks. Certain medications come with more risks, others with very few. Wellbutrin (bupropion) hasn't been proven harmful during pregnancy when taken in the right doses and is probably the best choice, assuming your condition will respond to it. Paxil (paroxetine), and perhaps other SSRIs (selective serotonin reuptake inhibitors)

Checking Up on Dad

Sure, you're not going to be the one doing the actual baby carrying (at least not for the first 9 months – you'll make up for it later), but you will be contributing half of the essential genetic material that makes a baby. To get your body into prime baby-making condition – so you can make the best contribution possible – you should see a doctor for a top-to-bottom checkup. After all, making a healthy baby takes the participation of two healthy bodies. A thorough physical can detect any medical conditions (such as undescended testicles, testicular cysts or tumours, or depression) that might interfere with conception or a healthy pregnancy, as well as ensure that any chronic conditions that might interfere with fertility (such as diabetes) are under control. While at the doctor's office, ask about the sexual side effects of any prescription medication, over-the-counter, or herbal drugs you might be taking. Some of the commonly prescribed medications that could affect fertility and/or libido include SSRIs like Prozac (you might be happier, but your sperm won't be), beta blockers and other drugs for hypertension, some ulcer drugs, and some prescription pain killers (like oxycodone). Ditto for steroids and testosterone pills. They'll bulk you up but will cut back sperm production. Viagra could possibly lower your chances of conception, though the jury's still out on that one (ask your doctor for the latest). If any of the meds you take regularly are potentially fertility unfriendly, talk to your doctor about changing your treatment plan to fit your baby plans (in most cases, a different medication will do the trick). You should also consider tagging along for some genetic screening – especially if you have a family history or other indication that calls for such testing.

Need to lose weight, get blood pressure or blood sugar under control, cut down on alcohol, or seek treatment for a condition that may stand between you and that baby you and your partner are planning? Now – before the baby making begins – is the time to do it all.

---

may carry a small risk for a developing baby, and Prozac (and still other SSRIs) use during the latter half of pregnancy has been linked to withdrawal symptoms in the baby after delivery.

Now, before you become pregnant, is definitely the best time to make any treatment changes. If you and your practitioners decide that you should wean yourself off your meds or try different and safer kinds, start at least 3 months before you begin trying to conceive so you've got plenty of time to see how it goes – and how you're feeling. If you notice the signs of depression coming back – sleep and appetite changes, anxiety, inability to concentrate, mood swings, and lack of interest in sex (which definitely won't help your baby-making plans) – talk to your medical team again about trying a different approach. Report in with them, too, about any changes in your condition once you become pregnant (the hormonal upheavals of pregnancy trigger mood swings in every expectant mum, but depression or anxiety that's consistent and interferes with functioning isn't normal).

And keep in mind that there are plenty of alternative therapies – from psychotherapy to light therapy, meditation to biofeedback – that can boost your emotional state naturally, and can be used instead of or in conjunction with medications. Eating plenty of foods high in omega-3 fatty acids (like salmon and walnuts) may moderate mood swings, too, as may taking a pregnancy-safe DHA supplement. And don't forget the mood-lifting powers of exercise. Those feel-good endorphins that are released with a brisk walk or a swim can do your body – and your mind – good.

Genetic Screening

"Is going for genetic screening a good idea before we conceive – even if we have no reason to believe we're at any increased risk?"

What will you and your partner be passing along to your baby-to-be besides curly hair, thick eyelashes, athletic ability, a flair for figures, or a way with words? That's what genetic screening can tell you before that baby-to-be is even conceived – and with news that's almost always reassuring. Not every couple who's in the baby-planning stages needs to contemplate genetic testing, but if you or your partner has a family history of particular conditions, or are of certain ethnic backgrounds, screening may be a good idea – and a great way to put your mind at ease. If either one of you knows (or even suspects) that you may be a carrier of a genetic disorder, talk to your practitioner about what screenings, if any, might be necessary. He or she can refer you to a genetics counsellor who'll walk you through all the odds and options. Keep in mind that many genetic disorders are recessive, which means that both you and your partner would have to test positive for your baby to be at any risk at all of being affected (and that if one of you tests negative, there's no need for the other to be tested). If neither you nor your partner have any genetic red flags, you may be able to skip this part of the preconception process.

Who might consider prepregnancy genetic testing?

- Women of African descent are often screened for sickle-cell anaemia, a blood disease in which blood cells are sickle shaped and have difficulty travelling freely through the blood vessels, causing pain and anaemia.

- Those of Mediterranean, African, and Far East Asian descent may be screened for thalassaemia, a group of genetic blood disorders all related to haemoglobin, the part of red blood cells that carries oxygen.

- Those of European Jewish (Ashkenazi) descent, and those of French Canadian, Irish American, or Louisiana Cajun descent are usually tested to make sure they don't carry the gene for Tay-Sachs disease, which affects the nerve cells of the brain and is inevitably fatal.

- Those with a family history of inherited disorders – such as cystic fibrosis, muscular dystrophy, or haemophilia – may be tested for specific risks.

- Women with previous obstetrical difficulties (such as two or more miscarriages, a stillbirth, a long period of infertility, or a child with a birth defect).

- Couples who are blood relatives.

Your Lifestyle Prep

Next up in preconception prep: a look at your lifestyle. Now that you're talking baby, will you have to say "later" to your morning lattes – and "nighty-night" to your nightcaps? Will you have to work out less, or (shudder) more? Can you still spend time in hot water – or hot saunas and tanning beds? How about your monthly highlights – will making a baby send you back to your roots? In the case of some lifestyle choices, the choice will still be yours (at least until baby's on board). In the case of others (those four-shot espresso drinks), some tweaking will definitely be on the menu (make half those shots decaf, and you're good to go TTC).

Caffeine

"Do I have to cut out coffee now that I'm trying to conceive – or can I wait until I'm pregnant?"

Lust after that latte? Crave that cappuccino? Must have that morning macchiatto? There's no need to drop Joe from your life entirely now that you're making room for Junior. In fact, depending on how much coffee and other caffeinated beverages you depend on, you may be able to continue your caffeine habit as usual even as you're trying to conceive that baby, especially if you're a light coffee drinker.

Have a hefty habit? You'll probably have to trim it down to baby-making size. Not only because you'll have to cut back anyway once you're pregnant, but because keeping caffeine intake sensibly moderate now may actually help you get pregnant – and stay pregnant. Some studies have linked downing too much caffeine with lowered fertility and an increased risk of miscarriage.

Dear Joe

Wondering if you'll have to step away from the coffee-pot now that you're stepping up to the baby-making plate? You'll be relieved to hear, probably not. Although some research suggests that a heavy caffeine habit can lower male fertility, other (happier) research speculates that a little caffeine may actually help sperm swim faster – and faster swimming sperm may be more likely to hit their target faster. But until more is known, it's probably sensible for you to keep your caffeine intake moderate (no more than a few cups a day) until your conception mission is accomplished.

What's too much caffeine when you're trying to conceive? Technically, more than 200 mg a day. Too technical for you? Here are some caffeine stats to help you see how your intake adds up. That 200 mg will buy you about 350ml of brewed coffee a day (that's a "tall"), or about two shots of espresso (which is why four-shot lattes will definitely put you over the top). A can of caffeinated diet cola will cost you 45 mg, and a regular cola 35 mg. Tea contributes to that tally, too, with between 40 and 60 mg per cup (whether it's iced, brewed, or green), as do energy drinks (80 mg in a Red Bull), chocolate, and some over-the-counter cold and allergy drugs. Even coffee ice cream or coffee yogurt packs a modest caffeinated punch.

But here's some news that may lift your spirits (and your sagging afternoon energy levels): You won't have to cut back any further on your caffeine once baby's officially on board. Most experts believe that up to 2 cups a day (that same 200 mg) is fine throughout pregnancy (when you'll need that energy more than ever).

Action Plan

Baby in your plans? Time to put less coffee in your cup. While you're TTC (and expecting, too), limit your caffeine intake to no more than 200 mg per day. That's equivalent to a daily total of about 2 small cups of brewed coffee or about 4 diet colas. A bonus of cutting down on caffeine: You'll be more relaxed – a definite plus when it comes to conception.

If your calculations indicate that you'll need to do some cutting down on your caffeine (or if you'd like to cut it out altogether), slow is the way to go. Rather than shocking your system into extreme exhaustion (and lots of headaches and crankiness) by quitting abruptly, gradually lower your caffeine intake. Think baby steps. Substituting decaf for some of each cup you normally drink will start you on the weaning process. Keep reducing the amount of regular and increasing the amount of decaf until your ratio is where you'd like to see it. Or order your espresso drinks with one shot of regular, another (or another two) of decaf. Eyeing that large coffee? Order a small in a large cup, then fill it to the rim with milk (hot milk for hot coffee, cold for iced). You'll cut down on your caffeine while scoring a calcium bonus (and calcium is something you'll need to be getting more of, anyway).

Eating smaller, more frequent mini-meals (each of which should contain some protein and some complex carbs) will keep your blood sugar up – and that will help lift your energy level during this possibly challenging transition. Prenatal vitamins will also help you fill in some of the energy blanks without a caffeine fix, as will regular exercise.

Herbal Tea

"I'm not a coffee drinker but I love herbal tea. Is it okay for me to have some when I'm trying for a baby?"

That depends on what you're brewing. Some commercial herbal teas are considered safe to drink both during pregnancy and the preconception period (for instance, peppermint, citrus, and ginger), but others may not be. How do you pick a brew that's right for you while you're trying to conceive? Since there aren't many studies on the

Thinking of Going Green?

That cup of green tea may be brimming with health benefits, but should you go green when you're trying to make a baby? Maybe not. Green tea decreases the effectiveness of folic acid (ironically found in green leafies), a vitamin that's vital to the healthy development of your soon-to-be baby, and one of the nutrients that you should be getting your quota of during your baby prep phase. So it's smart to limit yourself to a cup a day (or a glass of iced) while you're TTC, or to switch to a black brew.

safety of herbal teas, it isn't easy. Check with your GP or a herb-knowledgeable practitioner who knows that you're trying to get pregnant for a list of herbs to avoid (among those usually making the list: red raspberry leaf, southernwood, wormwood, mugwort, barberry, tansy, mandrake root, juniper, pennyroyal, nutmeg, arbor vitae, and senna). Screen for those red-flag ingredients – as well as any that you're just not sure about – by reading the packaging carefully before buying (or brewing) herbal tea. Teas that are touted as fertility or pregnancy brews should also get the screening (because these claims are not regulated, it's a case of drinker beware). If there isn't any packaging (as in bulk teas sold at health food markets) or lists of ingredients, play it safe and skip it for now. For more on the safety of herbs when you're TTC, see page 118.

No need to read the tea leaves – or the tea leaf boxes – if you choose a traditional black tea, like Earl Grey or English Breakfast. Those are safe to sip, as long as you keep an eye on your total caffeine tally; each cup of caffeinated black tea will cost you 40 to 60 mg of your 200-mg daily limit.

Drinking

"I know I have to stop drinking once I get pregnant, but we've just started trying – and holiday season is coming right up. Can I keep drinking a little until I conceive?"

If you're planning for a baby, you're probably already planning to change your drink order from cocktail to mocktail. But when exactly should you start putting that new order in? There aren't any hard and fast rules about alcohol

Booze and Your Boys

Hoping to toast some big baby news soon? You might want to consider swapping your accustomed toasting beverage before that big news even comes through, or cutting back on how many toasts you make during conception season. Too much alcohol (as you may have been dismayed to discover at one point or another) can impair a guy's sexual function – a function you're now counting on. But worse than that, research indicates that daily heavy drinking can damage sperm as well as reduce their number (in some men, even one or two beers or glasses of wine is enough to temporarily keep the boys down). Too many rounds on a regular basis can also alter testicular

function and reduce testosterone levels (not a good scenario when you're trying to make a baby). Heavy drinking (equivalent to two drinks a day or five drinks in one sitting even once a month) by the dad-to-be during the month prior to conception could also affect your baby's birthweight. So for best baby-making results, your best bet is to drink only occasionally and lightly – or if you find that hard to do, cut it out altogether for now. And because the future mum in your life will also be laying off the libations as she gets her body ready for the long and happy baby haul ahead, those cutbacks will probably be easier to make (besides, it's not fair guzzling Guinness when she's sipping sparkling water).

Last Call

About to take the baby-making plunge, and committed to staying dry until that bundle arrives? Why not celebrate your decision with one last round (that is, if you normally drink socially – no need to start now if you don't)? Whether it's a festive get-together with friends (you don't have to tell them exactly what you're celebrating, unless you feel like sharing) or a romantic dinner-with-wine for two, toast your future with your favourite grown-up beverage one last time before you settle into your role as a designated mother-to-be.

order sooner rather than later. The timing of conception isn't a precise science. Since you won't be getting a "stop drinking" bulletin from your body the moment sperm and egg seal the deal – and chances are you won't have that fertilization heads-up for a couple of weeks after that momentous moment occurs – it's probably best to call it quits (or start cutting back a lot) once you're actively trying to get that baby on board. If you do opt for a cutting-back approach in the meantime (especially during that holiday season, or during the upcoming holiday), keep it on the light side – and when you do sip the real McCoy (or the real Merlot), sip with a side of food to slow the absorption of alcohol into your system.

drinking when you're in the baby-making stages (like there are for those already pregnant, who – most experts agree – should be total teetotallers). It is known, however, that heavy drinking can mess with your menstrual cycle – possibly interfering with ovulation and making it more difficult for a fertilized egg to implant in the uterus – and that can definitely put a crimp in your conception plans. And the more alcohol you consume, some research suggests, the less likely you'll become pregnant.

What about a glass of sauvignon blanc with your supper or a beer with your barbecue? What if you can't imagine ending the day without a nightcap? How about that holiday eggnog, now that you've got a different kind of egg on your mind? And what if it takes a few months to conceive – wouldn't all that preconception abstention be kind of wasted (especially with 9 alcohol-free months ahead of you)?

Well, maybe. But here's the reason you might want to put in that mocktail

Butt Out, Dad

Are you a nicotine nut? It's time to butt out – once and for all. Not only can your smoking be harmful to your partner's fertility, it can lower your sperm count, lower the quality of your sperm – and overall lower the chances that you'll make a healthy baby together. Plus, after baby's on board, secondhand smoke can hamper your little one's development. Same is true of so-called thirdhand smoke (the kind that lingers on clothes and hair, even if you're doing your smoking outside the house). Once baby has arrived, your smoking can pose significant health risks for that precious bundle.

If you both smoke, commit to quitting as a team. If you're the sole smoker in the house, call it quits now. Easier said than done? For sure, but you can do it – and the tips on the next pages can help.

Calling It Quits

Need to clean house of all your unhealthy habits now that you're planning to fill that house with a baby? A smoke-free womb is a very good place to start – but you may be wondering (especially if you've tried to quit before and were unsuccessful) exactly how to get started, not to mention finished. Here's how:

Give yourself props. First thing you need to do is pat yourself on the back – or on the belly you're dreaming of filling – for taking this momentous (and probably pretty daunting) step. Accept that the road ahead won't be without its bumps, but try to remind yourself that the baby bump you'll hopefully be sporting soon will make your efforts more than worthwhile.

Make a plan. Will it be cold turkey or gradual weaning? You know your body and your willpower best, so choose the method of withdrawal that you think you can live with. Pick a "last day" target that's realistic (don't choose a day that's likely to be high stress or a time of month when your willpower is already challenged) but not too far off – remember, the faster you quit, the faster you may be able to make your baby dreams come true. Plan a busy schedule for that day – preferably of fun activities in locales where smoking isn't allowed. Window-shop for baby clothes, treat yourself to a mani/pedi (or splurge on a new hairstyle), and then celebrate your accomplishment with dinner and a movie. And don't try to go it alone. Take company along to help keep you occupied – nonsmoking company.

Expect the worst, at first. Symptoms of withdrawal may begin after a few hours, and will get as bad as they're going to get by the second or third day – but they should gradually ease up, and should be mostly gone after about 5 smoke-free weeks. They may include dizziness, depression, anxiety and irritability, trouble sleeping or focusing, headaches, fatigue, and restlessness. Eating regularly and well (grazing on protein and complex carbs will keep you feeling your emotional and physical best), getting some exercise daily, and staying away from excesses of caffeine and sugar (which can make you more jittery) may help while your body adjusts.

Sublimate and substitute. Figure out what you can swap those cigarettes for. If it's for oral gratification, chew gum, suck on a straw or a lollipop, nibble on raw veggies. If you smoke for stress relief, try other ways of chilling out during times of high anxiety – visualization, deep breathing, listening to music on your iPod, a swim or a workout, a warm bath, a massage (and maybe some post-massage sex). If you smoke to keep your hands busy, play with a strand of beads or fiddle with a pencil, take a knitting class, work on a Sudoku puzzle, play video games, or squeeze a stress ball or some play clay (you'll have to brush up on your technique anyway, if there's a little one in your future).

Be tough. Cheer yourself on, but also know when you need a kick in the butt, too. Try telling yourself that stopping smoking is a non-negotiable issue. When you were a smoker, you couldn't smoke in a cinema or a restaurant or at the office – now you can't smoke at all, full stop.

Picture your baby. Whenever you feel like reaching for a cigarette (or whenever you're feeling sorry for yourself or sick from withdrawal symptoms), close your eyes and picture the baby of your dreams, cradled in your arms. Or flip through parenting magazines or websites full of cute baby pictures. Another reminder of your mission might help, too – a special bracelet, for instance, or locket you'll be able to fill later.

Don't play with fire (or smoke). Stay away from smokers and smoky locales – and even from places where you can buy cigarettes for now (send your partner to the shop, and do prepaid at the petrol station so you won't be tempted to duck into the shop for a pack). Visit with friends and family who don't allow smoking in their homes (preferably ones who have babies and children) for inspirational purposes. If you associate a certain activity or a certain food or drink with smoking, keep them off the agenda and off the menu for now.

Enlist help. It'll be easier to take one for Team Baby if your team has plenty of support. Enlist your friends and family as your cheerleaders – and to keep you honest (and smoke free). Look for empathy and advice from ex-smokers or co-quitters on message boards, particularly TTC boards (check out the Prepping for Pregnancy TTC board at WhatToExpect.com). If your partner also has to quit, join forces and quit together.

CAM do. Lots of smokers have become ex-smokers with the help of such Complementary and Alternative Medicine (CAM) therapies as acupuncture, aromatherapy, and meditation. Hypnosis can be especially effective in conquering those cravings.

See your doctor. You may get more than a pep talk (though that could help, too). Your doctor can recommend a nicotine patch, gum, or lozenge (if you haven't already tried nicotine-replacement therapies), or a medication such as Zyban, to fast-track your quitting campaign so you can start your TTC campaign sooner. All of these options work best when they're used as part of a smoke-cessation programme (you'll find plenty of these online or through the NHS). Go to http://smokefree.nhs.uk or call 0800 0224332.

Don't overwhelm your willpower. Need to quit smoking, but also need to drop a few pounds before you begin your baby-making efforts? Don't try to take on both campaigns at once – that will only make you more likely to fail at both. Smoking is potentially more harmful to your fertility and your future baby than those extra pounds, so cut that out before you try starting to cut calories. But do try to begin eating more healthfully in the meantime, if you can – nutritious foods can help sustain you best when your willpower gets wobbly.

Take one day at a time. Think about the weeks of withdrawal ahead of you, and you'll make yourself crazy. Instead, take 1 day – or even 1 hour – at a time. Each time you pass another 24-hour smoke-free day, commemorate it on a calendar (maybe with a cute baby sticker), and give yourself a nightly round of applause.

Try, try again. Be forgiving if you slip up and have a cigarette. Resolve to make that smoke your last. Don't beat yourself up, and whatever you do, don't give up. Hang in there. You can do it – and you've never had a better reason to!

Smoking

"I'm planning to stop smoking once I become pregnant – but can I keep smoking while I'm trying to conceive?"

Now's the time to kick butt. Smoking poses a whole pack of risks not only during pregnancy, but before – the most significant risk being that you'll have trouble getting and staying pregnant. Smoking can age your eggs (meaning that a 30-year-old smoker's eggs may act more like 40-year-old eggs), making conception more difficult, lowering the odds that a fertilized egg will implant in your uterus, and making miscarriage more likely. What's more, heavy smoking damages the ovaries as well as the uterus, potentially reducing fertility even further – and probably explaining why smokers are four times more likely to take longer than a year to become pregnant. A smoke-free womb is the very best gift you can give your baby-to-be, but kicking the habit now will make it more likely you'll conceive that baby-to-be sooner.

Pretty much the same applies to secondhand smoke (so if your partner smokes, it's time for him to quit, too – and it'll be easier if you join forces and quit together). Just spending time in a smoky room or with smokers who have tobacco by-products lingering on their clothes, hair, and skin (thirdhand smoke) can harm your health, your fertility, and your future family. To tip the conception odds in your favour, stay as far away from cigarette smoke as you can.

Marijuana

"Is it true that smoking pot can make it harder to conceive?"

Already have your hands full with all the habit breaking (and other behaviour changing) you'll have to do before you begin making that baby? Add giving up pot to your list. Here's why:

For one thing, birthweight is lower, on average, in babies of pot smokers. But getting that baby conceived in the first place may be tougher, too. Believe it or not, your pot smoking can affect the ability of your partner's sperm to fertilize an egg – whether he smokes pot or not. That's because THC – the active ingredient in marijuana – shows up in your vaginal fluids and reproductive organs (including your vagina, fallopian tubes, and uterus). When the sperm arrive, they've got the urge to merge with your egg, but they can't follow through because the THC they've been exposed

Action Plan

Now that you've learned some of the major don'ts of the preconception period (don't overdo the caffeine; don't drink a lot, if at all; don't smoke; don't use drugs), you may be feeling a little daunted about the work you *do* have ahead of you (especially if you have some significant quitting to do). Habits, especially long-standing or hefty ones, can be hard to break – no matter how motivating that healthy baby reward might be. If you're having an especially hard time breaking a habit that might impair your fertility or put the baby you've been hoping for at risk (or both), get the help you need as soon as you can. Talk to your doctor and ask his or her advice. Join local support groups or online ones for the camaraderie (and help). A little company might provide all the motivation you need.

Say No to Pot Before You Say Yes to Baby

Thought you were the only one getting stoned when you smoke pot? Actually, your boys are too. According to research, the sperm of pot smokers don't behave the way they're supposed to or the way they need to in order to be good little fertilizers. Though sperm normally get washed into the cervix, going along for the ride until they approach their target (when the strength they've saved up is used to swim to the egg and forcefully penetrate its hard shell), sperm under the influence of THC (the active ingredient in marijuana) swim frantically at first, then fizzle out by the time they reach Egg Land. Sluggish and unmotivated, they're less likely to get the job done – or even to be in the right place at the right time. Meaning they get wasted – and then wasted.

What's more, THC can cut the total number of boys on your swim team, sometimes significantly. It lowers levels of that all-important hormone of male reproduction – testosterone – and can reduce sperm count, as well as seminal fluid. Though it's definitely possible for pot smokers to conceive a baby (and many have discovered this inadvertently), it's clear that smoking does handicap fertility – which means that it could put a man with a borderline fertility issue over the top. Avoiding smoking pot just before you have sex doesn't alleviate these fertility challenges (THC can stay in your system, stored in your body fat, for a surprisingly long time), so aim to quit entirely now – before your boys start aiming for that egg. Say good-bye to pot smoking so you can say hello to a healthy baby (and seek professional help if you have trouble going it alone).

to impairs their normal function, making these under-the-influence sperm too sluggish to get the very challenging job of fertilization done. The THC stays in your system, too, which means that avoiding a slacker sperm problem isn't as easy as skipping having a smoke just before you have sex.

Clearly, pot smoking and baby making don't mix. Though you may conceive even if you do continue smoking while you're TTC, it's also possible that your fertility will be compromised. Plus, while the risks of continuing to smoke during pregnancy aren't fully documented, there's plenty of speculation about how marijuana might affect an unborn baby. To be on the safe side – and the most fertile side – now's the time to quit smoking pot.

It may go without saying, but it needs to be said anyway: Using any illicit drug, including cocaine, crack, or heroin, can make conception more difficult and pregnancy much more risky, for both mother and baby. If you need help breaking any addiction, seek it before you begin your baby-making efforts.

Exercise

"I'm in pretty good shape and I work out just about every day. Is it okay to keep that up while I'm trying to get pregnant?"

You don't have to be fit to be fertile (and lots of mums conceive without ever putting in a single day at the gym), but it may help. In fact, some research has suggested that a few laps around the

Your Workout and the Baby Race

If you're a sports nut – and not just the kind that watches other people play – it's time to take a look at your sports and workout routine now that you're about to play in the baby-making big leagues. Playing any kind of rough sports (including football, soccer, basketball, hockey, horseback riding) without wearing protective gear to prevent injury to your genitals tops the list of must-don'ts, for obvious reasons (you'll need those genitals in their best operating order). Too much cycling (and that includes spin class or cycling on the stationary bike) also makes that list because the constant pressure from a bicycle seat on the genitals may, according to some experts, damage essential reproductive arteries and nerves. Occasional, leisurely bike rides are probably not a problem, but more than 12 hours a week in the saddle (including the horseback-riding kind), especially if you're mountain biking – and you could be spinning your fertility wheels.

And though a regular workout routine probably boosts your fertility by boosting your testosterone levels (a good reason to hit the gym before you hit the sack), it's probably smart not to take it to the max when you're trying to maximize your baby-making potential. Heavy-duty workouts that leave you exhausted can actually change your hormone levels and lower your sperm count – plus put you in the mood to collapse on the couch, not for love. Ditto for workouts – and post-workout hot tubs, saunas, or steam rooms – that overheat you (and those precious family jewels).

Have spectator sports always been more your speed (as in watching the game from the sofa)? You might want to jump in the game, or at least find your way to the gym or the running trails, now that you're trying to make a baby. Guys who don't work out at all – especially if they're also sporting plenty of extra padding – may be more likely to encounter fertility challenges than guys who are more fit.

track – or in the pool, or even around the shops – can put you on the right preconception track. A moderate exercise programme that promotes overall fitness (about 30 minutes a day of aerobic exercise, strength training, stretching, and/or daily activities that get your heart going) can boost fertility, just as being in overall good health can. This may be especially true if you're packing a few extra preconception pounds you're trying to lose to increase your odds of conception (and to improve your overall health). And that's not all: The right kind of exercise helps release those feel-good endorphins, making your mind and body feel its relaxed best – which, in turn, can make baby-making efforts more productive (relaxation is a key component of any conception campaign; see page 24).

That said, you can get too much of a good thing when it comes to exercise and the conception connection. Take exercise to the extreme (and what's extreme varies from woman to woman – there are no hard-and-fast rules about how hard or fast you should exercise when you're trying to conceive) and your workouts may actually work against your fertility. Regular prolonged strenuous exercise can disrupt the delicate balance of hormones needed for ovulation and conception, especially if it reduces your body fat too much (some body fat is needed to keep those female reproduction functions functioning). Clearly, if your exercise routine has been keeping you from having regular periods, conception will be challenging, at best. Even if your periods seem to be regular, in some women regularly strenuous workouts appear to throw hormone levels off enough to interfere with ovulation or implantation. If that seems to be the case with you, your body may need to slow down – and maybe trade in some of those cut muscles for a little maternal padding – before it can trade in those toned abs for a baby bump.

What's the best workout plan when you're planning a baby? Keep it moderate – keeping in mind that what's moderate for you might depend on your current fitness level (for an athlete, a 5-mile run may be like a walk in the park compared to her usual routine; for a confirmed couch potato, even that walk in the park might be challenging for starters). Though many women maintain a rigorous routine and conceive easily, others find that they need to cut back a little, or a lot. Not sure whether your workout will work with

Action Plan

It's time to exercise your right to make a baby. And there's no better place to start than exercising. Aim for 30 minutes a day combined of aerobics (to get your heart pumping), strength training (to tone your muscles), and stretching (to get yourself in shape for the pregnancy to come). No need to become an Olympic athlete, but the better shape you're in, the better your chances for conception and a healthy pregnancy.

your TTC plans? Check with your practitioner.

Keep it cool, too – avoid overheating when you work out (or anytime). Raising your core temperature excessively (to 38.9°C/102°F or above) isn't harmful to your fertility but it can be harmful to your pregnancy – and when you're actively trying to become pregnant, you won't know right away when

Keep Your Cool, Dad

There's nothing more relaxing after a long day or a long workout session (and nothing more mood enhancing before a baby-making session) than a soak in a hot tub. But, sad to say, a hot tub can put your baby-making plans in hot water. Male fertility plunges with frequent dips in the hot tub because sperm production is impaired when the testicles become overheated. That's why your testicles hang low – they prefer to be a couple of degrees cooler than the rest of the body. So hot tubs, steam rooms, and saunas (and even electric blankets or exercise that excessively raises your core body temperature) are off limits until mission conception has been accomplished. The same might be said about tanning beds, which send your body temperature soaring while they bake your skin (plus set you up for premature aging of the skin and a significantly increased risk of skin cancer – so who needs them, anyway?).

you've succeeded. It doesn't mean that you can't work up a sweat, just that you shouldn't exercise in hot environments (as you would in Bikram yoga).

And speaking of yoga, keep it relaxing. Choose a workout that's noncompetitive, conditions your whole body and gets your heart pumping, that's stress reducing, and that's pregnancy appropriate (so that you'll likely be able to stick with it after you conceive). Yoga definitely comes to mind (and spirit) – and it seems to provide an especially beneficial preconception (and post-conception) workout because it focuses not only on relaxation breathing but also on body awareness (and this is definitely one time you want to be aware of your body). It's good for overall body toning, but it's not physically draining – plus it's very low impact. What's more, the meditation you'll do during a yoga session may help chill you out, too. Finally, yoga can increase flexibility – so you'll be able to wrap yourself into some more interesting baby-making positions.

Yoga not your thing? Try swimming, dancing, Pilates, mild cardio workouts, light weight training, stationary bicycling, and other low impact workouts – all of which are not only TTC appropriate but pregnancy appropriate (which means you'll likely be able to stick with the routine of your choice once you're exercising for two).

Hot Tubs

"I heard it's not safe to use a hot tub when TTC. Why's that?"

You heard right – sort of. The no-hot-tub recommendation is actually aimed at the dad-to-be in your life, because he needs to keep his nether regions cool to keep them reproductively functional (see shaded box, previous page). As for you, it's safe to take

the plunge before you've conceived (and the heat won't affect your chances of conceiving). But once baby's on board, you'll need to keep your cool, too – staying out of hot tubs, saunas, and other environments (like tanning beds) that can overheat. Because you never know for sure when that sperm and egg will actually get together, you might want to play it extra safe during the active TTC phase by sticking to warm tubs.

Skin Care

"Are any skin care products off limits in the preconception period?"

Time to face the happy face facts: There are very few skin-enhancing products or processes (from facials to procedures to the creams and lotions

A Day at the Spa?

Looking for a way to chill out before baby making heats up in the bedroom? Melt tension and stress away with a good massage or another spa indulgence. There's nothing in the spa that's off limits right now (though once you're actively trying you might want to play it extra safe and skip those treatments that raise your temperature significantly in case sperm meets egg before you realize what's happened) – so detox and destress to your heart's (and soul's) content. A little relaxation might even bring you closer to your baby-making goal, since too much stress can actually impede fertility. No room in your budget for professional pampering? Try an afternoon of do-it-yourself treatments at home.

Time for a Mummy Makeover?

Have your heart set on a new set of veneers? Or a brightened, whitened smile? Or maybe it's laser eye surgery you'd like – the better to see your baby, once he or she is a bundle on your lap, and not just a gleam in your eye? Whatever elective procedure you've elected to try, you'll need to consider timing when you're TTC. Most cosmetic dentistry procedures (like veneers and whitening) aren't recommended during pregnancy – so you'll want to have your smile adjustment completed before baby's on board. As for laser eye surgery, not only isn't this procedure recommended during pregnancy, it's not recommended for 6 months prior to pregnancy and 6 months after giving birth. So if you're actively trying already, you'll need to stick with the glasses or contacts until halfway through baby's first year (or 6 months after you stop breastfeeding).

And just in case you're wondering, before-baby isn't the time to consider breast augmentation or reduction. After all, your breasts will be seeing enough changes in the 9 months following conception, and in the months after birth, if you'll be breastfeeding (and, in fact, some breast surgery can impact your ability to breastfeed exclusively). If you're thinking about making any surgical adjustments, think about waiting until your baby-making days are done.

you slather on each night) you can't indulge in now. In fact, you might as well indulge now – once baby's on board, many of your favourite treatments may need to be shelved for the duration (including Botox and fillers, chemical peels, lasers, and a variety of skin care products).

But there is one very significant exception to this skin care free ride during the preconception period. The acne treatment Accutane can cause serious damage to a developing fetus. Not only is it strictly off limits during pregnancy, but for at least a month before you actively begin trying to conceive (stay on those two forms of birth control required with Accutane until that waiting period is over). Topical Retin-A, which is prescribed for both zit zapping and wrinkle smoothing, usually gets the red light during pregnancy and may, too, once you're officially TTC.

If pimples are your problem, you can try to keep your complexion all clear with over-the-counter and prescription-strength topical acne fighters (including some that may have to stay out of reach during pregnancy). It'll also pay to learn more about natural tactics for taming breakouts, since you'll likely be relying on them more once you're officially expecting: Eat well (foods high in essential fatty acids, vitamin C, folic acid, iron, and vitamin B_6 can help your skin look healthier), keep your face clean, and follow every wash with an oil-free moisturizer.

As for those wrinkles you'd rather do without, treat away for now (some treatments will be tabled after you've successfully conceived). Just keep in mind that because fill-ups or follow-ups won't be possible once you're expecting, the effects will likely wear off before you can safely repeat the procedures. Ask your practitioner about any that you're unsure about – and if you don't get the go-ahead, look at the bright side. Once you're pregnant, you'll be retaining enough fluid to fill in all those laugh lines – without a drop of collagen or Botox.

Hair Care

"What about hair colouring – should I quit that now, too?"

Ah, what mums won't do for their babies – even before they're mums. From giving up their favourite beverage to selecting a salad (when they'd really rather choose a chilli cheeseburger) to skipping their regular hair colouring appointments, hopeful mums-to-be will do (or not do) just about anything it takes to get pregnant and have a healthy baby.

Fortunately, when it comes to hair maintenance, no preconception sacrifices are necessary. There's absolutely no reason why you'd have to go back to your roots – or give up those straightening treatments or perms – while you're trying to conceive. In fact, there isn't even any consensus about whether colouring or other chemical processes should stay off the salon menu once you're expecting (most doctors either green-light colouring or ask that you hold off until the second trimester).

If you feel more comfortable quitting your colouring once you're actively trying to conceive – because you never know when you're going to hit baby bingo – go ahead. You might want to change your routine anyway (based on your practitioner's advice) now that you're looking to get pregnant. Processes that are mostly natural or that don't come into contact with the scalp – such as highlights or lowlights – are widely considered safe. So rather than have roots to contend with in a couple

of months, consult with your stylist about a prepregnancy hair colour plan that will blend in with those pregnancy guidelines.

Tanning

"Can I continue going tanning while TTC?"

There is a dark side to preconception tanning. While there isn't any proof that tanning can keep you from reaching your fertility goals (no evidence exists on either side, actually), tanning beds can raise your body temperature to a level that can be dangerous to your developing baby when you do conceive – and there's no way of telling when you'll conceive once you begin actively trying. Plus, tanning beds aren't great for your skin or your health in general (think extra wrinkles and significantly increased risk for skin cancer). Still a fan of the tan? Sunless tanning lotions and sprays are probably fine while TTC.

Stress

"I'm a stresser by nature, so naturally I'm already stressing about how stress is going to affect my chances of getting pregnant. Help!"

Don't stress about your stress. Scientists are still trying to make sense out of the stress–conception connection, but studies so far have only linked *extreme* stress to fertility difficulties – and that's not the kind of stress that most women have (even big-time stressers like you).

How exactly does *excessive* stress impact fertility? Potentially, in several ways. First, being under lots of stress can cause the brain to release neurotransmitters that affect the hormones controlling ovulation – which in turn can delay or

Chill Out Before Things Heat Up

Stress can keep a good man down, at least when it comes to fertility. Too much stress can, as you probably already know, limit libido and bring down the curtain on performance – but it can also lower testosterone levels and sperm production. So after a busy day, and before you get busy – unwind a little (or a lot), using the tips on the next few pages or your own best stress busters. The less you worry about conceiving, the more easily you're likely to conceive.

disrupt ovulation. In fact, women who are under extreme emotional stress sometimes don't ovulate at all, even if they're getting their periods regularly. Second, extreme stress can cause fertile cervical mucus (the thin mucus that helps sperm swim to their target) to dry up altogether – making it difficult not only to pinpoint ovulation but also to conceive. And perhaps the most obvious reason why a super-stressed life can put a crimp in conception plans: Too much stress can keep couples from having frequent-enough sex (the key, after all, to getting pregnant).

Fortunately, the body is really good at adapting to just about everything – including stress. Average everyday stress is probably something your body's already used to (who isn't stressed these days?) – which means that if your stress is manageable, it's not likely to be affecting your fertility. And even if the normal stress in your life – especially once it's combined with the potential stress of TTC – does seem to

wreak havoc on your cycles (you don't seem to be ovulating on time, or your periods are less regular than usual), there's still no reason to stress over it. Chances are that as your body (and mind) learns to deal with the monthly challenge of TTC, it'll get used to this new, more stressed reality – and your cycles will normalize accordingly.

But that doesn't mean you should keep the stress up – at least not at levels that are stressing you out. Learning how to reduce stress now can help you in your conception quest – and help you handle the (happy) stress that inevitably comes with pregnancy and parenting later. So relax, take a deep breath, and check out these de-stressing tips.

☐ Schedule in a chill pill. Yes, one of the reasons you're probably stressed is there's not enough time in the day

Action Plan

So you know you should lead a less stressful life, especially now that you want a baby in your life. One way to bring on the relaxation whenever and wherever: breathing exercises. Breathing is quick, it's free – and you have to do it anyway, so you might as well do it in a way that's relaxing. Pause a moment any time you're feeling hyped up (heck, pause a moment even when you're not) to do this exercise: Take a series of three deep, smooth breaths in through your nose and out through your mouth. Allow your head to rise with each inhale and drop your chin to your chest with each exhale (to stretch your neck muscles).

Sleeping Like a Baby to Make a Baby

Dreaming of a baby? Then you'll want to spend more time dreaming. Believe it or not, sex isn't the only in-bed activity that can contribute to conception. There's something else you should be taking care of when you hit the sack – getting some serious shut-eye. Just like all those other well-known keys to overall good health (eating well, exercising, getting regular medical care), catching enough z's can help improve your chances of producing a little one – who, in an ironic twist, will be the one keeping you and your z's apart once he or she is born. In fact, skimping on sleep can mess with your hormones, which can lead to irregular periods – something a hopeful mum-to-be certainly doesn't need. Not spending enough time in the sack can step up stress, too, which can also undermine your fertility (via hormonal high jinks that can delay or prevent ovulation). Plus, if you're charting your basal body temperature to help better understand your cycle (you'll read more about that in Chapter 5), you need adequate, consistent slumber to get the best results.

So take advantage of your still baby-free home (and bed), and seek the sleep your body craves. Nap when you can, turn in early, and stay in bed late (unless you're charting, in which case it's better to maintain regular nod-off and wake-up times) – with the goal of catching 6 to 9 hours of shut-eye per night. If sleep proves elusive, turn to tried-and-true home remedies such as a consistent bedtime routine, an evening bath (add some lavender-scented bubbles), or a warm-milk or chamomile-tea nightcap. Avoid caffeine and chocolate (especially dark chocolate) during the afternoon so you're not wound up when you're trying to wind down. And if it's stress that's keeping you up, check out the relaxation tips on these pages.

Still wide awake? Ask your practitioner for help breaking out of your slumber slump. He or she can help you find a safe yet effective solution to your sleepless nights (some prescription, over-the-counter, or herbal sleep aids, including melatonin, can suppress fertility or endanger a newly conceived baby). Once you settle on a settle-down strategy, remember the advice of many an experienced mum: Store up that sleep now because you'll never get enough once your baby's on board – or in house.

(especially once you've added in all those hours of TTC activities). Still, making time for occasional R&R breaks can really pay off, not only in helping you de-stress, but also in helping you be more productive in everything else you're doing – including all that baby-making sex (aka baby dancing). So take those breaks, and do whatever relaxes you. Read a few pages of a book you're enjoying, flip through a guilty pleasure magazine, or catch up on the latest celebrity shenanigans on a gossip site. Listen to music that soothes your soul (take your iPod to coffee breaks and lunch, or even use it while you work, if that's feasible) – or to nature sounds, if that's what gets your calm to kick in. Take up knitting – a great way to unwind and hone your skills for those booties you'll want to start whipping up soon. Start keeping a journal (you can use the one on page 256) or scrapbooking or blogging your baby-making journey. Or just take a walk.

- Cut back where you can. If you're like most women these days, you've probably got a lot on your plate – make that way too much. So try to cut back on those heaping servings of stressful activities, starting with those that aren't high priority (this is something you're going to have to do big time, anyway, once you have a bigger priority – a new baby). Obviously, your baby-making activities are high on your to-do list now, so rather than trying to squeeze them into a too-tight schedule – which is only going to make doing them more stressful – decide which other responsibilities can be postponed or delegated to someone else. Learn to say no to new projects before you reach overload (another skill you're wise to cultivate prebaby). If your job is adding to an unmanageable stress level (and seems to be affecting your TTC work), see if there are reasonable ways to reduce workplace stress. If not, a change of jobs or careers might be something to consider now (finances and opportunities permitting), before pregnancy weighs you down. Just be aware that this might affect your entitlement to Statutory Maternity Pay or Maternity Allowance (see 'A Guide to Maternity Benefits' on the Department for Work and Pensions website www.dwp.gov.uk).

- Unload whenever you can. Of course, the TTC process can be an emotional roller-coaster ride – you're up (maybe we did it this time!), you're down (AF . . . again?). Letting those letdown feelings out is the best way to make sure that they don't keep you down. So vent away. Start with your partner. Try to spend some time at the end of each day sharing feelings that need to find the nearest exit – you might be surprised to hear that he's feeling some of the same baby frustrations you are (just don't bring those feelings into the bedroom, where they could definitely derail your lovemaking). Vent to anyone else who will listen, too, especially to those who best understand what you're going through (unload workplace stress on a co-worker; dump TTC baggage on a friend or relative who's been down that road before; share with your practitioner your concerns about stress affecting your baby-making plans). Possibly one of your best potential venting outlets: a TTC message board. There you'll find plenty of other hopeful mums who are riding that very same roller coaster at the very same time. Knowing that you've got lots of company won't necessarily make your stress go away, but it can definitely make it easier to cope with.

- Turn off. Chances are you don't get a lot of quiet time these days – surrounded, as you probably are, by the constant chatter of computers, mobile phones, BlackBerries, TVs, iPods, and other accessories of the high-tech, fast-lane life. So every now and then, unplug. Power off your mobile phone (you'll survive!), ban the BlackBerry, log off your instant messenger, and turn off the radio and TV. Get reacquainted with the sound of silence – and you're sure to regain some of the calm you and your body are craving.

- Sleep. Bringing stress to bed? Stress can keep you from sleeping – and not sleeping can make you more stressed. See the box on the facing page for more on getting the sleep you need.

- Stretch. Or swim. Or run. Exercise relieves stress and boosts your mood (even when you're not in the mood for it). Plus it can help you work out some of those frustrations. Build some moves into your busy day every day.

☐ Yoga. Or tai chi. Or Pilates. Any of these natural stress-relief techniques can help bring you that inner serenity you're seeking. Continue with them during pregnancy (and beyond) to stay relaxed and refreshed.

☐ Massage it away. Head to a day spa (budget permitting) for a soothing laying on of hands – or book your partner for a couple's massage (he kneads you, you return the favour). It'll de-stress you, and hopefully put you both in the mood for baby making.

☐ CAM do. Explore the many Complementary and Alternative Medicine (CAM) therapies that can promise inner calm – among them biofeedback, acupuncture, and

hypnotherapy. Meditation and visualization can melt the stress away, too – and you can try them at home (or at your desk). Taking a couple of minutes to daydream about a place that makes you feel safe and soothed can provide many of the benefits of actually being there. Close your eyes and visualize somewhere you've felt at peace – an ocean beach, a tranquil forest, a mountain trail, your grandma's kitchen. Mentally linger there, taking in the view, summoning up the smells and sounds – or even taking a bite of one of grandma's warm-from-the-oven chocolate chip cookies – and relax.

☐ Have some scents. Your nose knows what scents you find soothing. Let it lead you to essential oils, lotions, or bubble baths with relaxing aromas (lavender is especially soothing). Put a few drops of the oil into a bottle

Your Other Job

So how does your day job affect your nighttime (or early morning) job of baby making? That depends on your day job. Most workplaces are fertility friendly for dads, especially with a few precautions. Jobs that involve radiation or chemical exposure are a key exception. High lead levels, as well as some organic solvents (such as those found in paints, glues, varnishes, and metal degreasers), pesticides, or other chemicals can compromise male fertility, so avoid these or limit your exposure as much as possible in preparation for conception (you don't want those sperm zapped). Contact IOSH (Institution of Occupational Safety and Health; www.iosh.co.uk) to find out if you need to be careful at your job site and how you can best play it safe.

If you're a road warrior – or you often tote a computer notebook for work – here's another preconception precaution you'll want to take: Keep your laptop off your lap. Research has found that men who use a laptop (on their laps) have lower sperm counts. That's because the heat from the laptop can raise the temperature in the testes, lowering sperm count and potentially reducing fertility. No need to pack up the laptop until baby's on board; just treat it like a desktop until you and your partner conceive.

And one more thing to avoid on the job – no matter what the job – when you're in baby-making mode: excessive stress, which can take a toll on your fertility, too.

Non-Traditional Conception

Most babies are born the old-fashioned way (boy meets girl, sperm meets egg). But what if you're a girl on your own? Or a couple of girls – or a couple of guys? Today's reproductive technology makes parenting possible in just about any lifestyle scenario.

What should your preconception plans include if you're a same-sex couple (or singleton) pursuing parenthood? That all depends on the route you're planning to take. If one female partner will be carrying the baby-to-be, her preconception prep should mirror any other wannabe mama's. If conception will be occuring the natural way, no further prep may be necessary. But if intrauterine insemination (IUI) or in vitro fertilization (IVF) plus donor sperm will be involved, Clomid and/or hormone shots may be on the agenda. If a pair of potential papas is planning to make a baby using a surrogate and sperm from one of the partners, his preconception prep should be focused on getting his boys in the best possible shape before they go to work. Either way, you'll find more about the assisted reproductive therapies (and more and more of them are available) that can help make your baby dreams a reality beginning on page 160.

of unscented lotion and rub it onto your hands, shoulders, and arms. Or purchase an electric aromatherapy diffuser to fill your rooms with a soothing scent. (Don't stock up on that scent, though: Once you do become pregnant, a relaxing fragrance can suddenly become a nauseating one.)

◻ Wash it away. A warm bath is an excellent way to relieve tension. Try it after a hectic day or whenever you're stressed out (and at home). Add some soothing aromatherapy oil or salts to complete the spa experience. If there's enough room in your tub, invite your partner to join you to get clean before you start messing around.

Stress still getting the best of you? Feeling unreasonably anxious? You might want to consider getting some professional counselling to help you learn some coping strategies that can really help you relax – and maybe even help you realize your baby dreams sooner.

Work and Fertility

"Could conditions at my job make it harder for me to get pregnant?"

You may have your work cut out for you making a baby, but that doesn't mean you'll have to cut out work to do it. Luckily, most 9-to-5 (or even 8-to-7) jobs are preconception compatible – and the vast majority of workplaces are perfectly safe when baby's on board, too. Even those jobs that might present some potential risks when it comes to conceiving and/or carrying a baby (X-ray technician, for example) can be made safer with some precautions. Here's how to play it extra safe when you're at work:

◻ Health care work. If you work in health care or dentistry, steer clear of exposure to dangerous chemicals and radiation (ask for a change of duties if possible or exercise extra caution by shielding yourself from any radiation and by wearing a special device that keeps track of daily radiation exposure to make sure it doesn't exceed safe levels). Be certain to take precautions (as any health care worker should) when treating patients with diseases such as HIV, hepatitis B, and CMV. Gloves, hand washing, and wise judgement are good bets for protecting yourself, as is making sure all your immunizations are up to date.

- Office work. Putting in a day at the office before you put in a night of baby making? No reason why not – even if your workday keeps you in front of a computer for hours at a time. Luckily computers don't pose a threat to fertility or fetuses (some studies have linked very high levels of radiation from older-model computers to fertility difficulties, but newer computers emit lower levels and aren't implicated). If you'd like to take some easy extra precautions anyway, push the screen as far back on your desk as you can and take breaks often so you're not in front of the computer all day long (your eyes and back will be grateful for these changes, too).

- Animal work. If you work with cats, you're probably aware that toxoplasmosis, an infectious disease that can be passed to humans through cat faeces, is something pregnant women need to be concerned about. And that means pregnant-to-be women should be aware of it too (since you never know when you might become pregnant, especially if you're already trying in earnest). If you're not sure whether you're immune to the disease, ask your practitioner to test you. If you turn out not to be immune, stay gloved when changing cat litter and remember to wash well after.

A Last Hurrah

Beyond excited about getting those baby plans under way, but feel like you have an adults-only holiday you need to get out of your system first? Pack your bags and go. Whether it's Sex on the Beach (the cocktail, that is) that you're craving, along with a couple of days of sun and sand, or a wine-and-cheese tasting in France, or that weekend in Monte Carlo you never got around to before (enough said) – now, before conception efforts begin in earnest, is the best time for that last hurrah. Or turn your last hurrah into a conception-moon and start your baby-making efforts with some sex on the beach (minus the cocktail).

- Industrial work. Some chemicals (though far from all and usually only in very large doses) are potentially harmful to your eggs before conception, and later to a developing embryo or fetus. Though the risk in most cases is slight or even just hypothetical, play it safe by avoiding potentially hazardous exposure on the job. Take special care in certain fields (art, photography, transportation, farming and landscaping, construction, hairdressing and cosmetology, dry cleaning, and some factory work). Because elevated lead levels when you conceive could pose problems for your baby, you should be tested if you have been exposed to lead in the workplace or elsewhere. Contact IOSH (Institution of Occupational Safety and Health; www.iosh.co.uk) for the latest information on job safety and pregnancy. In some cases, it may be wise to ask for a transfer to another position, change jobs, or take special precautions before trying to conceive.

Whatever your workplace environment, common sense should always be your first order of business. Wash your hands frequently, put on protective clothing as appropriate, and wear a mask or respirator when necessary. Talk to your doctor about your specific workplace circumstances – he or she will be able to let you know what might be dangerous and what you needn't be concerned about.

A final word on workplace issues and fertility: Extremely stressful work conditions, no matter what type of job you have, can contribute to fertility difficulties. For tips on how to try to minimize stress in your life, see page 24.

Your Financial Prep

Your body might be ready for a baby, but what about your wallet? Have you thought about how a baby is going to affect your bottom line (hint: a lot)? Or your career path or priorities? Planning now for the financial changes and business decisions that'll be coming your way long before your family officially expands (from the cost of prenatal care to the cost of a nursery, from health insurance to life insurance) is a smart component of your preconception prep. So open up the balance sheet, whip out the calculator, and start doing the baby maths. And while you're at it, consider issues that can come up at your workplace (like maternity leave).

Baby Costs

"Every time we hear about the costs of raising a baby, we wonder if we can really afford it. Is there anything we can do now to prepare financially?"

Little babies do come with a hefty price tag. Factor in all the big-ticket items (including a cot, a buggy, a car seat, and, possibly, childcare) plus the small ones (like baby food and nappies), and that baby bottom line adds up faster than you'd think. Before you conceive is the perfect time to start getting your financial rubber duckies in a row and plan for the financial changes you'll experience once baby makes three.

No need to tackle every budgetary line item at once (don't stress out about how you'll pay those university bills – yet), but anything you can start taking stock of now (including your stocks) will make budgeting down the road easier on your wallet and your sanity. Start small:

Tally it up. Make a list of your current expenses and then make a list of items you'll be calculating soon: nappies, bottles, formula (if you don't plan on breastfeeding or if you'll be combining breast and bottle), baby clothes, baby gear, baby food, baby toys, and so on, so you can get a clearer accounting of what your expenses really will be once your family starts to grow. Remember, there's a good chance you'll be getting plenty of those baby necessities and niceties as gifts; others you'll be able to borrow from friends and family.

Rebalance the budget. Think of ways (big and small) to cut corners and generate savings. Cut back on luxuries

When There's a Will, There's a Way

No one likes to contemplate mortality, especially when you're just about to begin a new life that's likely to be a very, very long and happy one. But planning for a baby should also mean planning for that baby's future security – and that includes planning for your baby's care in the highly unlikely event that you and your partner die. A will can provide for the financial security of your child (all your assets can go to your child, and depending on his or her age at your death, be managed by a responsible and trustworthy adult). But when an underage child is involved, there's more to your will than just money. If both of you die without a will, you will have no choice in who will raise your child. And that could be a bad thing – especially if you have serious issues with your in-laws or your sister's husband and that's who is chosen.

So think about drawing up that will soon – and definitely by the time your baby arrives. Choose a guardian who you believe will raise your child with values that best match your own, who will love your child as you would, and who will provide the healthiest and happiest environment for your precious one (and who is willing to take on the job – you definitely should ask first). And then don't give it another thought.

you can live without (passing on that morning mocha can save you at least 10 pounds a week; bringing a sandwich to work instead of eating out can save a lot more). Divert some of your current savings/investments into an interest-bearing baby fund and get serious about saving even more. Look critically at monthly expenditures for home and mobile phone plans, cable, gym memberships, and the like, and see if you can switch to cheaper ones (often just calling to threaten a switch will secure you a lower monthly cost). Negotiate discounts on whatever you can (more businesses and services are open to this option), and if you have a skill or a service that you can barter, save more cash by trading.

Crunch your credit. Still throwing away your hard-earned money on credit card interest payments? Stop (or at least slow down) the financial bleeding and reduce credit card debt by avoiding late fees, paying more than the minimum each month, and rolling balances onto low-interest cards. Once you get out of debt, consider staying that way. Pay your full balance each month and you'll save a yearly bundle on interest – a bundle you can invest, instead, on your bundle of joy. Living within your means definitely has its rewards (and may eventually help those means grow significantly). Reconsider your rewards cards, too – now may be the time to opt out of one that offers holiday perks (how practical will that trip to Bora Bora be when you're toting baby baby?) and swap it for one that'll help put you in the driver's seat of a family-friendly car or that'll score you savings on baby gear.

Start laying that egg. No, not *that* egg, but the egg that will keep your fledgling-to-be cosy and secure in the years ahead: your nest egg. If you've been saving up for something you'd love to have but can live without (that big-screen TV, perhaps), consider socking the cash away in a savings vehicle instead (a high-interest savings account, mutual funds, or bonds) so that your little nest egg can turn into a bigger one. Choose one that maximizes growth over the long term. If you haven't started saving yet, now's the time. Set aside a small amount from your monthly paycheque to start or add to your account (paid off by those skipped lattes or bagged lunches). If your savings self-discipline is lacking (or nonexistent), enrolling in an automatic savings programme may give you the tough financial love you need. Almost all banks allow you to authorize monthly (or even weekly) deductions from your current account to your investment account. Unexpected funds land in your lap (from a tax refund or a bonus – or a lucky scratch-card)? Sure, that pair of strappy sandals would be a fun way to unload the windfall, but a smarter move would be to drop that spare change into your nest egg before you're tempted to hit the shops (besides, once you're expecting, you won't be able to squeeze your swollen dogs into those sandals,

anyway). And speaking of spare change, don't forget the oldest savings trick in the book – the jar. Drop those annoying pennies (and other coins) into a jar, convert them periodically at a supermarket coin changer, and add the found money into your savings account. Fattening up your piggy bank now will help you handle the bigger expenditures that are just around the corner – plus, it'll get you in the savings habit (a habit that will definitely come in handy when you have a little someone else to save up for).

Be smart with your money. Look for tax-saving vehicles, such as ISAs. Such accounts allow you to sock away money that can be used for medical expenses (such as prenatal vitamins and ovulation kits).

"What about life insurance? It never occurred to me, until we started thinking about getting pregnant."

Life insurance is probably something you've always associated with the much older set – or at least, the all-settled set. But there's no better time to think about a life insurance policy than when you're thinking about starting a new life. Although no amount of money will replace a lost parent or spouse, every parent should be insured so that his or her surviving dependants will be financially protected. You don't need a policy with a huge payoff, but rather one that will cover costs of living and raising your child with one less salary. There's another reason (unfair as it may be) why shopping for a life insurance policy prepregnancy is worthwhile: Some insurance companies charge higher rates for pregnant women. It might be even harder to get a good premium later if you end up developing a complication during pregnancy that could develop into a chronic

Action Plan

Savings plan? Check. Balanced budget? Check(book). Sounds like a lot of financial planning to prepare for a baby you haven't even conceived yet – and pretty overwhelming if you're a finance newbie – but there's no better investment in your time right now than investing in your family-to-be's fiscal future and security. It's also a good way to avoid sticker shock down the road.

Mobile Sense

Are you living the wireless life? Of course you are – who isn't? But even the best mobile phone or texting plan can come at a cost when you're a hopeful father, and we're not talking roaming charges. Believe it or not, preliminary evidence links *excessive* mobile phone use by a man with the potential for fertility difficulties. The more the guy uses his mobile phone, apparently, the lower his sperm count is likely to be.

Researchers speculate that the electromagnetic radiation from a mobile phone alters sperm cells, lowering their count and making them less healthy and less able to fertilize an egg. Stress might play some role, too (after all, wireless junkies tend to be

. . . well, more wired). So what's a guy (who wants to become a dad) to do? Though moderate mobile phone or BlackBerry use is fine, you might want to consider cutting back if you're a certifiable addict. And instead of keeping the phone in your trouser pocket (where it'll be closer to the package you're trying to protect), keep it in your jacket pocket or holstered to your belt, away from those jewels. Do these precautions apply to a beeper as well? No evidence at all yet, but because it functions in a similar way to the mobile phone, the theoretical link is there. If you want to play it extra safe while staying connected, stash your beeper in your jacket pocket as well.

condition postpartum (for instance, preeclampsia – or pregnancy-induced high blood pressure – could lead to chronic hypertension after delivery). Again, not fair, but a pretty common insurance practice.

Maternity Leave

"My friend at work (who knows I'd like to get pregnant soon) told me I should find out what my company offers for maternity leave. Is it too early to look into it?"

Maternity leave may not be right around the corner (after all, you're not even pregnant yet), but now's actually a good time to take a peek around that corner – and find out everything you can about your company's maternity leave policy. The sooner you know what's in store for your career and your income once baby's born, the

easier it will be to figure out your post-delivery back-to-work plan and financial picture.

First, review your company's maternity leave policy (ask someone at Human Resources, or if you'd rather be more discreet about your TTC plans, check the benefits handbook). Find out how long your company's maternity leave is, whether or not you'll be paid (and at what rate) during your leave, if you're allowed to add accumulated sick, holiday, or personal days, and if any other work conditions are required for you to qualify for maternity leave (such as being an employee for a certain amount of time before the benefits kick in).

Then decide as best you can at this point (keeping in mind that little babies can bring big changes, even before they're born), what your financial and career situation can bear, as well as what your preferences are, given a choice.

You may qualify for either Statutory Maternity Pay or Maternity Allowance (there are user-friendly guides to both on www.direct.gov.uk) which can be paid for up to 39 weeks. But consider: after that period, will your budget allow you to take more time off? Or will you be returning to work as soon as possible, either for financial reasons (the cost of childcare factored in) or career reasons? Will both of you have to work full time, or will it make financial sense (given the high cost of childcare) for one of you to stay home with the new baby? Are there other options such as flexitime, job sharing, working from home, or working part time that you can start exploring now (rather than right before your maternity leave is over and you're forced to make a decision you may not be happy with)?

Combining parenting (already a full-time job) with another full-time job will take plenty of juggling and, most likely, some shifting of priorities. But giving it some thought now, before the decision heat is on, can get you started on finding that happy (if not perfect) balance of work and home that will work for you and your family.

CHAPTER 2

Weighing In Before You're Expecting

SO YOU PROBABLY FIGURE THAT you'll be in for some weight changes once you're expecting (and maybe you're really looking forward to watching those numbers on the scale creep up, especially if you've spent your whole adult life trying to keep them down). But maybe you didn't realize that making some weight changes before you're expecting can actually help you expect sooner – and expect a healthier and more comfortable pregnancy, too. That's right – getting your weight as close as you can to that elusive "ideal" should definitely top your preconception to-do list (and it's something you should definitely try to do before you start trying to make that baby). Whether you've got a little (or a lot) to lose, or a little (or a lot) to gain, weighing in before you're expecting can help you zoom in on conception – and fast-forward to the pregnancy starting gate.

Not sure where your weight should be, or how to get it where it should be in the most fertility-friendly way possible? Check in with your practitioner for some guidelines, and read on for tips on how to tip the scales in conception's favour.

Your Weight and Your Fertility

Are you overweight, underweight, or just the right weight to make a baby? There's a strong connection between weight and fertility, but it's a complicated one, too – and it's much more than just a numbers game. Getting to the bottom of your bottom line is one of the most important steps you can take when you're getting your body ready for the baby making big time.

Body Fat and Hormones

"My doctor mentioned that there's a connection between my weight and my hormones. What's that all about?"

Oestrogen – the reproductive hormone responsible for helping eggs to mature, building up the uterine lining, and producing thin cervical mucus – is produced primarily in your ovaries. But did you know that more than 30 percent of the oestrogen in your body is produced by your fat cells? It's true. The same cells you thought served no purpose at all (besides sitting around your bum and thighs) are closely tied to your fertility. And whether that's a good association or not is in the numbers. If you have about the right amount of fat cells (no need to count them, just take a look at your body mass index, or BMI; see the next question), then you're likely producing just the right amount of oestrogen. If you have more than the normal amount of fat cells (because your BMI is high), those fat cells will be producing more oestrogen than necessary. If you have far fewer fat cells than you should have (because your BMI is very low), your body will be oestrogen starved. Because a delicate balance of hormones – which includes the perfect supply of oestrogen – needs to be maintained for your reproductive cycle to work the way it's supposed to, too much or too little oestrogen (from too many or too few fat cells) can throw your fertility off kilter. In fact, it's suspected that more than 10 percent of all fertility problems stem from weight issues.

Have too few fat cells, or too many? Give your hormones the best shot at conception by getting your weight on track. If you need to gain, see page 48; if you need to lose, see page 47.

Prebaby BMI

"How do I figure out whether I'm at the ideal weight for TTC?"

Bodies, in case you haven't noticed, come in all kinds of packages. Tall, thin packages; short, chubby packages; more muscular packages; more fleshy packages; top heavy; bottom heavy; nowhere heavy; everywhere heavy. And when it comes to figuring the "ideal" size for your TTC body, a lot really depends on the kind of package it comes in.

That's exactly why most practitioners don't rely on scale numbers alone in determining whether your weight is at – or close enough to – that preconception ideal, or whether you'll have some gaining or losing to do before you get busy TTC. They still use the scale (before you get excited about skipping your office weigh-in), but they factor it into a calculation known as body mass index, or BMI, which describes the relationship between weight and height and provides a better measure of body fat content than the scale alone. Remember, body fat is the key to fertility: Too little fat could mean too little oestrogen, whereas too much fat can mean too much oestrogen. Either scenario could spell fertility trouble.

The formula for calculating your BMI is: weight (kilograms) ÷ height (metres)^2. For example, a woman who weighs 65 kilograms and is 165 centimetres (1.65 metres) will have the following BMI equation: 65 kilograms ÷ 1.65 × 1.65 metres (2.7225 metres) = 24.

Once you've calculated your BMI (or if you don't want to do the maths, or have left those skills back in your school algebra class, just check the chart on the next page), you can determine what category you fall into.

- Have a BMI less than 18.5? You're considered underweight – and you'll need to put on some weight before TTC.

What's Your BMI?

Height (feet and inches)

Weight (pounds)	5'0"	5'1"	5'2"	5'3"	5'4"	5'5"	5'6"	5'7"	5'8"	5'9"	5'10"	5'11"	6'0"	6'1"	6'2"	6'3"	6'4"	Weight (kilograms)
100	20	19	18	18	17	17	16	16	15	15	14	14	14	13	13	12	12	45
105	21	20	19	19	18	17	17	16	16	16	15	15	14	14	13	13	13	47
110	21	21	20	19	19	18	18	17	17	16	16	15	15	15	14	14	13	50
115	22	22	21	20	20	19	19	18	17	17	17	16	16	15	15	14	14	52
120	23	23	22	21	21	20	19	19	18	18	17	17	16	16	15	15	15	54
125	24	24	23	22	21	21	20	20	19	18	18	17	17	16	16	16	15	57
130	25	25	24	23	22	22	21	20	20	19	19	18	18	17	17	16	16	59
135	26	26	25	24	23	22	22	21	21	20	19	19	18	18	17	17	16	61
140	27	26	26	25	24	23	23	22	21	21	20	20	19	18	18	17	17	63
145	28	27	27	26	25	24	23	23	22	21	21	20	20	19	19	18	18	66
150	29	28	27	27	26	25	24	23	23	22	22	21	20	20	19	19	18	68
155	30	29	28	27	27	26	25	24	24	23	22	22	21	20	20	19	19	70
160	31	30	29	28	27	27	26	25	24	24	23	22	22	21	21	20	19	72
165	32	31	30	29	28	27	27	26	25	24	24	23	22	22	21	21	20	75
170	33	32	31	30	29	28	27	27	26	25	24	24	23	22	22	21	21	77
175	34	33	32	31	30	29	28	27	27	26	25	24	24	23	22	22	21	79
180	35	34	33	32	31	30	29	28	27	27	26	25	24	24	23	22	22	82
185	36	35	34	33	32	31	30	29	28	27	27	26	25	24	24	23	23	84
190	37	36	35	34	33	32	31	30	29	28	27	26	26	25	24	24	23	86
195	38	37	36	35	33	32	31	31	30	29	28	27	26	26	25	24	24	88
200	39	38	37	35	34	33	32	31	30	30	29	28	27	26	26	25	24	91
205	40	39	37	36	35	34	33	32	31	30	29	29	28	27	26	26	25	93
210	41	40	38	37	36	35	34	33	32	31	30	29	28	28	27	26	26	95
215	42	41	39	38	37	36	35	34	33	32	31	30	29	28	28	27	26	98
220	43	42	40	39	38	37	36	34	33	32	32	31	30	29	28	27	27	100
225	44	43	41	40	39	37	36	35	34	33	32	31	31	30	29	28	27	102
230	45	43	42	41	39	38	37	36	35	34	33	32	31	30	30	29	28	104
235	46	44	43	42	40	39	38	37	36	35	34	33	32	31	30	29	29	107
240	47	45	44	43	41	40	39	38	36	35	34	33	33	32	31	30	29	109
245	48	46	45	43	42	41	40	38	37	36	35	34	33	32	31	31	30	111
250	49	47	46	44	43	42	40	39	38	37	36	35	34	33	32	31	30	114

150 152.5 155 157.5 160 162.5 165 167.5 170 172.5 175 177.5 180 182.5 185 187.5 190

Height (centimetres)

☐ Have a BMI between 18.5 and 24? You're considered average weight – and at the ideal weight for TTC.

☐ Have a BMI between 25 and 29? You're considered overweight – and ideally, you should lose some weight before TTC.

☐ Have a BMI of 30 or higher? You're considered obese – and it's time to get serious about losing weight, before you start trying for a baby.

Keep in mind that your BMI doesn't always tell the whole story when it comes to weight and body fat. For example, if you've been a regular on the training circuit (especially the weight-training circuit), you may be on the heavier side on the BMI chart because of all those extra muscles (muscles weigh more than fat). But as long as you're packing a normal amount of body fat (even if your muscles weigh you down on the scale), your body's likely to produce just the right amount of oestrogen to keep your cycles regular – and keep your fertility high. On the other hand, if you're on the heavier side largely due to soft padding around your belly and your thighs (and not thanks to rock-hard abs and quads), your body may produce too much oestrogen, which could undercut your fertility.

Are you thin? The same principle could apply on the flip side. You could be very thin (or even underweight by standard BMI measurements), but still nicely padded – with much of your weight coming from fat, not muscle mass. Chances are that the padding you have (as minimal as it might be, compared to a heavier woman) will be enough to generate the oestrogen your body needs to keep your reproductive cycle running smoothly. Thin and athletic, with much muscle, but precious little fat? Even if you weigh the same as someone who's thin and padded, you might produce much less oestrogen – which could disrupt your cycles and undermine your fertility.

Overweight

"I'm overweight. Will that affect my fertility?"

Extra weight can definitely weigh you down when it comes to fertility – and it takes less extra weight than you might think. Obese women (those with a BMI over 30) have a significantly lower chance of becoming pregnant compared to average-weight women. But even being moderately overweight (with a BMI of 25 to 29) can slow down – or even sabotage – your baby-making efforts. Extra kilograms (in the form of extra fat) trigger extra oestrogen production. And though having extra female hormones sounds like a good

---

What Fruit Are You?

Are you an apple (shape) or a pear (shape)? These two fruit-shaped body types not only dictate what bathing suit you should choose, but they may also have a connection to your fertility. Researchers have found that overweight women who are apple-shaped – those with a high waist-to-hip ratio – have a harder time (on average) getting pregnant, whereas overweight pear-shaped women – those with a low waist-to-hip ratio – have an easier time (on average) conceiving. It seems that where your excess body fat is located on your body may be just as important as – if not more important than – how much extra body fat you have.

Weighing In on Male Fertility

Extra weight doesn't impact just a woman's fertility; it can weigh heavily on a man's, too. Overweight men tend to have more fertility problems than normal-weight hopeful dads – with a 10-kilogram overage increasing a guy's chances of infertility, research suggests, by about 10 percent. That's because excess fat converts the male hormone testosterone into the female hormone oestrogen, possibly suppressing sperm production and lowering overall sperm quality. It can also negatively impact libido (the more body fat you have, the higher your levels of a natural chemical that binds existing testosterone, making less available to stimulate desire) – and it almost goes without saying that libido is something you'll need in spades while you're TTC. What's more, obese men are more likely to have erectile dysfunction (vessel-clogging fatty deposits form in the tiny arteries in the penis, causing it to shut down), certainly a problem you don't want to bring to bed when there's baby making on the agenda.

To make sure you reach optimum baby-making potential once you and your partner begin trying to conceive, try to reach your optimum weight first (or as close as you can get to it). As with mum hopefuls who have preconception weight to shed, it's smart to go on a sensible diet plan – one that decreases calories and fat, but doesn't short-change you on nutrients you'll need. If you have a lot of weight to lose, it might help to check in with your doctor first for some guidelines and suggestions – as well as to set a realistic goal. Getting some exercise, which boosts testosterone levels, can also boost both function and libido (a good reason to get busy in bed after you've just been busy at the gym).

If you're significantly overweight, and haven't had any luck dropping the kilos through diet and exercise, you may have considered bariatric or lap-band surgery – but may also have wondered how such a procedure might affect your chances of becoming a father. Good news: So far, the research has shown that a significant weight loss from weight-loss surgery can actually improve fertility for obese men, as well as for obese women. Many of the conception problems that a very heavy man may have faced prior to such surgery may resolve post-op, often delivering a return of libido and sexual function.

thing when you're trying to make a baby (after all, isn't it the most fundamental of female functions?), the opposite is actually true. Too much oestrogen can keep you from ovulating regularly, or even ovulating at all (30 to nearly 40 percent of obese women have irregular menstrual cycles) – decreasing your chances of becoming pregnant.

Even if you're overweight but have normal periods, you're still not out of the weight woods completely. Studies show that overweight women have a harder time getting pregnant even if they have normal periods.

And there's more to the weight story than just weight: Being obese or overweight is associated with polycystic ovarian syndrome (PCOS), another fairly common cause of fertility issues (see pages 42 and 142). Too much weight can also cause insulin levels to rise and too much insulin, in some women, can cause the ovaries to overproduce testosterone, a male hormone that definitely doesn't help in the female fertility department.

Plus, here's another weighty issue to contemplate while you're contemplating conceiving: Not only can being overweight compromise fertility, but it can also be problematic once you do become pregnant – even if you don't gain too much weight during pregnancy. Those extra kilograms can increase the risk of miscarriage, gestational diabetes, pregnancy-induced hypertension (pre-eclampsia), a longer labour, and a caesarean delivery. What's more, children born to overweight or obese mothers are at increased risk of becoming obese or diabetic during childhood and as adults. And prepregnancy obesity can also raise the risk of neural tube and other birth defects, especially if mum wears much of her weight around her middle, rather than on her hips.

So getting closer to the recommended weight range for your height and body type (aiming for a BMI of 20 to 24, if possible) before you conceive may help speed your baby-making success – and may help keep your pregnancy safer. But any amount of weight loss in obese or overweight women can improve fertility, and studies show that spontaneous ovulation will reoccur in 60 percent of women who reduce their overall body weight by 5 to 10 percent. So if getting to your goal weight before you start your conception campaign isn't a realistic goal, just aim to lose what you can (see page 47 for tips how).

"I'm about 30 kilograms overweight, and I know I'm supposed to lose it before I get pregnant, but I just don't want to wait that long. Can I just go ahead and try to conceive?"

Ideally, every woman would conceive when her weight was right about where it was supposed to be – giving her the optimum chances of conception, and the optimum chances of a healthy, comfortable pregnancy, a healthy baby, and a safe delivery. But conception doesn't always wait for the ideal circumstances, and sometimes waiting for conception isn't ideal, either, especially if you're over 35 (timing can be everything when you're planning a family).

It's possible that you'll have more trouble getting pregnant if you're significantly overweight (the statistics definitely support that possibility). But it's also possible that you won't. Though it's best to have a normal BMI when you TTC, overweight women get pregnant all the time – just as underweight ones do. If your cycles run like clockwork, and if you appear to be ovulating regularly, your odds of conceiving may be pretty good.

Of course, improved fertility isn't the only reason why waiting for that ideal prepregnancy weight (or something approaching it) makes sense. Being overweight at the beginning of pregnancy poses a number of potential risks that can weigh down your pregnancy and even impact your baby-to-be's future health (see previous answer). Keeping your pregnancy weight gain to a minimum, under close supervision by your practitioner, can help reduce the risks significantly, if not eliminate them

Action Plan

If you're overweight, aim to bring your weight down so your BMI is in the 20 to 24 range. Can't get that low – or get that low quickly enough for your preferred conception timetable? Even a weight loss of just 5 to 10 percent (that's 3¾ to 7½ kilograms for someone who weighs 75 kilograms) can help regulate your cycle and get you pregnant faster.

Double the Weight, Double the Baby-Making Trouble

The couple who eats too much together, it appears, may also have a tougher time making a baby together. Though fertility can be impacted when just one mate is overweight, conception challenges multiply when both partners are packing extra pounds. In fact, making that baby can take three times longer for heavy couples than for average-weight ones. To help ensure that you and your partner reach your baby-making goal together, try reaching your weight loss goals together first. After all, it's always easier to shed pounds when you're not trying to do it alone (and when nobody's chowing down on chips while you're nibbling on veggies and dip – or slumped on the sofa while you're trying to get motivated to take that morning jog). Eating right and exercising together will make it more likely that you'll both hit your goals (and the baby jackpot) faster. Go Team Baby!

---

entirely. So can getting regular exercise (again, with your practitioner's input) and eating as well as you can. And don't wait (if you decide to move ahead with your TTC plans) to make those adjustments to your lifestyle – getting on a balanced eating plan and an appropriate exercise programme now can not only improve your fertility, but it can get your body in the best possible shape for pregnancy. Who knows, maybe you'll even lose a good chunk of weight while you're waiting (or not waiting) to get pregnant.

Before you make any decisions about your TTC timing, though, talk to your practitioner about your plans – and about ways to help optimize your conception and pregnancy success, even if you're not waiting for that optimum weight.

Polycystic Ovarian Syndrome and Overweight

"I have PCOS. Is that why I'm overweight and have so much trouble losing weight?"

It definitely could have something to do with it – or even everything to do with it. Polycystic ovarian syndrome, or PCOS, is a condition associated with irregular periods, lack of ovulation, elevated levels of male hormones, and, very often, obesity and/or persistent, sometimes unexplained weight gain. Women with PCOS may find that losing weight is a losing battle, even when they're giving dieting everything they've got. In fact, studies show that women with PCOS tend to gain more weight than women without PCOS, even if they eat the same foods and amount of calories. Definitely unfair, but at least it explains what you're up against and why.

So what's the biological connection between PCOS and weight gain (and trouble losing weight)? First, women with PCOS often have insulin resistance. Normally, insulin transports glucose (sugar) out of the blood and helps convert it to energy. But with insulin resistance, the body is unable to use insulin properly. Thinking that there's not enough insulin to get sugar out of the blood and into the cells, the body reacts by producing even more insulin to get the job done. Too much insulin, however, causes the glucose to be stored as fat instead of being converted to energy. Extremely high levels of insulin also turn off a fat-metabolizing enzyme, preventing you from burning stored fat – and making shedding the kilos frustratingly difficult.

Second, some women with PCOS are hypothyroid (they don't make enough thyroid hormone). This thyroid dysfunction causes a lower metabolic rate (the rate at which you burn calories), and it makes losing weight even tougher.

Even with all the weight-loss cards seemingly stacked against you, there are treatments that can help you in your efforts, so that you can lose weight and regain your fertility. Some women with PCOS are prescribed metformin, an insulin-resistance medication that seems to help reduce the effects of PCOS, often making weight loss possible. A diabetes-friendly low-glycaemic type of diet – your doctor (and perhaps a dietitian) can put one together for you – plus exercise can also help get your weight under control, giving your chances of conceiving a needed boost. And if you haven't yet, make sure you're tested for thyroid dysfunction. Treatment for a thyroid condition is simple (as easy as taking thyroid replacement hormone) and effective, and it can help you melt that weight off. For more on PCOS, see page 142.

Diabetes and Weight

"I have type 2 diabetes and I'm overweight. If my diabetes is under control, do I have to worry about my weight too?"

Pat yourself on the back for getting your diabetes under control – no easy job (as you know), and yet such an important one when you're hoping to make a baby. But it shouldn't be the only priority on your preconception to-do list. Being overweight – whether those extra kilos are causing your diabetes or not – is still a risk factor for decreased fertility and increased pregnancy problems. Which is why your next step should be a concerted effort to get your weight down to where it should be (or close to that ideal).

And that goal may be easier to reach now that your diabetes is under control. It's true that having insulin-resistant diabetes makes you more prone to being overweight because the excess blood sugar in your body is stored as fat. Excess insulin also turns off a fat-metabolizing enzyme, not allowing stored fat to be burned off, and creating a double weight-loss whammy. But controlling your diabetes may help you get your weight under control – and getting your weight under control may help you keep your diabetes under control. With well-controlled blood sugar, a good diet (usually low-glycaemic, which keeps blood sugar level), and regular exercise (shoot for 30 minutes a day of cardio, strength training, and stretching), you should be able to get your weight down. Yes, it'll take plenty of effort, loads of dedication, and more than a little sweat and sacrifice (so long, couch and crisps; hello, Stairmaster and healthy snacks), but the rewards don't get any better. Not only will this strategy help put conception within reach, but if you continue it after conception, it'll help ensure an uncomplicated pregnancy and a healthy baby.

Underweight

"I'm underweight. Will that make it harder to get pregnant?"

Often, women with a very low BMI – usually under 18.5, but sometimes

Thin Isn't in When You Want a Baby

Here's the skinny on another weighty issue: underweight. Men whose BMI is less than 20 may be more likely to encounter fertility challenges than average-weight guys. It seems low weight in men is linked to lower sperm count and decreased sperm function. So if you're on the extra-lean side, you might want to think about adding a few healthy kilos before you and your partner start trying to add to your family.

that benchmark can be a little higher or a little lower – tend not to have regular periods (or any periods) or to ovulate regularly (or at all). Irregular (or nonexistent) cycles can, to state the obvious, make conception tricky or impossible. Which means that you may have to add some bulk to your body before you can add a baby to your body.

There are other reasons to consider filling out your frame before filling up your uterus, besides avoiding conception problems. Women who are underweight when they become pregnant have an increased risk of severe nausea and vomiting during the early months of pregnancy, and severely underweight women (those with a BMI less than 18) are much more likely to miscarry than those of normal weight. These extremely underweight expectant mums also run a higher risk of having a premature or underweight baby (though excellent nutrition and good weight gain before and during pregnancy can definitely reduce those risks).

Talk to your practitioner about whether you should pack on some pounds before beginning your baby-making efforts – and how many you should aim for. Every body is different (and some naturally extra-lean bodies conceive and handle pregnancy with ease), but chances are you'll be advised to shoot for a BMI of at least 18.5 but preferably between 20 and 24, the range widely considered optimum for baby making. Not only may a boost in BMI boost your chances of getting pregnant in the first place, but it will allow you to enter pregnancy at an ideal weight – so you'll be able to gain that 9-month standard of 11 to 16 kilos later without worrying about playing weight gain catch-up first.

"I've always been thin – and definitely underweight for my height – at least according to the charts. But my doctor says I shouldn't be concerned about my fertility. Why's that?"

There's often a thin line between thin and too thin. And that line may be different for different women. The weight that's right for you may be off the "normal range" charts – especially if it's a weight you've stayed at pretty consistently through your adult lifetime, without resorting to dieting or overexercising, if you're otherwise in good health, and if you have healthy lifestyle habits (including healthy eating habits).

That's why weight alone doesn't tell the whole story, particularly when it comes to fertility. You may be thin, but you may have just the right amount of body fat to keep your reproductive health humming along perfectly (regular periods, regular ovulation, and so on) even if your weight – and even your BMI – is on the low side. So if your doctor isn't concerned about your weight affecting your chances of becoming pregnant, you shouldn't be, either.

Eating Disorders and Fertility

"I've battled on and off with an eating disorder for years, and lately I've been doing much better. I'm thinking about getting pregnant, but I wonder whether having had an eating disorder might affect my fertility."

Fighting an eating disorder can be a real struggle – as you know all too well. So first of all, congratulations on the hard-earned progress you've made – that makes your pregnancy prognosis very promising. Putting your eating disorder in the past will almost certainly help you put a baby in your future.

Untreated eating disorders are a very different story, however, and a story that's not as likely to have a happy reproductive ending. Fertility can definitely be compromised – sometimes seriously so – by an eating disorder, especially an active one. In fact, as many as 1 in 5 women treated for infertility have either anorexia or bulimia. Not surprising, actually, since such disorders can disrupt the balance of hormones necessary to make baby making happen.

Here's how: With anorexia, drastically reduced calorie intake and excessive exercising leads to dramatic weight loss and significant reduction of body fat (usually to levels way below normal). These factors can combine to result in a complete shutdown of a woman's menstrual cycle – no ovulation, no periods – which can obviously make conception virtually impossible. If anorexia continues for years untreated (or treated unsuccessfully), her reproductive system may be permanently damaged, and in some cases, her period may never return. Even if she does manage to get pregnant, extremely low levels of body fat can increase the risk of miscarriage.

Bulimia can have a devastating effect on a woman's fertility, too – even if she manages to keep her weight relatively normal. In fact, about 50 percent of bulimics don't have regular menstrual cycles (which, again, makes conception less likely). But infertility issues are also possible in bulimics who have regular menstrual bleeding, since the bingeing and purging can lead to deficiencies in circulating hormone levels.

A nutritionally deprived diet, common for both anorexics and bulimics, can also lead to lowered libido, reduced egg quality, poor uterine environment, and ovarian failure – all of which can make a healthy pregnancy more elusive. Psychological stress (from constant anxiety about food and weight monitoring) is another potential fertility thwarter for those who suffer from eating disorders.

The good news? Taking steps to bring an eating disorder under control – as you've already done and are committed to keep doing – can help you take charge of your fertility and make your baby dreams a reality. Talk to your practitioner about your plans, and be completely up front about the problems you've had (and any you're still grappling with, even if they're minor compared

Action Plan

If your BMI is under 18.5, you may need to pack on some poundage before you begin your TTC campaign. Talk to your practitioner about the weight-gain goal that's right for you (you may be advised to aim for a BMI of 20 to 24, though every body is different). Filling out your frame a little may actually make it easier for you to fill your belly with baby.

to those you've struggled with in the past). If you still need treatment before you take the pregnancy plunge, now's the time to get that help – from either a programme or a therapist who specializes in eating disorders. You may even want to consider continuing the therapy while you're expecting to make sure that normal pregnancy body changes don't trigger a relapse. Enlisting a dietitian can also help you reshape your eating habits, so you can continue nourishing your body, and hopefully soon, your baby-to-be's. Support groups (you can find them online, too) can also help you get your nutritional status back where it should be, as well as help you cope with new body image issues that might come up during pregnancy.

The best news of all? Approximately 80 percent of women whose eating disorders are successfully treated will regain their ability to conceive. You can do it, too.

Weight-Loss Surgery and TTC

"My doctor said I need to lose at least 30 kilos before I can get pregnant – but dieting isn't getting me anywhere, and I'd really like a baby sooner than later. Should I think about weight-loss surgery?"

When you're seriously overweight – and a lifetime of dieting and exercise haven't helped you melt off the kilos you're desperate to lose – gastric bypass or lap-band surgery may seem the answer to your weight problems. Especially when baby fever has you sweating the kilos that stand between you and conception. But do weight-loss surgery and baby making mix?

Actually, they can mix – and pretty successfully. In fact, such procedures can pave the quickest path to pregnancy for women who are too heavy to conceive. Women who've undergone weight-loss surgery often see a return to regular menstrual cycles within months of the operation, even if they haven't yet come close to their ultimate weight-loss goal. Fertility may return, too, sooner than expected. Some women are able to conceive just months post-op.

But while the surgery may well fast-track your fertility, you may not get the baby green light as quickly as you'd like – even if your cycles are back up and running. Some doctors suggest that women who have had weight-loss surgery put the brakes on their post-op conception plans until their weight has been stabilized for a year – not only so their bodies have time to adjust (dropping so much can be a big adjustment), but so they have time to replenish nutritional reserves that may have been drained by rapid weight loss. Still, regardless of when they conceive, women who become pregnant after gastric surgery can have healthy pregnancies and healthy babies – and, in fact, healthier than they would have if they hadn't lost weight at all.

If you're contemplating weight-loss surgery – or you've already had it, and wonder how it might affect your pregnancy plans – talk to your doctors (if you haven't already) about the best baby-making timing for you. Also keep in mind that you'll have to be extra vigilant to make sure your nutritional needs are met during the preconception period and during pregnancy, to prevent shortfalls of vital baby-making nutrients. That's tricky after bariatric surgery because your food intake will be drastically reduced, but it's definitely possible with some extra effort, the right vitamin supplements, and guidance from your medical team.

Reaching Your Ideal Weight

Okay, it's one thing to have a weight loss – or gain – goal, it's another to actually make that goal a reality. Dieting to lose weight is never easy (and for the super skinny, eating enough to gain may be tricky, too), but it can be particularly challenging when those kilos need to be shed sensibly, as they should be when conception's next up on your agenda. Need a plan to get those numbers where they need to be in the fastest yet most baby-friendly way possible? Read on.

Losing Weight

"I'm around 14 kilograms overweight and I want to start a family. What's the best way for me to lose weight?"

Losing weight is easier said than done – even if your baby-making plans are making you especially motivated – but it's definitely doable. Your first stop (even before you stop at the market to stock up on yogurt, fresh fruit, and carrot sticks) should be at your practitioner's office. Together, come up with a sensible weight-loss goal and a sensible plan for reaching it – and discuss, too, any health issues that might be contributing to that extra weight, such as a thyroid condition or insulin resistance. It's best to reach your goal about 6 to 8 weeks before you start trying to conceive so your body can get used to its new shape before it starts changing again (in case you haven't heard, pregnancy is definitely a big-time shape changer).

Resist the urge to sign up for a crash diet – even one that's high protein, low carb – because it can too easily deplete your body's stores of vital baby-making nutrients (and after all, it's weight you want to lose now, not nutrients). Steer clear, too, of liquid diets, diet pills and supplements, or anything that promises a quick fix ("lose 12 kilograms in 2 weeks!"). Weight loss that's too quick can also lead to fertility issues – this time disrupting ovulation by decreasing progesterone production. Rapid weight loss can also lead to rapid weight gain a few months later, and studies show that yo-yo dieters have a lower rate of fertility than those who lose the weight sensibly. Slow and steady may not have you winning any weight-loss races, but it's definitely the best diet plan when you're planning a baby. A gradual weight loss will give your reproductive hormones ample time to readjust to your new weight reality.

Stick to a well-balanced diet that's lower in calories and fat but doesn't overrestrict them, and one that focuses on a healthy balance of those sensible standbys: lean protein, lowfat dairy products, veggies, fruits, and whole grains. Sensible doesn't make many diet headlines, but it's more likely to get the job done – and keep it done. Practise portion control (fill up on low-calorie salads, eat petite when it comes to more calorie-dense foods), and get in the habit of grazing on small amounts of food more frequently (a good eating strategy for pregnancy, too). Drink lots of water, and don't forget to take your prenatal vitamin (to help fill in any nutritional blanks that dieting may create). Cut down on – or if it's easier for you, and it is for some serious junk food fans, cut out – puddings, fizzy drinks, and other junk food. If you haven't been exercising, start fitting in fitness. Even 30 minutes of walking a few days a week is a great way to shed some weight while helping to jump-start your journey to a healthy pregnancy.

Some women find that a side of camaraderie helps them stay motivated to lose weight (and stick to that side salad, instead of that side of chips). If that's the case with you, check out TTC message boards (you'll find them on WhatToExpect.com) – to see if you can team up with other hopeful mums who are anxious to lose weight and gain a baby. Or consider joining Weight Watchers or another balanced diet plan that offers support along with those carrot sticks.

And if you're feeling discouraged about the weight loss you have ahead of you, here's an encouraging bulletin that's sure to put a smile on your face (and maybe a piece of healthy fruit in your mouth): A loss of just 5 to 10 percent in overall body weight in overweight women (particularly obese women) who haven't been ovulating results in spontaneous ovulation in 60 percent of women. And you know what ovulation can bring you: baby bingo!

Gaining Weight

"My doctor says I should gain some weight before I start TTC. Where do I begin?"

Gaining weight – like losing weight – is about calories in, calories out. So, first, start packing those calories in. If you tend to be a meal skipper, you may also be skimping on your day's quota of calories. Instead, get into the regular-eating habit. Try sitting down for three squares a day, but supplement those with healthy, calorie-dense snacks (especially important if a smaller-than-average appetite keeps you from eating too much food at one time). Though the obvious weight-gain formula might be fast food and lots of it (Super Size Me Mum?), remember that the goal isn't just to gain – but to gain on foods that provide baby-friendly nutrients (chips, not so much). A better way to add those extra calories: Add more "good" fat foods into your diet, including nuts and seeds (add some dried fruit for extra calories and extra nutrients), avocados, and flaxseed oil, which can tip the scale in your favour while pumping up your nutritional stores. Focus on complex carbs, too (think whole-grain pasta, whole-wheat bread – the denser the better – and beans). And while you're at it, top them all with some cheese (calcium is your preconception pal, and so are the calories in cheese). Don't skip the fruits and veggies, even though they're low in calories because they do provide essential baby-making fuel (but do try taking some of your fruits in a healthy higher-calorie smoothie, too). And of course, dig into that ice cream – you'll get a calcium bonus with those calories.

What about calories out – the ones you're burning through activity? If you're able to gain weight without cutting back on your fitness routine (if you have a fitness routine), great. The exercise may even fuel your appetite for more calories. But if you're taking more calories in, yet seeing no results when you step on the scale, take a look at your activity level. If you're exercising strenuously or often, you may just be burning too many calories. Taking your routine down a notch (or maybe two) will still keep you fit, but will allow you to keep more of those calories you've taken in . . . in. And a little extra soft padding on top of that lean frame of yours may be just the ticket to mamahood.

As with hopeful mums who need to lose weight before they step up to the preconception gate, you're wise to make slow and steady your motto, too. Gain weight gradually, and be sure to give your body some time to adjust to its new weight before trying to conceive (about 6 to 8 weeks should do the trick).

CHAPTER 3

Eating Well Before You're Expecting

HOPING TO BE EATING FOR TWO soon? You may want to look at how you're eating (for one) now. That's because growing evidence suggests that your fertility may be impacted by your diet – possibly (depending on what that diet consists of) improving it, or possibly impeding it. Scientists are learning more and more about how what you eat can put you on the right path toward conception, which means that getting your eating plan up to baby-making speed may help you get closer faster to that pregnancy you're hoping for. The right preconception nutrition can even help your soon-to-be embryo get a healthier start in life while helping you enjoy a more comfortable pregnancy. Best of all, it's easier than you might think, and not that different from any sensible eating plan – or from the balanced baby-friendly eating you'll be doing once that baby's on board (which means you won't have to do much reshuffling of your eating habits later).

Your Preconception Eating Habits

Are you a chocolate kind of girl? A breakfast skipper? A crisps snacker? A cola sipper? Is your idea of a fresh vegetable the slice of tomato on your double bacon cheeseburger – or that side of onion rings (they were cooked fresh, weren't they)? When was the last time you ate something loaded with omega-3s? And are you wondering what exactly an omega-3 is? If you answered "yes" or "huh?" to any (or all) of these questions, it's time to take a hard look at your eating habits. That's because your fertility (like the rest of your health) may be impacted by what you eat – and what you don't eat. Plenty of folic acid and the right kind of carbs, for instance, may boost those baby odds. Too much junk food, on the other hand, may trash your conception plans. Bottom line: Filling your stomach with the right foods may help you fill your belly with baby.

Pretty content with the content of your diet (and the contents of your refrigerator)? Good for you – you're ahead of the game. All you'll have to do is balance your already balanced diet with some especially fertility-focused foods. Never met a vegetable or fruit you liked – or a chocolate bar or pastry you didn't? You may have some work cut out for you. Just remember, any nutritional change for the better improves your chances of healthy baby making, even if it's just adding a daily piece of fruit to your lunch, or switching your bread to whole wheat, or trading in your Frosties for muesli. Or finally finding out what omega-3s are and where they can be found (you might be surprised).

How Well Do You Eat?

So maybe you think you eat really well already. Or maybe you're pretty sure your eating habits are about as bad as they could be (that is, without officially moving into Wimpy). Or maybe you'd rate your diet somewhere in the middle – not too shabby, nothing to brag about. But the truth is, the only way to evaluate your eating habits accurately is to take a good, honest look at them – and the best way to do that is to keep a food diary.

A food diary takes the guesswork out of assessing your diet, and it can also be a real eye-opener (particularly if you're a mindless eater – the kind

Action Plan

Over the course of 7 days, write down everything you eat and drink (including the amount and approximate calorie count, especially if you'll need to be dropping some preconception weight). You can use the food diary on page 200. Note in the diary the number of portions you consume in each category on each day. Once your chart is complete, you'll be able to figure out where your eating habits are – and where they need to be to boost your baby-making profile.

who tends to nibble your way through a bag of crisps while watching TV, realizing it only when you find yourself at the bottom). So try keeping a diary for a week, writing down everything you eat (including the handful of M&M's you snagged from your boss's desk, those chips you stole off your husband's plate at dinner). Be as specific as possible. And be truthful, too (don't give yourself credit for a side salad you ordered, but didn't end up eating). Remember, no one's going to see your food diary but you, so there's no reason to cheat.

Seems like a lot of effort? It is, but it's an effort worth making as you begin your baby-making efforts. What you'll have when you're done is a complete picture of how you eat, the first step in figuring out how to eat better. You'll see where you're already hitting (or even exceeding) your mark, where you're falling somewhat short, where you're coming up empty – and how changes, either big or small, may be just the ticket you need to help you get that tiny (and cutest) passenger on board.

Making a Change for the Better

So now you know what your eating habits look like (the good, the bad, and the fried) and hopefully, what you'd like them to look like (you'll get the lowdown on what a balanced preconception diet should look like beginning on page 53). Now all you have to do is make a change for the better – which should be easy as pie (or as easy as switching from pie to fresh fruit), right? Well, maybe not so much. Changing your habits (whether it's eating habits or any other kind of habit) can be challenging – and even if you're fully up to the challenge, it's not likely you'll completely transform your diet overnight. So give yourself some time, take your efforts one day – or one meal – at a time, and be realistic in the goals you set so you can set yourself up for success. Keeping your eye on the prize – a healthy baby on board – will also help you make those changes for the better. So will these tips:

Think positive. Unfortunately, the word "diet" doesn't usually stir up positive thoughts – just flavourless flashbacks of rice crackers, celery sticks, and dry boneless chicken breast. Fortunately, eating well for your fertility doesn't have to mean denying yourself eating pleasure. Even if you have serious weight to lose before you conceive, restrictive eating isn't the way to go. Focusing on a wide, well-balanced, and delicious variety of fertility-friendly foods (that will later on be baby friendly) is. And that's a positive change.

Think small. As committed as you are to healthy baby making, thinking too big can be daunting ("I have to change my diet completely to make a baby, then continue the changes through 9 months of pregnancy?"), and can make you want to give up before you've really got going. So stop thinking about it that way. Think, instead, of working your way toward your goal (appropriately) in baby steps. Need an example? If your food diary shows that you're not getting any whole grains in your diet, think small changes: Switch from cornflakes to a whole-grain cereal at breakfast the first few days, then start ordering your sandwich on whole-wheat bread a couple of days later. Drop that mid-morning cinnamon roll the following week, adding a whole-grain muffin in its place. Before you know it, most of the grains you eat will be whole – and the change will have come so gradually that you'll barely have noticed. Do you have a snack habit at work that propels you to the vending machine? Give the machine 2 weeks' notice, cut back on your visits (once a day instead of twice), and in the meantime try to develop a taste for cheese, fresh fruit, and cereal bars (it's been done!).

Get rid of preconceptions (about food). Quick – what do you think of when you think of green vegetables? That they're good for you, but not so good to eat? Whole-wheat bread? Something you want to eat . . . or something you feel you should eat (but wouldn't, given the choice)? Oatmeal? A chewy, satisfying breakfast (especially when cinnamon and raisins find their way on top) . . . or something mum made you eat when you would have rather dug into a bowl of Frosties? Maybe it's time to rethink those preconceptions and take a fresh look at food. Instead of serving spinach in the form of your childhood nightmares (that nasty boiled mound that stood between you and dessert), eat it raw in a sprightly spinach, red onion, and peach salad; lightly steamed as a bed for grilled salmon; stuffed with cheese inside rolled chicken breasts; or chopped up in lasagne. With a new perspective and new preparations, you may find the healthy foods you had some misgivings about aren't bad at all – making the change for the better all that much easier.

Plan ahead. The very definition of a habit is that it's something you do all the time, without thinking. Which is why habits can be tough to change – especially when they're long standing (skipping breakfast since school, for instance). So start thinking and planning ahead. Instead of waiting until your stomach is growling in hunger (and that chocolate bar starts calling you by name), have an eating-well plan in place. Stock up on healthy snacks (think dried apricots and toasted almonds, individual containers of yogurt, cut-up raw veggies and dip) and keep them within nibbling distance (in your bag, at your desk, in the car) so you won't be as tempted to make a dietary detour (to the drive-through for chips, to the corner shop for a bag of crisps). Instead of leaving your shopping list up to impulse (and the seductive powers of Sara Lee), compose it ahead of time (leaving Sara off), and stick with it (unless a sudden healthy impulse has you reaching for fresh strawberries or a whole-grain cereal you've never seen before). Plan a healthy breakfast the night before so you're not left scrambling in the morning when you're late for your lift; pack a healthy lunch (also the night before) so you're not tempted to add your name to the KFC order. And have a plan for a nutritious dinner, too – even if it's nothing more ambitious than one of those healthy frozen dinners and ready-made salads you were clever enough to add to your shopping list – so that you won't be tempted to veer into McDonald's on the way home.

Keep it real. When you're making your change for the better, take into account the limitations of your lifestyle (and real life) – otherwise, those new habits won't stand a chance. If mornings have you running to catch an early commuter train, a full-on, sit-down breakfast probably isn't in the cards. Instead, blend yourself a strawberry-mango-yogurt smoothie, to be sipped on the train. If you just can't get behind a bowl of cereal (or other traditional breakfast foods), break with breakfast tradition and heat up a slice of veggie pizza or toast a grilled cheese and tomato. If you know the chances of your making a sandwich to take to work are slim to none, find a deli that will make it for you, then pick it up on the way. Or get your last licks of sushi (it'll be off the menu once you conceive) picking up a ready-made package of salmon rolls at the supermarket, alongside a salad bar selection. If you're certain that willpower won't hold you back from the

Action Plan

It's never too late to begin making healthy changes to your diet when you're making a baby, but it's never too early, either. So start your diet makeover as soon as you can, and preferably at least 3 months before you plan to get earnest in your baby-making efforts. Not only will beefing up your nutritional status (and shedding any extra weight) help you boost your fertility, it'll help you provide the baby you hope to make with the healthiest possible start in life. Getting enough of the right nutrients (with the help of a prenatal supplement) can even help you avoid some of pregnancy's most miserable symptoms, too (like morning sickness).

fast-food chips, visit the grilled chicken place instead of the burger joint.

Don't deny it. If you've ever tried to stick with a diet before (and who hasn't?), you know that too many restrictions lead to crumbled resolve (and a big slab of crumble coffee cake, when all you meant to order was a nonfat latte). So don't go there. Craving a bowl of ice cream? Fine, eat it. Just don't eat three of them. Longing for a chocolate bar? Munch on a mini instead of a king-size – and enjoy every bite. Just keep the balance of healthy foods higher than the unhealthy ones – and find ways to make the less-than-wholesome food a little healthier (add walnuts instead of chocolate chips to your brownies). Recognize your limits, though, too. If you know you won't be able to stop once the lid's off the pint of ice cream, don't open it (or better still, don't stock it in your freezer – buy single-serve cups or lollies instead).

A Fertility-Friendly Diet

Since you're not pregnant yet, there's no need to start eating like you are (though if you'd like a preview of expectant eating, check out *What to Expect When You're Expecting* and *Eating Well When You're Expecting*). Still, not surprisingly, the very same kind of balanced diet that best nurtures a baby who's already on board can also best help you get that baby there. Eating well now, while you're in preconception mode, may increase the likelihood that you'll get pregnant – plus it sets the stage for a healthier pregnancy once egg and sperm meet up.

But a balanced diet – as important as it is, not only to fertility, but to general health – is just the beginning when you're trying to make a baby. Putting specific foods (and types of foods) on the menu can actually help jump-start a pregnancy by boosting your fertility. Here's what you need to know to make sure your eating plan is fertility friendly.

Full Fat for Full Fertility

Though standard nutritional recommendations have long dictated that lowfat or nonfat is the way to go when it comes to dairy products, some research suggests that full-fat versions may offer some fertility perks – possibly offering protection against ovulation-related infertility. But before you grab that pint of ice cream and a can of whipped cream and get busy, keep in mind that just one serving of high-fat dairy – as in one glass of whole milk – will net you any potential fertility benefits without the obvious, definite drawbacks (extra weight, which can actually decrease fertility). What's more, if you're trying to drop a lot of preconception weight, you should probably get all your dairy the fat-free way (check with your doctor).

Fertility-Friendly Nutrients

Already found balance in your diet? That's definitely a good place to start when you're hoping to eat for two. Want a little more direction to point you toward the baby goal line? Look no further than these six fertility-friendly nutrient categories. Each contributes a little something to the baby-making process – but put them together, and they pack a powerfully proactive preconception punch.

Bone up on calcium. You already know it's fashionable to sport a milk moustache when you're pregnant. But upping your calcium intake even before you conceive is smart, too – especially because it might help you conceive a lot sooner. Boning up on calcium will help ensure the proper functioning of your reproductive system, the system you're understandably most focused on right now. Plus, it'll help stock up your stores of this bone-building mineral – important not only for your future baby's bone health, but for your future bone health. If your calcium stores – and intake – fall short during pregnancy, your body will

tap into your own bones to build baby's, possibly setting you up for osteoporosis later on in life. And if that's not reason enough to raise your glass of milk in a preconception toast, consider that getting enough calcium in your system now will help strengthen your fetus-to-be's developing teeth and bones, as well as help muscle, heart, and nerve development.

The most well-publicized source of calcium is milk, but it's just as easy to find in other dairy-case favourites (including cheese and yogurt), as well as in some surprising sources (calcium-fortified juice, almonds, sesame seeds, green leafy veggies, tofu, and other soy products). You'll even cash in on calcium when sipping on a smoothie (made with milk or yogurt), and net a modest amount when dipping into a bowl of frozen yogurt.

Can't be sure you're hitting your calcium goal? Or just want to give your bones (and your fertility) every edge? Pop some calcium supplements – aim for 1,500 mg a day – along with your prenatal vitamin. Three Tums or three calcium chews will net you the same total.

Power up on protein. When you think of protein, what usually comes to mind (or lands on your plate)? A juicy burger? A slab of meat loaf? A sizzling sirloin steak or pork chop? It's true that such animal proteins can definitely be an important component of any healthy human diet, helping build muscle and ensuring an adequate supply of essential amino acids. But they're not the only way to fill your plate with protein – and when it comes to fertility, sticking exclusively with those steak house favourites (especially if you're eating supersize servings of them) may not be the best strategy.

Protein can come from two sources: animal (meat, poultry, fish) and plant

---

Action Plan

How much calcium do you need in your preconception diet? Aim for three servings of calcium-rich foods daily. One serving is equivalent to 30 g grated or shredded cheese; 220 ml milk or calcium-fortified juice; 220 ml yogurt; 330 ml frozen yogurt; 110 g canned salmon with bones; 115 g cooked greens; 210 g cooked edamame (soybeans); 3 tablespoons sesame seeds.

Action Plan

Where's the beef? Where it probably shouldn't be is heaped high on your preconception plate, at least if it isn't lean. Current recommendations advise the fertility focused to get about two to three servings of protein daily – with one of those servings preferably being a plant protein, and most animal proteins coming from lean sources (the exception would be fatty fish, like salmon, which comes by its fat the healthy omega-3 way). Each protein serving is surprisingly small – equivalent to about the size of a computer mouse. Choose from these (and many other) offerings: 110 g (before cooking) poultry, beef, or pork; 110 g fish or seafood; 100 g canned fish (see page 63 for information on fish safety); 210 g cooked beans, lentils, split peas, or chickpeas; 140 g cooked soybeans (edamame) or quinoa; 85 g peanuts; 110 ml miso; 225 g tofu; 170 g nuts (such as walnuts, pecans, and almonds); 30 g sunflower or pumpkin seeds.

(legumes, nuts, seeds). According to some research, too much high-fat animal protein (the kind we tend to favour) may hurt your chances of getting pregnant (not to mention hurt your waistline and your overall health), so it's best to cut back on those hunks of marbled beef or greasy burgers when you're trying to conceive. Instead, order up lower-fat animal protein more often – lean beef and buffalo, lean pork (such as loin), poultry, fish, and shellfish. Just don't chow down on too much animal protein, even if it's lean, or make it the major ingredient in your preconception diet.

It's best to limit yourself to 50 to 75 grams of even lowfat animal protein, or two to three modest servings a day, when you're TTC. More than 100 grams per day, or four servings, can actually adversely affect fertility (which means a high-protein/low-carb diet isn't your best bet; see page 66).

Other research finds that swapping out even one serving of animal protein (lean or high fat) in your daily diet for one serving of plant protein may help give fertility a boost (which means beans are good for your heart *and* your baby-making prospects). So instead of plunking that rib eye front and centre on your dinner plate, think about opting instead for a pilaf of vegetables and quinoa (one of the best sources of protein in the plant kingdom) or a main of high-protein pasta. Swap a veggie burger for the traditional beef at lunch. Wrap yourself around a black bean enchilada instead of a carne asada. Spoon up a bowl of split-pea or white bean soup instead of beefy chilli.

Pump up with iron. Each month your iron stores are depleted by your period – especially if your flow is heavy (the more blood loss, the more iron loss). Pumping up the iron before you conceive will give your body a chance to replenish those stores before they're needed during pregnancy (it'll take a lot of iron-rich blood cells to nourish and grow that baby-to-be). Pumping up now also makes it less likely that you'll suffer from iron-deficiency anaemia during pregnancy (nature takes care of baby's iron needs first, which can leave mum short on her supplies), and after delivery.

But there's even more to the iron story – and in fact, the story begins before sperm meets egg. Researchers have found that women whose iron stores are adequate have a higher fertility rate than

Order Up Some Omega-3s

Never thought fat could be your friend? Well, here's a fat you should definitely get to know – and get to love: omega-3 fatty acids. These fabulous fats, most notably DHA, will be essential to your baby-to-be's brain and eye development, so they're definitely a must-have-often during pregnancy, as well as while you're breastfeeding.

But the omega-3 benefits don't just begin once you've conceived your baby. Rewind to the preconception phase (now), when these essential fatty acids are essential to your overall health, and perhaps to your fertility, too. Omega-3s help regulate hormones, including, possibly, the ones that induce ovulation. They may also increase blood flow to the reproductive organs (for both sexes), always a good thing when baby making's on the agenda. What's

more, omega-3s are deservedly touted for their mood-balancing effects, which means that getting your fill may help relieve emotional stress (definitely a fertility plus – and absolutely a pregnancy one).

It's easy to get in the omega-3 habit, especially if you're fond of salmon and other fatty fish (such as anchovies, sardines, and herring), all stellar sources of this super fat (see page 63 for a safe fish list). Not a fish fan? Get your omegas in walnuts, seeds, flaxseed and flaxseed oil, DHA (or omega-3) eggs, chicken, and even rocket (random, but true).

And while you're feeding yourself these phenomenal fats, don't forget to feed your partner some, too. The preconception perks of an omega-3 rich diet are even greater for hopeful dads (see page 59).

women who are iron deficient. Plus, women who develop iron-deficiency anaemia tend to have disruptions in their menstrual cycles, which might be the body's way of protecting against further blood loss – and further depletion of iron stores. Messed-up menstrual cycles, not surprisingly, make it more difficult to conceive.

To pump up your iron, turn to leafy greens (kale, spinach), beef (just keep it lean), dried beans, peas, dried apricots, and oatmeal. Couple your iron with foods rich in vitamin C to help with iron absorption (so sip some OJ with that oatmeal, or toss some tomatoes with those beans). If your blood test reveals that you need more iron than your diet (and a prenatal vitamin with iron) can serve up, your practitioner may recommend adding an extra iron supplement. But since far from every

woman needs extra iron – and you can get too much of a good thing – don't add a supplement without that go-ahead.

Consider carbs carefully. A carb is a carb is a carb, and all carbs are bad – right? Wrong. Though carbs have had a bad rep of late (thanks to the popularity of high-protein diets), it's important not to lump all carbs together in the same bread basket, especially when you're trying to get a bun in your oven. There's a world of nutritional difference between carbs that are complex (whole grains, beans, legumes, fruits, and vegetables) and those that are simple, or easily converted to sugar (such as white bread and other refined baked goods, white rice, white potatoes, sugared fizzy drinks, chocolate bars, and so on). And that difference apparently extends to fertility, too. Researchers have found that women who eat more complex carbs have higher fertility rates than those whose diets include more of those easily digested carbs. What's the connection, and since when is easy digestion a minus? Rapid digestion of noncomplex carbs leads to an increase in blood sugar (as in that sugar high you get after you polish off a doughnut) and an increase in insulin. Insulin – besides being a factor in diabetes – also helps regulate ovulatory function. Too much insulin in your body can disrupt the delicate balance of reproductive hormones, throwing your menstrual cycle off kilter, and making conception much more elusive. On the other hand, eating complex carbs that take longer to digest (that bowl of whole-grain cereal and strawberries) doesn't adversely affect insulin levels – and can actually improve your body's ability to ovulate regularly and improve your ability to get pregnant.

Need another reason to order up your sandwich on whole wheat, to

Carbs and PCOS

Opting for complex carbs is an especially important nutritional strategy if you have polycystic ovarian syndrome (PCOS), a hormonal problem that's related to high insulin levels. To keep your insulin from spiking and your reproductive system from going off track, shun those refined carbs and slow down your digestion with whole grains, fresh fruit and vegetables, beans, and legumes. See page 142 for more on PCOS.

reach for the brown rice instead of the white, or to toss some beans into your soup, especially when you're trying to conceive? Complex carbs contain an impressive variety of fertility-friendly nutrients – from antioxidants to iron

Action Plan

What's the plan for complex carbs in your fertility diet? Aim for:

▢ Six servings of whole grains. Sound like a lot of dough, or a hill of beans? Keep in mind that whole grains are often stellar sources of plant protein, too, so they perform double nutritional duty. Plus, a serving is a lot smaller than you'd think (a serving of whole-grain pasta, for instance, would only fill an ice cream scoop). Equivalent servings of whole grains include 1 slice whole wheat bread; 55 g whole-grain cereal; 70 g cooked bulgur, couscous, buckwheat, barley, brown rice, or quinoa; 28 g (before cooking) whole-grain pasta; 70 g cooked beans, lentils, split peas, or soybeans (edamame).

▢ Two to four servings of fruit, with each serving equivalent to (among many others) ½ grapefruit; ½ orange; ½ mango; 60 g berries; 220 g diced watermelon; 2 fresh apricots or 6 dried apricot halves; 1 banana; 110 ml fruit juice; 2 plums; 1 apple or pear.

▢ Three to five servings of vegetables, with each serving equivalent to (among many others) ¼ red, yellow, or orange pepper; 60 g broccoli or cauliflower; 1 tomato; 55 g raw spinach or green leafy lettuce; ½ carrot or sweet potato; 110 g raw mushrooms; 60 g cooked courgette; 30 g cooked winter squash.

Feed Your Boys

You've probably heard that you are what you eat – but did you know that your sperm are, too? It's true. The healthier your diet, the healthier your sperm – and the more easily you'll likely conceive.

So what foods can give you the fertility edge? A balanced diet, one that includes plenty of fresh fruits and vegetables, whole grains, and lean protein, will almost certainly get the job done. Want more specifics? Here are some key sperm-friendly nutrients, as well as the foods you can easily find them in:

▢ **Vitamin A.** This A-list vitamin is essential for the production of good swimmers; in fact, deficiencies in vitamin A in men have been linked to lowered fertility due to sluggish sperm. You can find plenty of this nutrient in green leafies (dark green lettuce, broccoli, spinach, kale) and orange and yellow vegetables and fruits (carrots, sweet potatoes, red peppers, mangos, apricots, yellow peaches, cantaloupe), as well as in dairy and other animal products, and in oatmeal and other whole grains. Getting your A is as easy as having a V-8, tossing back a salad topped with red peppers and carrots, or starting your day with the breakfast of swimming champions: a bowl of oatmeal topped with dried apricots. Or, heck, earn yourself an A+ by eating all three in the same day.

▢ **Vitamin C.** This essential nutrient affects sperm motility and viability – and it's easy to find. Look no further than the obvious sources (grapefruit and OJ), but also look to asparagus, broccoli, cauliflower, kale, red peppers, mangetouts, sweet potatoes, tomatoes (they're especially good for you cooked – so pour on that tomato sauce), melon, kiwis, peaches, straw-

berries, and watermelon – to name a tasty few. You'll find many C's overlap with A's, giving you extra credit.

▢ **Vitamin D.** This is actually a nutrient that many people don't get enough of these days. Fortunately, it takes a severe D deficiency to lead to lowered fertility, in the form of deterioration of testicular tissue. But because you want to give your baby-making effort every edge, stock up on the D in your diet. It's actually as simple as pouring yourself a glass of milk or fortified OJ, scrambling up some eggs (it's in the yolks), or chowing down on some sardines (okay, it's an acquired taste). Easier still – score all the D you need by getting a few minutes of sun each day. Vitamin D is manufactured in the body from a chemical reaction to the ultraviolet rays in sunlight – but skip the sunscreen during those few minutes, otherwise you'll be blocking out some of the rays you want to be soaking up.

▢ **Vitamin E.** So you've heard a lot about antioxidants, but do you really know what they do? They're substances found in vitamins that serve to protect cells in your body. When it comes to your fertility, they're busily protecting your boys. Researchers suspect that antioxidants from vitamins A and E (and others) protect sperm DNA from being damaged, ensuring that they stay vital, vigorous, and up to the job of fertilizing an egg. Get your E the easy way, from vegetable oils (choose rapeseed, flaxseed, olive, or sunflower oils), sweet potatoes (yes, the same sweet potatoes that made the A and C lists – so bake a couple tonight for you and your sweetie), mangoes (ditto – share a mango smoothie for dessert), avocados (yes, as in the guacamole you love), spinach, almonds, and sunflower seeds.

◻ **Folic acid.** There's plenty of buzz about the importance of folic acid for hopeful mums (and expecting mums), but it's a nutrient that's vital for hopeful dads, too – and their boys. Inadequate amounts of folic acid in a man's diet can lead to low sperm quality – and may even be linked to birth defects since men with folate deficiencies have a higher rate of sperm with chromosomal abnormalities. Plus, prospective fathers appear to need even more folate than their partners. Researchers suggest that guys who consume 700 mcg to 1,000 mcg of folic acid daily show the most benefit when it comes to healthy sperm. Find your folic in leafy green vegetables (time for another salad), most fruits (and another smoothie), avocados (there's that guac again), and beans (while you're having the guac). There's also folic aplenty in whole grains, as well as in refined grains (it's added in during processing).

◻ **Zinc.** How important could a nutrient called zinc be to the baby-making process? Actually, incredibly important. Inadequate amounts of this mineral can lead to low testosterone levels and diminished sperm count. Fortunately, chances are excellent you've already got lots of zinc on your menu – it's found in beef (finally, some good news about burgers!), turkey, yogurt, oatmeal, eggs, seafood, and corn. But if you really want a load of zinc (and maybe a really hot night), load up on oysters. Apparently what they've always said about the oyster's amorous effects is true.

◻ **Omega-3 fatty acids.** Fat's got a bad name – and, in fact, too much of the wrong fats can really mess with fertility. But here are some fats you can feel good about loving – and eating – in large amounts. DHA and other essential omega-3 fatty acids help improve blood flow to the genitals and increase sexual function (you'll need to be rising to the occasion a lot to make a baby). Plus, they also naturally lower blood pressure (which is good for the heart and good for your performance). And here's another reason to reach for these phenomenal fats: Fertile men's sperm contains more of this essential fatty acid than the sperm of infertile men. Find your omega-3s in salmon and other fatty fish, like sardines and anchovies (so order a Caesar salad with your anchovy pizza), walnuts, omega-3 eggs (you can buy them in most supermarkets, and they taste great), rocket, crab, shrimp, flaxseed (look for these nutty-tasting seeds in many whole-grain breads), and even chicken (and everybody likes chicken).

◻ **The whole vitamin-mineral gang.** Even if you eat well (and especially if you don't), a good vitamin-mineral supplement acts as a nutritional insurance policy. Buying this insurance (and taking it daily) will help you be sure that you get adequate amounts of the nutrients most essential for fertility and healthy sperm. Just remember that too much of a good thing can actually be a bad thing. Megadoses of some vitamins and minerals in supplement form can have a negative impact on fertility and sperm production (though don't worry about getting too much from foods; you can't overdose on naturally occurring vitamins and minerals). For example, too much supplementary zinc can be toxic to sperm. So stay balanced, stay moderate – and you'll stay on track for baby making.

to those baby-boosting B vitamins. Refined carbs have had many of those naturally occurring vitamins and minerals stripped away in processing.

And the reasons to get more complex with your carbs keep on coming. Once that bun is in the oven, opting for whole grains and other complex carbs will, among other things, provide essential baby-growing nutrients, fibre to help fight constipation (a common pregnancy symptom; stay tuned), vitamins you'll need to ease any early pregnancy quease, and blood sugar regulation to combat fatigue, mood swings, and more.

Give me an "A" . . . give me a "C" . . . give me a "B$_6$". . . What does it spell? A healthier pregnancy – and possibly, a sooner one. You may not be pregnant yet, or even actively trying to conceive, but adding a daily prenatal vitamin to your diet is already a smart move. That's because the same nutrients that will eventually help you grow a baby can also help you conceive that baby – which makes stocking up on them now doubly important.

What makes a prenatal supplement so perfectly suited to the preconception set? It's the carefully selected team of vitamins and minerals it contains. Here are just a few examples. Many of the B vitamins, most notably folic acid, appear to increase fertility. B$_{12}$ is another B vital to healthy reproduction, and in fact a B$_{12}$ deficiency (more common among vegetarians) has been linked to ovula-

Action Plan

Start taking a prenatal vitamin as soon as you start thinking about getting pregnant – and at least 3 months before you start trying (starting a year before is even better, if you're planning that far in advance). Not only will it get you into the habit of taking a daily pill (so that it'll become second nature by the time you're actually pregnant), it could also get you on the expectant express faster. Plus, it'll help ensure a healthier baby and a more comfortable pregnancy. So get popping!

tion issues and even repeat miscarriages. Vitamin D (hard to come by unless you take a supplement or soak up a lot of sun, which means many women don't get enough) is also a fertility friend, particularly for those who have ovulation problems. Iron can give fertility a boost, too, especially if you're low on stores. And the benefits of taking a prenatal continue – from the right amount of A (a baby-friendly antioxidant) to zinc (another notable star in the fertility field). A zinc deficiency can slow the maturation of good-quality eggs, something you definitely want to have in your reproductive basket right now – and all the more reason to toss that prenatal in your shopping cart. And as if that isn't enough incentive to start popping your prenatal today, consider this. Take a prenatal that's chock full of B$_6$ now, and you're likely to experience fewer episodes of nausea and vomiting during your first trimester of pregnancy.

Look for a vitamin that has at least 400 mcg (micrograms) of folic acid, 1,000 mg of calcium, 30 to 40 mg of iron, plus fertility-boosting nutrients

What About Herbs?

They're touted for their ability to boost fertility, but could herbs be more of a bust? Check out what's known about herbs on page 118.

such as zinc and manganese. If you find pills hard to swallow (literally, especially when they're horse-size pills), choose one with a slicker coating. Chewable prenatals are also an option – but don't expect great taste (you'll still be chewing vitamins and minerals along with that "zesty tropical flavour"). Most important, stay with the recommended dosage and don't take extra supplements of any kind unless your doctor recommends them. More isn't better when it comes to vitamins, unless they're the naturally occurring kind (the ones you find in the food you eat).

It's true you can get vitamins and minerals aplenty from eating a healthy, well-balanced diet – and you should definitely try to. But a good prenatal supplement serves as a nutritional insurance policy, making sure that your intake of those vital nutrients is always up to snuff, even when your diet . . . not so much.

Factor in the folic. You've probably already heard how important it is to take the B vitamin folic acid (or folate) during pregnancy – it's a vital vitamin in the fight against crippling neural tube defects, such as spina bifida. But studies show that getting enough of this crucial nutrient before you conceive (for a year before even) lowers the chances that your baby will develop a neural tube defect and possibly cardiac defects and may lower your risk of premature delivery. Even more relevant in your short-term plans: An adequate intake of folic acid has been linked to increased fertility.

Where can you find folic acid? Most leafy green vegetables and whole grains are naturally full of it – plus, it's added to most refined grain products (by law). Want extra insurance? You're already covered if you're taking a prenatal supplement, which you should be. And that's a good thing – because

you can't be too careful when it comes to folic acid (after all, a three-salad-a-day habit is a worthy goal – but not one you'll always manage to reach, especially in those queasy early days of pregnancy). Choose a prenatal supplement with 400 to 600 mcg of folic acid to be sure you're getting your fill. And while you're at it, stop by the salad bar for a folate fill-up – more is more.

Fertility-Friendly Foods

Though old wives have practically been put out of business by Internet legends, the tales they told for generations are still making the rounds (more efficiently than ever, thanks to Google). And one category of tales that seems to have the most legs: foods that make you fertile. You've heard them, you've read them, you've probably told some – and still you're probably wondering, could they possibly be true? Could there really be foods that enhance fertility – a breakfast (or dinner) that's sure to serve up a fertilized egg? Maybe . . . and maybe not. So far there really aren't any well-documented studies to back up the claim that putting any one food in your tummy will put a baby in your belly – but there haven't been any done that rebut them, either. With that in mind, take the following fertile food recommendations (and any others you stumble on during your TTC mission) with a grain of salt – and maybe a side of salad (hey, you can't go wrong with salad). Still, there's definitely no harm in adding these to your balanced diet (they're all healthy foods anyway), and in the case of some there could actually be some pretty substantial fertility perks.

Yams. Since populations that eat wild yams as their staple food seem to have

Fertile Food for Fathers-to-Be

Hungry for fatherhood? Some evidence indicates that you can feed your fertility by feeding yourself certain foods (and maybe, get yourself a little closer to having that extra little mouth to feed). Though the scientific jury is still out on just how much nutritional input can affect your output (of sperm), there's no downside to adding these healthy foods to your balanced diet, and there could be a significant upside – in more ways than one.

◻ Oysters. No doubt you've heard that slurping a plateful of these bivalves can raise the libido roof, but oysters may also hop up your fertility. That's because they're loaded with zinc, a mineral that helps fuel semen and testosterone production. Can't acquire a taste for oysters? Pumping up your intake of other zinc-rich foods will also help pump up your sperm. Though none can even come close to the oyster's colossal content, you'll find some zinc in beef, turkey, nuts, legumes, and in a good vitamin-mineral supplement (which you should be taking preconception anyway).

◻ Honey. Put this sweet treat on your "honey-do" list (and add it instead of sugar to tea, hot cereal, yogurt, and more). It's packed with boron, a mineral believed to increase the production of testosterone, a hormone that comes in very handy when you're TTC. Enjoy some before you enjoy your honey.

◻ Fruits and veggies. Mum was right about eating your broccoli – except she probably didn't have this benefit in mind: The more fruits and vegetables a man eats, the less sluggish his sperm will be. The antioxidants in vibrantly coloured produce (such as red peppers, carrots, blueberries, peaches, pink grapefruit, sweet potatoes, tomatoes, and greens of all kinds, except for iceberg lettuce) give sperm a boost, potentially giving you a fertility edge.

◻ Pomegranate juice. This juice is making a splash in the nutrition headlines as a powerful antioxidant (its naturally occurring potent purple colour can clue you in), but it's also making waves when it comes to male fertility, at least in the laboratory. Pomegranate juice has been shown to increase sperm count and boost sperm quality in mice – probably because of that high antioxidant content. Researchers are trying to determine if these benefits are reproducible (so to speak) in humans. Until then, it can't hurt to chug-a-lug some PJ every now and then – or even to swap it for your morning OJ (they're actually pretty tasty in combo).

◻ Pumpkin seeds. Naturally high in zinc and essential fatty acids, pumpkin seeds can give your boys a boost as they swim off on their conception quest. So snack on a handful every now and then.

a higher rate of twin pregnancies, some have suggested that yams have fertile properties. In fact, research has shown that yams contain a substance similar to progesterone, which just might help stimulate ovulation. Even if they don't turn out twins, they're definitely a fertile source of nutrients – all the more reason to serve them up all year round.

Nuts and seeds. Walnuts, almonds, and pumpkin seeds (to name a few) are all abundant sources of omega-3 fatty acids, which research shows is not only vital to productive baby making but also to a healthy baby. That's because these fabulous fats (yes, fats can be fabulous!) help regulate hormones (and it's hormones that induce ovulation, after all). Which means that snacking on some trail mix (instead of, say, crisps) may help get you on the road to conception. Clearly, this is one fertility food theory that isn't nuts.

Oysters. You've almost certainly heard that oysters can heat things up between the sheets, but did you know that these tasty bivalves can fuel your fertility, too? That's because oysters are off-the-charts rich in zinc, and any food that's rich in zinc can help maintain a healthy menstrual cycle. Zinc deficiency, in fact, has been linked to decreased fertility because it can slow the production of good-quality eggs – something that's obviously essential for conception. Is it a month without an "r" in its name? Do the oysters' slimy texture turn your stomach? No food comes even remotely close to oysters in the zinc competition, but you'll find smaller amounts of this fertility-friendly mineral in other kinds of seafood (such as crab and lobster), as well as in beef, turkey, dairy products, nuts, and legumes.

Berries. Berries (think blueberries and raspberries) are berry, berry good sources of those headline-making antioxidants, which can prevent cell damage and aging. How does this relate to fertility? By protecting eggs from damage – especially important for those that have been on the shelf longer (as is true for older mums who are expecting to expect), but helpful for all who want to give their eggs an extra edge. So go berry crazy – toss them on your cereal, in your smoothie, over your ice cream.

Fertility-Unfriendly Foods

So now you know what foods make the conception cut – and you're likely chowing down on some already. But what about foods – and drinks, and supplements – that can act as fertility busters? Are there any you should be minimizing on your preconception menu? Though scientists are still trying to figure out the science behind fertility-boosting and fertility-busting foods, being sensible about certain foods (cutting back on some, eliminating others) while you're trying to conceive may help get that baby on board faster.

Mercury. This heavy metal is a pretty insidious substance – especially because it can accumulate in your body and linger there, without you even knowing it. What's the connection to fertility? Not only do men and women struggling with infertility tend to have higher mercury levels in their blood than those with normal fertility, but having high mercury levels at the time of conception can be harmful to your baby-to-be's development – even if you're careful to steer clear of the toxin during pregnancy. So it's a good idea to limit mercury in your diet.

Fish is the major dietary source of mercury, and probably the only one you need to be mindful of when you're in baby-making mode. If you're pregnant, nursing, trying to conceive, or even thinking about trying to conceive, experts suggest avoiding entirely any fish that's typically high in mercury, such as shark, swordfish, king mackerel, and fresh tuna, and limiting your intake of other fish (such as salmon, trout, shrimp, pollock, and canned light tuna) to a total of 340 grams a week. Albacore (white) tuna is higher in mercury, so choose it less often, and don't eat more than 170 grams a week. But don't take fish off the

A Side of Perspective

Of course you want to get pregnant – that's why you're reading this book. And you're almost certainly in a hurry to get that baby on board (the sooner to snuggle that little bundle!). You'll probably do just about anything – or eat just about anything (or not eat just about anything) – to make that baby dream a reality. But speaking of realities, keep this reality check in mind as you fill your plate. Much of the research that's been done on the connection between diet and fertility – and there really hasn't been much yet – is preliminary, and much of it isn't yet fully substantiated. Some if it may apply more to hopeful mums (and dads) who are already experiencing infertility issues – such as ovulation problems – than to those who are facing no reproductive challenges.

Maybe eating less meat, or switching out the bread on your sandwich from white to wheat, or cutting back on the chocolate in your life will make you a mama faster – or maybe it won't. Either way, all of the potentially (but not necessarily) fertility-friendly dietary changes suggested in this chapter are definitely good for your general health, and absolutely good for the baby you hope to be nurturing soon.

Just remember to order up a little perspective along with your salmon, broccoli, and brown rice. A healthy diet, as much good as it can do, doesn't guarantee a healthy reproductive system or rapid conception success. Fertility can be affected by many factors – from weight (though that's another compelling reason to eat well), to age, to genetics, and much more. There's definitely no downside to eating well before you're expecting – and potentially a lot of benefits. So, if you're experiencing trouble conceiving, eat as well as you can (it can only help), but also speak to your doctor about other steps you can take at the same time to boost your fertility.

---

menu altogether (if you're a fish fan). Fish is packed with lean protein and vitamin D, and loaded with the most fabulous of all fats, omega-3 fatty acids (especially such fatty fish as salmon, herring, and anchovies). So go fish, but just fish selectively. And as you do, here's one fish favourite you may want to go wild with now: sushi. There are no restrictions on enjoying raw or rare fish or seafood while you're trying to conceive – only after you're pregnant. So belly up to the sushi bar before you've got that belly – just skip the tuna rolls.

Too much of the wrong kind of fats.
Plenty is still not known about the effect of dietary fats on fertility, so stay tuned. In the meantime, some preliminary research

has suggested a possible reproductive downside to eating too much saturated fat (from fatty cuts of meat, butter, full-fat cheeses), though the connection isn't clear. One fat more closely implicated as a culprit in decreased fertility is trans fat. According to researchers, the more trans fats you have in your diet (you'll see it listed on food labels as hydrogenated or partially hydrogenated oils), the greater the likelihood you'll have trouble conceiving. Fortunately, avoiding trans fats is becoming a lot easier because many restaurants and food manufacturers have eliminated or reduced the amount of trans fats they add to their foods.

Still, while it makes sense to be fat-aware, there's no need to be completely fat-phobic. Women who eat too little fat can have a harder time conceiving – especially if their own body fat is low. What's more, once you do become pregnant, your baby will need the essential fatty acids that dietary fats provide to grow and develop properly (there's a reason why they call them "essential"). Stick to monounsaturated and polyunsaturated fats for the most part (olive or rapeseed oils, fats from healthy foods like nuts and avocados) and omega-3 fatty acids (found in salmon, walnuts, and DHA-rich eggs).

Too much sugar. Before you start trying to imagine life without chocolate, no, you won't have to surrender your favourite sweet treats entirely now that you've got plans to bake that little bun. But limiting your intake of sugar (from biscuits, doughnuts, cake, sweets, sugared fizzy drinks, and just about anything else you might grab from the vending machine, the corner shop racks, the snack aisle . . . you get the picture) isn't only good for your waistline. It's also good for your chances of expanding that waistline with a baby bump. Why? Because too much sugar can disrupt the delicate balance of reproductive

hormones vital to making your reproductive dreams come true.

Too many refined grains. How could your bread choice affect your fertility? A diet that's heavy on refined grains (that white bread, that white rice, that white pasta, those white pancakes, that refined cereal) can come with potential baby-making drawbacks. Carbs that are fast to digest (yup – the white, refined ones) can raise your blood sugar and insulin levels, in some cases causing a disruption of ovulatory functioning. Refined grains are also missing those naturally occurring B vitamins so vital to reproductive function – and the making of a healthy baby and a healthier, more comfortable pregnancy.

Too much soy . . . maybe. Soy is an excellent source of protein and also a phenomenal source of phytoestrogen (also called isoflavones) – a plant form of oestrogen that mimics your own natural hormone. So what could be wrong with soy when you're trying to conceive? After all, aren't reproductive hormones a significant ally in your baby-making campaign? Those hormones are your

---

Soy and Your Sperm

Is soy your joy? If it is, you might want to consider containing it while trying to conceive. That's because there's some – though still inconclusive – research showing that eating too much soy may reduce your sperm production. The link? It could be due to the phytoestrogens in soy that mimic natural oestrogen (the female hormone) – and extra oestrogen is never a good thing when it comes to sperm production. The soy–sperm link is more pronounced in overweight and

obese men, according to researchers, probably because overweight men already produce more oestrogen than thinner men, on average.

Never ate a soybean (knowingly) or piece of tofu in your life? Keep in mind that not all soy looks or tastes like health food. Just about all protein bars (including those gooey chocolate peanut ones you consume before you hit the gym) and some protein shakes contain lots of soy protein, so you may be getting more soy than you think.

fertility friends, for sure, but some research has shown that eating *large* amounts of soy may throw off your hormone levels, increasing cycle length, and in turn, affecting ovulation.

Does that mean you should skip soybeans, soy milk, tofu, and other soy products while you're TTC, at least until more research weighs in? Not at all. In fact, some evidence indicates that swapping a serving of animal protein in your diet for a plant-based source (like soy) may improve ovulatory function. And even moderate amounts of soy haven't been implicated in fertility problems. But if you're having trouble conceiving – or if you're just a very big consumer of soy – you might want to consider cutting back somewhat. You should also steer clear of soy supplements when trying to conceive.

Action Plan

If you have any reason to believe you may have been exposed to high levels of mercury (for instance, you're a big fish eater, and have been for years, or you've had a lot of silver cavity fillings – especially if they've been broken or drilled out in the past), check with your doctor about whether you should be tested for mercury before you try to conceive. If your levels of mercury do test high (and don't try to test yourself because many at-home tests are inaccurate), discuss ways of bringing those levels down before you start your baby-making engines.

Fertile Eating Your Way

Now you know how to eat well before you're expecting, but maybe you're not sure how to apply those general guidelines to your specific eating style. Fortunately, with just a little finessing and fine tuning, any eating style can become fertility friendly.

Low-Carb Diet

"I've been on a low-carb diet to lose weight – and it's working, but I have a lot more to lose. Can I stick with it now?"

Low-carb/high-protein diets may be effective when you're trying to lose weight, but when you're trying to gain a baby – maybe not. Low-carb diets aren't just low on carbs (from fruits, vegetables, cereals, and breads), but they're also low on the fertility-friendly nutrients found in carbs – especially the most essential preconception nutrient of all, folic acid. These diets can also send your protein consumption through the roof (a girl's got to eat something, right?) – and that's definitely not the best way to give your fertility a boost. In fact, eating more than 100 grams of protein a day – which a high-protein dieter can easily knock back by lunchtime – can result in a fertility dip. Excesses of soy protein (if you're big on those protein bars and shakes featured in many low-carb diet plans) may also be a fertility buster.

The same goes for any eating plan – or weight-loss plan – that stresses one food group over others or eliminates a food group entirely (unless that food group is "deep fried" or "frosted").

Good nutrition is a balancing act, especially when you're trying to maintain the complex balance of reproductive hormones that'll help you get that baby on board faster. Not only can nutritionally unbalanced dieting make conception more elusive, it can also result in a nutritional deficit – definitely not the best way to start your pregnancy. So aim for a daily diet that taps into all the food groups when you're aiming for conception.

Getting your weight to where it should be before you conceive is a smart move, and one that should make conceiving (not to mention pregnancy) a lot less complicated. Definitely keep your weight-loss efforts up, but transition to a balanced weight-loss plan to send those numbers down. For more on weight loss, see page 47.

Vegetarian Diet

"I'm a vegetarian. Will that affect my chances of getting pregnant?"

You definitely don't have to eat meat (or poultry, or fish, or even dairy) to make a baby. Vegetarians – including vegans – get pregnant all the time and go on to have healthy pregnancies and healthy (meat-free) babies. That said, as a vegetarian, you'll have to be a little more conscious and conscientious about what you eat while you're on your conception campaign, and also once you've conceived that baby. That's because, though vegetarian diets are often heavy on many fertility-friendly nutrients (notably, the ones found in whole grains, legumes, and fresh fruits and vegetables), they're sometimes light on others (notably, the ones found most plentifully in animal products). Getting enough calories for optimal baby making can be tricky, too.

One key nutrient that you'll have to keep an eye on – especially if you're

Can Dads Veg Out, Too?

Hey, vegetarian dad-wannabes: Is your plate heaped high with brown rice and veggies, instead of meat and potatoes – or granola and fruit instead of bacon and eggs? No need to make a dietary change while you're trying to make a baby. But you will have to make a special effort to get enough sperm-boosting zinc (usually found in animal products, including eggs, but also plentiful in wheat germ, oatmeal, potatoes in their skin, and corn). A multivitamin can fill in the blanks if these foods aren't a regular part of your diet. If you're a big soy eater (as in those big protein bars), read up on the potential pitfalls of soy excesses for guys on page 65.

a vegan – is zinc, a well-known fertility booster. Zinc is found most plentifully in animal products, and if you aren't eating animal products, you may be skimping on zinc. If you're an ovo-lacto vegetarian, you can get your fill of zinc by dipping into some yogurt or cracking open some eggs. If you're a vegan, concentrate on vegetable and grain sources of zinc (potatoes with their skins on, black-eyed peas, corn, oatmeal, wheat germ). Either way, a daily prenatal vitamin will fill in any shortfall.

Another nutrient you'll need to be mindful of now that you've got baby on the brain is vitamin B_{12} – a very important vitamin when it comes to fertility. B_{12} occurs naturally only in animal products. So if you eat dairy and eggs, you'll be filling your baby-making quota, but if you're a strict vegan, you'll need to turn to fortified foods (many cereals have B_{12} in them) to give you what you need.

Once again, that prenatal vitamin can fill in any blanks.

Iron can be dicey, too, for the non-meat eaters because many sources of this essential nutrient are off the vegetarian menu (such as red meat). You'll get some iron if you eat your spinach, dried beans, dried apricots, lentils, and oatmeal, but that prenatal vitamin can come to the rescue if you don't. If a blood test shows that your iron stores are on the low side, your practitioner may also prescribe an iron supplement.

One nutrient you've probably got an edge on is folic acid, found in many leafy greens, whole grains, and other vegetarian-preferred foods. In fact, vegetarians tend to consume more folate-rich foods than meat eaters, without even trying (though you should still take that prenatal vitamin for extra insurance – you can't get too much folate that way, even if you're getting a tonne from your diet).

Something you may possibly be able to get too much of is soy, in any of its forms (tofu, tempeh, soy milk, soybeans). Soy proteins – which are understandably popular among vegetarians – can, according to early research, have an oestrogenic effect in some women that may prolong the menstrual cycle and cause disruptions in ovulation, potentially leading to fertility issues. If you've been going soy crazy, this research suggests, you may want to take your intake down a notch, particularly if conception has been elusive. How much soy is too much soy? A whole lot – more than, say, 30 millilitres of soy milk a day; see page 65.

Fortified Foods and Prenatal Vitamins

"I eat fortified cereal each morning plus fortified energy bars during the day. I also take a prenatal vitamin. Can getting too many vitamins prevent conception?"

It's hard to avoid fortified foods these days (unless you mill your own flour, bake your own bread, milk your own cows, and make your own cheese). Fortunately, you don't have to; there's absolutely no harm in eating fortified or enriched foods, even if you take a prenatal vitamin – and even if you're totally energy dependent on energy bars. In fact, the scientists take into account all the nutrients that likely already find their way into your diet (either naturally or from packaged foods) when they formulate those pills. You'd have to take megadoses of nutrients (way more than what's in your prenatal vitamin, which you shouldn't be doing anyway) to mess

A New Pill to Pop

Obviously, you've stopped popping those daily birth control pills now that you're trying to get pregnant. But you're not off the pill-popping hook. Every wannabe mum benefits from taking a daily prenatal vitamin during the preconception period, but if you were on birth control pills for a while, you may benefit even more. That's because taking oral contraceptives for an extended period may put some women at a nutritional disadvantage. Make sure all your nutritional stores are fully filled now by popping that prenatal vitamin, as well as by eating a diet that's chock-full of baby-making vitamins and minerals.

with your fertility or have any other negative health effects.

All that said, keep in mind that processed foods – the ones that tend to have the most fortification because those extra vitamins and minerals are tossed in to compensate for the ones stripped away on the assembly line – run a very distant second to wholesome natural foods, nutrition-wise. It's fine to supplement your diet with them – especially when they're made with worthy ingredients, like whole grains – but smart to balance them with nature's finest. So top that fortified cereal with fresh blueberries, and enjoy that energy bar after you've had a sensible salad for lunch, not instead of it.

Organic Foods

"Will eating organic produce help me get pregnant faster?"

Organic produce isn't necessarily more nutritious than conventional produce (you'll get the same fertility-boosting vitamins and minerals from regular produce), but organically grown fruits, vegetables, and other foods will likely be as close to pesticide free as possible – a definite plus once you've got baby on board since the pesticides you consume through your diet when you're pregnant are shared with your baby in utero. What's more, eating fewer pesticides now will mean you'll have less stored up later, a very good thing for your pregnancy and beyond, if you're planning to breastfeed (since stored-up chemicals can ultimately make their way into your milk).

Whether the pesticide-free pluses will add up to increased fertility is, so far, unclear. Some research has suggested that women who ingest a lot of pesticides and other chemicals through their food (and that's definitely not the majority of women) may find their fertility somewhat reduced, but the jury's still out – like it almost always is in the ever-changing fields of fertility and nutrition.

So there's no downside – and potentially, a lot of upside – to going organic during your preconception prep period and beyond. Still, it's no secret that organic food is usually more expensive than conventional, and sometimes harder to track down. If you have to pick and choose, focus on organic meat and dairy (conventionally raised animal products contain higher concentrations of chemicals that could disrupt your fertility hormones) and the fruits and vegetables you eat most often. Many types of produce – such as bananas, kiwis, mangoes, papayas, pineapples, asparagus, avocados, broccoli, cauliflower, corn, and onions – don't contain pesticide residue on them, so there's no need to go organic with them if you can't afford to. Instead, spring for organic when it comes to produce that typically wears the most pesticide residue (the so-called dirty dozen of apples, cherries, grapes, peaches, nectarines, pears, raspberries, strawberries, peppers, celery, potatoes, and spinach). For a lower price on organic foods that are also likely to be more nutritious than the ones you'll find in a market, visit the local farmer's market if you're lucky enough to have one. The fresher off the farm those fruits and veggies are, the more nutrients they'll have retained, and the more you'll retain when you eat them.

Meal Skipping

"I skip meals a lot – sometimes breakfast, sometimes lunch, sometimes both. Do I have to eat more regularly while I'm TTC, even though I'm trying to lose weight?"

Not only should you think about switching over to regular eating, you should think about trading in those one or two big meals a day for five or six much smaller ones.

There's no better way for an expectant mum to eat than a little at a time, a lot of times a day – in other words, to graze. The Six-Meal Solution (you'll read all about that once you've graduated to *What to Expect When You're Expecting*) minimizes or eliminates a plethora of pregnancy symptoms, from headaches to heartburn, morning sickness to mood swings. And it's an easy concept to swallow. Instead of sitting down for three squares (or one or two, as meal skippers like you do on a regular basis), you simply nibble on five or six mini-meals or snacks, each containing a source of protein and a source of complex carbs (whole-grain crackers and a cheese wedge; a smoothie made with yogurt and fruit; a half a turkey sandwich and a peach).

But how does the graze craze apply to the not-yet-pregnant? How can eating less more frequently boost your fertility? And why would you eat more often if you're trying to lose a few pounds before pregnancy starts packing the pounds on?

Here's the how and why. As far as fertility is concerned, keeping your blood sugar on an even keel can definitely improve your reproductive outlook, especially if you have insulin issues (you have PCOS or you're diabetic, for example). And one of the most efficient ways to regulate blood sugar is – you guessed it – to graze on small amounts of protein and complex carbs throughout the day, instead of gorging once or twice a day.

And though it sounds counterintuitive (when has eating more often ever led to weight loss?), grazing can make it easier to drop that preconception weight, which in turn can help your fertility campaign. Just make sure that the foods you choose to nibble on are mainly healthy, lowfat ones and that you don't overdo the calories over those five or six mini-meals (otherwise you could end up minimizing your weight loss, or even netting a gain).

PART 2

Making a Baby

CHAPTER 4

The Biology of Baby Making

CHANCES ARE YOU ALREADY HAVE a pretty good idea of how to go about making a baby (insert part A into part B; repeat as needed). But how much do you really know about the science of conception beyond the basics of baby-making biology? If you're like most hopeful mums- and dads-to-be, probably not a whole lot.

So before you begin your baby-making efforts in earnest, take a moment to marvel at the incredible and improbable process of conception. How two tiny cells, one from you and one from your partner, beat the seemingly insurmountable odds stacked against them to meet, greet, and form a perfect union – a unique human being whom you'll soon call baby. Learning about the science of conception – one of the most amazing biological feats in the body's remarkable repertoire – isn't only fascinating stuff, it's practical stuff. It'll arm you with all the biological know-how you'll need to get the job of baby making done – and also give you a new appreciation for the miracle that's about to take place in your body.

Anatomy 101

Remember when you were in year six? When your teachers said you'd be getting "the talk"? The boys got an extra period of gym. And the girls – you got an extra period to learn about your period. And about how each month your ovaries, uterus, fallopian tubes, and cervix (not to mention a bunch of hormones) gear up for baby making – even when there's no baby making on the agenda. Did you pay attention? If you did – great! Go to the head of the class.

If your basic anatomy is a little rusty, and if the mysteries of your body are still, well, mysterious, then find a comfortable spot on the couch and read on. Because knowing what all those reproductive organs inside of you do (and equally important – where they're located) will give you a leg up on understanding how your reproductive cycle works, which in turn can help you get that reproductive process started sooner and get that baby on board faster.

Inside You

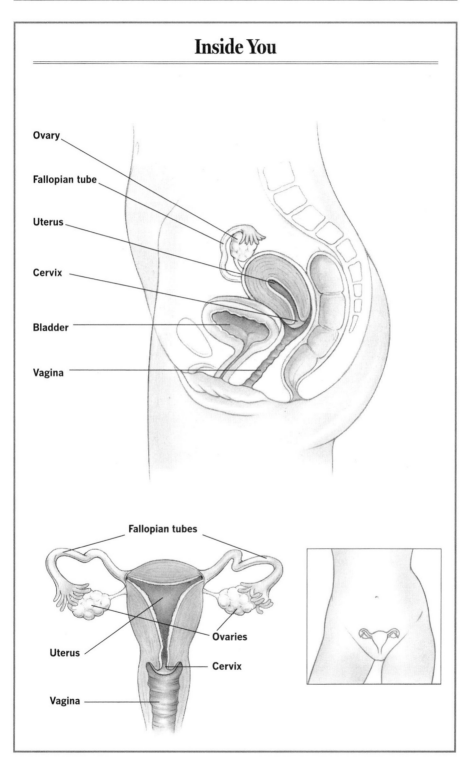

Ovary

Fallopian tube

Uterus

Cervix

Bladder

Vagina

Fallopian tubes

Ovaries

Uterus

Cervix

Vagina

Your Body Basics

Let's get the basics out of the way. As you can see in the illustration on the previous page, your internal reproductive organs include the ovaries (you've got two of them – one on each side), the fallopian tubes (ditto), the uterus, the cervix, and the vagina. You probably already know that you have them – and that they come standard issue to the female of the species. But now it's time to learn a little more about these baby-making must-haves:

■ **Your ovaries** are where your eggs (also called ova, or ovum for a single egg) are stored. Each month, one of those eggs matures inside an ovarian follicle and is released from one of your ovaries into a fallopian tube. Most often, your two ovaries take turns releasing eggs (left side one month, right side the next). The ovaries also produce the hormones oestrogen and progesterone – much more about these later – both of which are essential for conceiving and growing a baby.

■ **Your fallopian tubes** are 12½-centimetre-long narrow tubes (you have one tube on each side of the uterus) that connect the ovaries and the uterus. It is here – in one of these tubes – that egg and sperm meet up and fertilization takes place. Once conception occurs, the fertilized egg completes its travel through the fallopian tube and arrives at its destination: the uterus.

■ **Your uterus** (aka your womb) is the pear-shaped organ where your yet-to-be conceived baby will spend your pregnancy developing and growing – essentially, his or her first home. Each month, the lining of the uterus (known as the endometrium) builds up in preparation for a pregnancy – just in case a baby shows up. If a fertilized egg does implant in the endometrium, the cosy uterus incubates the fetus and, eventually, the muscles of this phenomenal organ contract during childbirth to push the fully formed baby out. If conception and implantation do not occur – as they don't, of course, most months of your reproductive life – the endometrium will shed in the form of your period.

How Many Eggs in Your Basket?

Ready to count eggs (before they hatch)? Wondering just how many you have in your basket? Consider these interesting egg number factoids: As a 16- to 20-week fetus, your ovaries were housing a mind-boggling 6 to 7 million eggs – way more than one woman could ever use, even if she had her eye on a really big family. From then on, those numbers were all downhill. Not that you would have missed them or used them, but by the time you were born, your egg count was down to about 1 to 2 million, the rest having fallen victim to normal attrition. The gradual attrition continued throughout your childhood, and by the time you reached puberty – and started tapping into those eggs each month through ovulation – you were hosting about 300,000 to 400,000 eggs. By age 37, you're down to 25,000 eggs. Definitely a lot fewer eggs than you started with, but still plenty to go around. After all, it takes only one egg to make a baby.

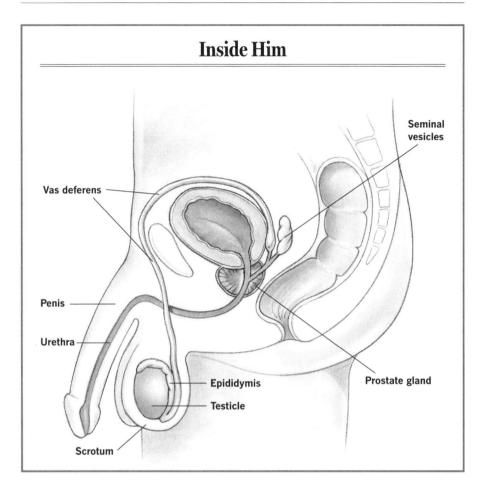

Inside Him

Seminal vesicles

Vas deferens

Penis

Urethra

Epididymis

Testicle

Prostate gland

Scrotum

- **Your cervix** is located at the bottom of the uterus and serves as its entrance. The cervix is shaped like the neck of a bottle (the bottle is the uterus) and will stretch up to 10 centimetres (about 4 inches) wide when it's time to birth a baby. The opening of the cervix (which internally is located at the top of your vagina) is known in medical speak as the "os". It's from here that cervical mucus is secreted (more about that super-significant component of fertility later on).

- **Your vagina** is the gateway to the reproductive tract. Here's where reproduction begins (when sperm is deposited in the vagina during intercourse) and ends (when the baby exits through the vagina during birth – that is, unless that vaginal exit is preempted by a caesarean delivery). Usually around 10 to 15 centimetres (4 to 6 inches) in length, the vagina is quite elastic (which is why it can feel snug around a slender regular tampon yet can stretch to accommodate the passage of a 7- or 8-pound baby).

His Body Basics

Though females take on the bulk of the reproductive responsibility – actually all of it, once conception takes place – it does take two to make a baby. Without the contribution of her partner's sperm, no female (human, that is) would get pregnant in the first place. Here's the lowdown on what goes on down below on a guy (for a peek inside his reproductive parts, see the illustration on the previous page):

- **The testicles.** Unlike his female counterpart, who has a lifetime supply of eggs already produced and ready to roll at birth, the male produces fresh sperm each day in his testes (or testicles), the pair of oval-shaped glands that hang below the penis. Ever wonder why the testicles hang – for the most part – outside the body? Sperm can only develop in a place that is 3 to 4 degrees below normal body temperature. The scrotum (the skin that surrounds the testicles) serves as a natural climate control, helping the testes stay consistently cooler by thickening and thinning in response to external temperatures (which explains why they hang lower in a hot shower and why they "shrivel" up after a dip in a cold pool).

His Olympic Swim Team

Ever stop to think about sperm? With all the fertility focus on your eggs (When will they be ripe? When will they be released? When will they be conception ready?), it's easy to forget about those incredible swimmers of his, who wait on the sidelines, eager to make their vital contribution to Team Baby. Sperm – those tiny tadpole-like cells with whiplashing tails dancing in frantic figure eights – are the smallest cells in the body, but each one potentially packs a powerful punch. A teardrop-shaped sperm head measures only two one-thousandths of an inch (in comparison, the egg – the largest cell in the body – is 30 times the width of a sperm cell).

What sperm lack in size (and who says size matters, anyway?), they certainly make up for in number. Each testicle produces 4 million new sperm per hour (yes, hour) – about 1,200 sperm per heartbeat! Add it all up, and a healthy male can expect to generate 12 trillion (yes, trillion) sperm over his lifetime (compared to the mere million or so eggs a female starts off with). If that number isn't impressive enough, consider this: In each ejaculate, there are on average 100 to 200 million (yes, million) sperm yearning to become half of a full-fledged human being (though to be fertile, a man needs only 15 percent of those sperm to be capable of fertilizing an egg; the other 85 percent are often abnormally shaped, sluggish, or otherwise unserviceable, and that's no problem).

Sperm also make up for their small size with their astonishing athletic ability and mind-boggling speed. The tail propels each sperm forward at the unbelievable pace of a fifth of a centimetre per minute. To put that into perspective, hop onto the treadmill and rev it up to 4 miles per hour. That's the human equivalent of a sperm's speed. Not too shabby for a microscopic cell.

Sperm need all the speed – and strength – they can get to swim from point A (vagina) to point B (waiting egg in the fallopian tube). If that doesn't sound like a big deal, consider that in sperm terms, the distance it needs to travel is equivalent to you swimming across the English Channel three (yes, three) times without stopping. Now that's some Olympic swim team!

Did You Know?

Did you know that sperm makes up only 1 to 3 percent of semen? The rest of that gooey goop consists of fructose and other complex sugars, protein, and trace vitamins and minerals that protect, feed, and fuel the sperm on their journey. Bon voyage!

- **The epididymis.** The sperm matures and learns how to swim – its most important skill – in the epididymis, a series of tightly coiled tubes located in the scrotal sac right on top of the testicles. It can take 12 to 21 days for sperm to pass through the epididymis in its maturation process. Sperm is stored in the epididymis and the vas deferens until ejaculation.

- **The vas deferens.** During arousal (aka an erection), sperm is pumped from the epididymis to the vas deferens, a pair of 38-centimetre-long tubes that wind from the top of the epididymis through the scrotum and up into the lower abdomen.

- **The seminal vesicles.** As the sperm travels through the vas deferens, a fructose-filled fluid from the seminal vesicles – called semen – is pumped into the tubes and mixes with the sperm. This will help push the sperm toward the prostate gland.

- **The prostate gland,** located in the lower abdomen under the bladder, adds an alkaline fluid to the semen (to protect it from the acidic environment of the vagina) as the sperm journeys toward ejaculation. From the prostate, the sperm-loaded semen is transported into the urethra (which runs through the penis shaft) and is then released through the tip of the erect penis during ejaculation – with the hope of meeting its match, in the form of a willing and able egg.

Your Cycle at Work

Ever since you hit puberty, your body has been going through an intricate monthly dance involving brain signals, hormones, and physical changes that ultimately ends with your period – that is, unless it ends with a pregnancy. Whether your periods arrive like clockwork or are a little irregular, your body goes through the same twelve-step programme during each menstrual cycle:

1. Your period. The first day of your period is considered the first day of your menstrual cycle – though logically, it's more like the end than the beginning (you'll see why when you read on). But forget about logic for now – and just remember this: Because a period is the easiest-to-predict, easiest-to-notice, and easiest-to-record reproductive event in the month (unless you count that sudden, uncontrollable craving for all things chocolate), the medical establishment has taken to calling the first day of your period the first day of your cycle. When you do become pregnant, this day will be crucial to dating your pregnancy – and figuring out your due date.

Over a period (so to speak) of approximately 5 days, the lining of your uterus sheds, causing menstrual blood to flow through the cervix and out your vagina (or into those tampons). While you're menstruating, your endocrine system (aka your hormones) starts gearing up for a fresh reproductive start.

2. FSH production. While you're busy bleeding, your pituitary gland (located at the base of the brain) is busy, too, secreting increasing amounts of the hormone FSH (follicle-stimulating hormone), which, you guessed it, stimulates 10 to 20 egg-containing follicles in your ovaries to develop, getting them ready for ovulation (the release of that egg of the month).

3. LH production. By the time your period is ending (around day 5), the pituitary adds another hormone to the mix, releasing increasing amounts of LH (luteinizing hormone). LH works with FSH to stimulate the ovarian follicles and help them mature.

4. Oestrogen production. As the follicles in the ovaries are stimulated (thanks to FSH and LH), they in turn begin to stimulate production of the hormone oestrogen. Oestrogen production stimulates further LH production (talk about positive feedback!), which helps the follicles mature even more.

5. The dominant follicle wins. Sometime around day 8 of your cycle, one of those maturing follicles emerges as the dominant one – the one destined for ovulation. As that top-dog follicle establishes its dominant position, the other follicles that had begun to mature in hopes of releasing their eggs, now begin to disintegrate instead. (Sometimes, more than one follicle continues to mature, resulting in multiple ovulation – and possibly, a multiple pregnancy.)

6. Endometrial cycle. As the dominant follicle continues to mature, it produces more and more oestrogen. This increased oestrogen production gets this month's reproductive party started in your uterus, and by day 12, the surge in oestrogen has caused the endometrium (the uterine lining) to build up anew (remember, that lining was cleaned out after the last period, a week and a half earlier).

7. Cervical mucus production. Oestrogen production has far-reaching reproductive effects, also impacting the glands in your cervix – triggering the production of cervical mucus. As the level of oestrogen rises to its highest point midcycle, the quality – and quantity – of cervical mucus changes, from cloudy and sticky (day 8 or 9) to wet, clear, and slippery (days 10 through 13). Read about this very important fertility sign on page 87.

Fertility by the Clock

What are your fertility numbers? That depends, at least in part, on the number of birthdays you've celebrated so far. A woman in her early 20s who isn't using birth control has a 20 to 25 percent chance of conceiving each month. By her late 20s, she has a 15 to 20 percent chance of hitting the baby jackpot each month. That number drops to a 10 to 15 percent chance per month in her early 30s, and an 8 to 10 percent chance each month by her late 30s. By the time the average woman reaches her 40s, that number gets lower still. But notice that, though the numbers do decline as you age, they decline relatively gradually, which gives most women plenty of time to clock in their baby making while that biological clock's still ticking strong.

8. LH surge. For reasons not exactly clear (the body works in mysterious ways), the hormone LH now surges to six to ten times its normal rate, peaking about 12 to 16 hours before ovulation. Within hours of this LH surge, FSH also surges, but not as dramatically. The surge of these two hormones temporarily shuts down the production of oestrogen in the now mature dominant follicle.

9. Ovulation. Midway through the menstrual cycle (around day 14 in a 28-day cycle, though it could be anywhere from day 12 to day 18 in a shorter or longer cycle), and courtesy of the LH and FSH surge, the dominant follicle in the ovary begins to swell and then rupture. From the ruptured follicle emerges that egg of the month, and the force of the rupture propels the egg through the ovarian wall and into the waiting fingers of the fallopian tube. Ovulation has just occurred.

10. The egg's journey. Once the egg leaves the ovary, the fimbria (the petal-like fingers of the fallopian tube) creates a safety net for the egg – catching it and coaxing it into the fallopian tube to begin its voyage toward a possible conception. If sperm has found its way into the fallopian tubes at the same time (and timing is everything when it comes to conception), fertilization might occur. But if there is no sperm around to meet the egg – or if the sperm miss their mark and fertilization doesn't occur – the egg will disintegrate within 12 to 24 hours.

11. Progesterone production. Meanwhile, the follicle that was emptied when the egg was released turns into the corpus luteum (translation: "yellow body"), which begins to secrete large amounts of the hormone progesterone and smaller amounts of oestrogen. The oestrogen continues to build up the uterine lining, and the progesterone acts to mature the

Give It Time

Of course you're anxious to make baby magic happen – and if you had your way, it would happen overnight (or at least, after your first round of make-a-baby). But while there's always the chance that you will get that lucky that fast, realistically, the odds are it will take a little longer. In fact, it can take a completely healthy, fully fertile couple 6 to 12 months of active trying before they hit the baby jackpot.

So try not to be a clock watcher. Keep an eye on the calendar, but don't obsess over it – and definitely don't stress about it. Instead, relax and enjoy your conception campaign.

uterine lining, readying the uterus for a potential pregnancy – and its potential occupant. Progesterone also alerts the pituitary gland to limit further production of FSH and LH (since those follicle-stimulating days are over for now).

12. Deterioration of the corpus luteum. If this cycle is destined to end in a period, not a pregnancy, the corpus luteum begins to deteriorate once the residual levels of LH diminish (usually around 12 to 14 days after ovulation). Without the corpus luteum to continue producing progesterone, levels of the hormone drop around day 27, triggering the shedding of the uterine lining – and the beginning of your period, activating the entire cycle all over again. If, on the other hand, conception has occurred, the pregnancy hormone human chorionic gonadotropin (hCG) will signal the corpus luteum to remain viable for a few more months to help sustain the pregnancy until the placenta gets up and running.

Conception 101

Sure you know how babies are made, but beyond those basic body mechanics, do you really know what will be going on inside of you after sperm and egg are introduced to each other? Here's the lowdown on Conception 101.

Ovulation

Ovulation, as you've just read, is when an egg (smaller than the size of the full stop at the end of this sentence) is served up from one of your ovaries and caught by the ends of the fallopian tube. The key to planning conception is knowing when the big O occurs. Why? Because to make a baby, you need to make sure sperm and egg meet up during a very tight window of opportunity – right around ovulation. And that window is even slimmer for an egg than it is for the sperm. Though sperm can hang around and get their job done (assuming they're in the right place) for 72 hours after ejaculation or even longer, eggs are only viable for 12 to 24 hours after ovulation. Once a released egg has expired without meeting its sperm match, the conception window closes down for the month. For more about predicting when ovulation will occur so you can time your conception efforts right, turn to page 84.

Fertilization

The journey to fertilization starts with sex. You're probably familiar with this part of the drill: With his climax, your partner's sperm shoot their way from his penis into your vagina in a sea of semen. What you might not know is what lies ahead for the sperm. Semen provides the perfect travel environment for the sperm as they set out on the long trip ahead, keeping them well fed and protected on their journey while helping deliver them safely to Destination Egg. Semen coagulates in the vagina right after ejaculation to prevent the sperm from getting off track and wandering too far in the wrong direction, such as right back out the vagina (and that's a good thing – you know how few guys are willing to stop for directions). About half an hour after ejaculation, the semen reliquifies (and usually ends up dribbling out of you, sometimes in a post-coital gush). But don't worry about any loss of semen at this stage of the game. Any sperm that haven't made it up through the cervix by then are clearly not worth saving. What's more, any sperm stragglers who find themselves left behind in the vagina for more than a few minutes don't have much of a chance of surviving anyway, thanks

---

Beat the Clock

It takes 30 minutes for sperm to reach the fallopian tubes after entering the vaginal canal. It takes another 15 to 20 minutes for the sperm to find the egg and start attempting penetration (of the egg, that is). And it takes a good 20 minutes for the winning sperm to drill its head through the tough shell surrounding the egg and officially get lucky – while officially kicking off conception. Add it up and you'll see that this incredibly intricate process – from sex to fertilized egg – can take as little as an hour. How's that for a game of beat the clock?

Conception Closeup

You've heard about sperm meeting egg, but have you ever wondered how the miracle of conception actually plays out – start to amazing finish? Take a look at this conception closeup.

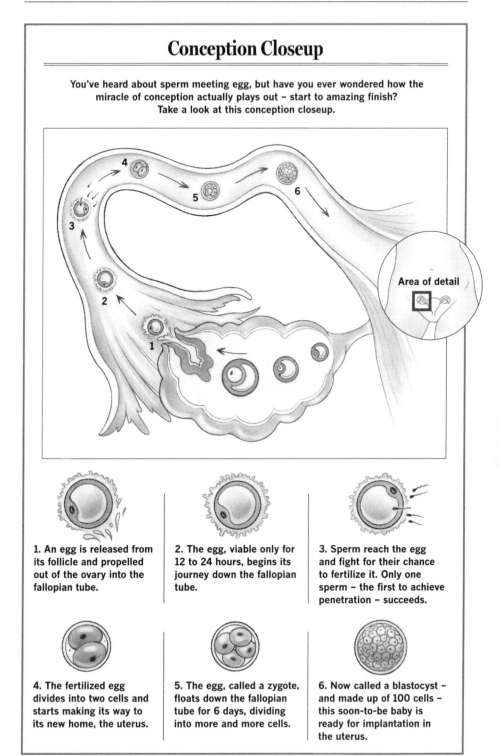

1. An egg is released from its follicle and propelled out of the ovary into the fallopian tube.

2. The egg, viable only for 12 to 24 hours, begins its journey down the fallopian tube.

3. Sperm reach the egg and fight for their chance to fertilize it. Only one sperm – the first to achieve penetration – succeeds.

4. The fertilized egg divides into two cells and starts making its way to its new home, the uterus.

5. The egg, called a zygote, floats down the fallopian tube for 6 days, dividing into more and more cells.

6. Now called a blastocyst – and made up of 100 cells – this soon-to-be baby is ready for implantation in the uterus.

(or no thanks) to the vagina's sperm-unfriendly acidic pH.

As the sperm quickly pass through the inhospitable vagina toward the more welcoming cervical canal that is awash in cervical mucus (the thin, clear mucus associated with ovulation is specially designed to transport sperm more efficiently), they undergo biochemical changes that transform them from sluggish slackers into tail-thrashing dynamos, ready to jump the starting gate and propel through the uterus and fallopian tubes toward their target – the egg.

But those boys are not home free yet. For starters, sperm have to get their

---

Phase Facts

And now, more cycle facts that can come in handy when you're trying to make a baby. The first part of the menstrual cycle – from the start of your period through ovulation – is called the follicular phase, and its length varies considerably from woman to woman, depending on the length of her cycle. The second part of the menstrual cycle (beginning at ovulation) is called the luteal phase and usually lasts 12 to 14 days, but no longer than 16 days. This second phase is more consistent from woman to woman, no matter how long or short her cycle is, making it easier to look to for fertility clues.

How can these phase facts help you in your quest for conception? By helping you pinpoint that all-important monthly event essential to baby making – the release of that egg of yours. If you have longer cycles (say 33 days or 40 days), it's likely to be because your follicular phase is longer than average – not because your luteal phase is. Chances are, you'll still be ovulating approximately 12 to 14 days before your next period. Likewise, if your cycles are on the short side, that's a sign that your follicular phase is shorter than average. Even if your periods arrive 24 days apart, figuring out your ovulation date is often as easy as counting back 12 to 14 days from the beginning of your period (most of the time; read on to learn when

that's not the case). If your cycles are irregular, you'll have to focus on other tools to help you pinpoint ovulation (such as those starting on page 85).

Though most cycles have a predictable luteal phase, about 10 percent of women – an equal number of fertile and unfertile – may have a luteal phase deficiency (LPD). With an LPD, the time from ovulation to the next period lasts about 10 days or fewer. A short luteal phase is associated with lower levels of progesterone (there's not enough time in the cycle for the progesterone to build up) and an inadequately prepared uterus (there's not enough time for the endometrium to sufficiently thicken). That, in turn, can make it difficult for an embryo to implant or stay implanted. Chronic LPD affects 3 percent of women with infertility, though 30 percent of all women can have an LPD in any given cycle.

Diagnosing an LPD is tricky, but one way is to chart your basal body temperature (see page 85). If you notice fewer than 10 to 12 post-ovulation high temperature days, there's a chance you're experiencing problems with your luteal phase. Your doctor can test your levels of progesterone and give you progesterone supplements, if needed, to increase your luteal phase and boost your fertility. Clomid (a fertility drug; see page 160) may also be prescribed in certain situations.

timing just right. If they reach the fallopian tube too early, they risk dying before the egg shows up. Too late, and the egg will be long gone – and the sperm will have missed their once-in-a-lifetime opportunity to fertilize one. They also need to pick a tube – and not just any tube. An egg is usually present in only one of the two fallopian tubes in any given month. Pick the wrong tube, and the sperm come up empty.

Even the sperm that are resourceful enough to reach the egg still have their work cut out for them. Hundreds of sperm will fight for the chance to fertilize the same egg, swarming around it and attempting to plough headfirst through its hard outer layer. The best man wins – as long as he's the first man to break into the egg's inner sanctum, too. As soon as the one lucky sperm cell succeeds in penetrating the egg, the egg immediately forms a barrier to keep the other sperm from getting through (who's your daddy?). Then without so much as a celebratory toast, the victorious sperm plunges into the egg's nucleus, releases its own genetic contribution – and the egg is officially fertilized. Within a matter of hours, the microscopic fertilized egg (called a zygote) divides, then splits again and again. It continues to divide and float down the fallopian tube toward the uterus – a journey that takes around 6 days – and by the time the cluster of cells (now called a blastocyst) reaches your uterus, it numbers around 100 cells strong.

So You Think You're a Stud?

Get ready for a reality check, courtesy of the animal kingdom. Consider this: A male pig ejaculates ½ litre (yes, litre) of semen each time he mates; the average human male ejaculates only ½ to 1 teaspoon of semen. Here's another stat that may leave you a little, well, deflated. The average bull ejaculate contains 10 billion sperm. In comparison, the average healthy man's ejaculate contains 100 to 200 million sperm. But before you start feeling sorry for yourself – or a little envious of those other male animals – remember that pigs and bulls don't get nearly as many opportunities to mate as humans do. So who's the stud now?

Implantation

When the blastocyst reaches its residence for the next 8½ months (your uterus), it wastes no time in making itself at home. First, it begins to burrow deep into the uterine lining (the endometrium) that was built up in anticipation of its tiny occupant's arrival, attaching itself firmly. Once snug and secure, the ball of cells you can't wait to cuddle (at least once they turn into a baby) differentiates into two groups. Half (now called the embryo) will become your baby; the other half will become the placenta, the amazing lifeline that channels nutrients to the fetus and carries waste away. As soon as the fertilized eggs implants, it starts to release hCG – the just-for-pregnancy hormone that will turn your home pregnancy test positively positive.

CHAPTER 5

Predicting Ovulation

O F ALL THE COMPLEX PROCESSES involved in the making of a baby – and, as you've read, there are plenty – there's no more important one than ovulation. Sure, knowing precisely when that egg will be ripe, released, and ready for fertilization definitely isn't necessary for conception. Many a baby has been made without any ovulation heads-up (typically it's just a matter of time before egg and sperm find themselves together in the right place at the right time), but it sure takes a lot of the guesswork out of getting pregnant. Whether you're just looking for some general guidelines to direct your baby-making efforts or you're looking to micromanage Project Conception by employing every ovulation prediction tool known to reproductive science, this chapter will point you in the right direction.

How to Pinpoint Ovulation

D uring each monthly cycle, your egg is open for the business of fertilization for only about 12 to 24 hours after ovulation – after which your reproductive shop shuts down until next month. But before you get discouraged by what seems like an impossibly short fertilization time frame, remember that sperm have a much longer shelf life than eggs do – and can live to fertilize for up to 3 to 6 days. Even though it's ideal to have sex the day you ovulate – giving sperm and egg the best chance of hooking up successfully – you may score a fertilized egg even if you have sex a couple of days before ovulation. After all, there may be plenty of viable sperm still hanging around in your fallopian tube waiting patiently for the egg when it finally emerges. And it takes only one Mr. Right to make a baby.

Even with that encouraging news from the sperm front, the goal of fertilization becomes a little more challenging when you factor in the very limited use-by date of each egg. Which is why pinpointing when ovulation occurs – and when that egg will be ready for the taking – is key to making a baby.

How can you pin down the big O, so you can pin each other down for some baby-making action? By tuning in to changes in your body – changes you may have largely ignored up until now. Mother Nature wisely drops clues each month that signal the imminent arrival of ovulation. Knowing how to read those clues will help you to better predict when that monthly egg will be released – so you'll know to grab your partner, time sex, and up the odds that your conception quest will end in success.

Cycle Length

The second half (luteal phase) of your monthly menstrual cycle – the time span between ovulation and the onset of your next period – is fairly predictable, lasting no longer than 16 days and usually between 12 to 14 days. Which means that if your period usually starts 30 days after the previous one started, it's likely that you ovulated between the 14th and 18th day of your cycle (in other words, halfway through the cycle). And if you have a fairly regular cycle and keep track of cycle lengths, you'll be able to estimate when you'll likely ovulate during your next cycle (so you can assume your baby-making position at just the right time).

As with everything reproduction related (you'll soon notice), there's a wide range of normal when it comes to menstrual cycles. Some women have short cycles lasting a mere 23 days or so (with ovulation most likely occurring on days 9 to 11); others have a long reprieve between periods – say, 35 days (with ovulation taking place anywhere from days 19 to 23). Most women find

Action Plan

Looking to schedule in baby making? Keeping an eye on your calendar now can help you pencil in that bundle of joy sooner. A few months before you plan to begin baby making (and after you've ditched the Pill, patch, or ring), grab the calendar and start circling the first day of each period. After a few months, you'll be able to determine your natural cycle length. Count back 12 to 16 days each month to get an idea of when you ovulated during the previous cycle. This will help narrow down when you'll likely be ovulating next cycle (and more important, during the cycle you're going to begin giving conception a try). You can start keeping track of your cycles on page 212, if you like.

their cycles fall somewhere in between. If your periods are irregular and there's no discernible pattern you can count on (one month you have a 27-day cycle, the next a 49-day cycle, the next a 33-day cycle, and so on), you won't be able to look to your cycle for fertility bulletins. Instead, you'll need to be more alert for other signs of ovulation.

Basal Body Temperature

You know all those hormones that make you feel, well, hormonal during your cycle? For most women, the ups and downs of those trademark female hormones – most notably oestrogen and progesterone – cause plenty of typically unwelcome emotional and physical changes (from crankiness to cravings, bloating to breakouts). But one by-product of those hormonal fluctuations that isn't as noticeable – unless you're really paying attention – is subtle changes in your body temperature. More precisely, your basal body temperature (BBT) – the baseline reading you get first thing in the morning, after at least three to five hours of sleep and before you get out of bed, talk, or even sit up (and definitely before you indulge in any early-morning loving). If you ever needed an excuse not to jump out of bed at the first sounding of the alarm, this is it (hey – you just bought yourself a few extra minutes under the covers).

During the first part of your cycle – before ovulation – oestrogen dominates. Once ovulation occurs, there is a significant surge in progesterone (the "pro" gestation hormone), which helps ready your uterus for a fertilized egg. With that bump in progesterone comes a rise in your body temperature – about a half a degree increase (think of it as nature's way of getting your body warmed up for baby making). In other words, your temperature will be lower before ovulation

The Art of the Chart

To make a baby, consider starting in bed – and not for the obvious reason. Taking your BBT with a digital basal thermometer each morning before you get out of bed (yes, even before you pee or take a sip from that glass of water on your bedside table) can help you figure out when during your cycle you ovulate – so you'll know when during your cycle you're most likely to succeed in baby making. Mark each daily reading on a graph and connect the dots (you can use the fertility charts starting on page 215).

You should see evidence of ovulation a day or two after it has occurred by noticing a half-degree jump in temperature. Over the course of a few months, you should be able to detect patterns of highs and lows, and you'll be able to pinpoint the dramatic increase in temperature, giving you a clue for the next month when ovulation typically takes place – about a day or two before that jump – and giving you a heads-up on when to hop back into bed for baby making. As an example, if your BBT jump occurs on day 16 each month, you're probably ovulating a day or two before that – on day 14 or 15,

which means you should be baby dancing (aka having sex) on days 13 to 16 (since sperm can hang around for a few days waiting for the egg to show up).

One thing to keep in mind when it comes to BBT: keeping track of it, especially once the novelty wears off, can be tedious. Make that a real drag. Especially on those mornings when you don't have time for lounging in bed (the alarm didn't go off, you have an early meeting, you have to pee desperately). A meticulously kept fertility chart can definitely provide some clues to better help plan your baby dancing, but remember that it can only issue that ovulation bulletin after the fact – at which point, it may be too late to put that just-released egg to good use. To make it a more effective conception-planning tool, you'll probably need to keep at the charting for at least 2 cycles so you'll know when to anticipate ovulation in the next cycle based on your ovulation history. Sick of taking your temperature after the second day – and can't imagine keeping it up for 2 months? Skip this preconception step altogether, and move on to other, less time-consuming ovulation clues.

A Confusing BBT Chart

Wouldn't it be great if BBT readings were reliably consistent from month to month, with clear, predictable patterns of highs and lows – and without any outlying (and confusing) temperature numbers? Unfortunately, rare is the BBT chart that is neat and tidy. Real life often gets in the way, making your real-life charts a little more mysterious than you might have thought – at least some of the time.

So what if you've been getting reassuringly regular-looking charts, but then one month you get a temperature reading that's much higher than it should've been, throwing off the pattern you've come to expect? Not to stress. Just remember that your BBT measures your temperature at total rest, and it's extremely sensitive to any change (which is why it's recommended you take the reading immediately after waking and around the same time each morning). Perhaps the day you noticed that elevated temperature reading was a Saturday and you'd slept in, taking your temperature at 10 A.M. instead of your usual 6 A.M. Since temperatures rise the later in the day it gets, that might account for your bumped-up reading. Or maybe that soup bowl-sized margarita you sipped with your enchilada plate last night caused a spike in your waking temp. Or maybe your body was busy fighting an infection that day (and fighting so effectively, you never got sick – but your temperature was temporarily elevated). Or your 5 A.M. trip to the bathroom (it was dark, so you thought it was still nighttime) caused the higher reading at 6 A.M. when your alarm woke you for real. Or you tossed and turned for hours before you actually got up. For best results from your BBT chart efforts, remember that you're looking for an overall pattern, rather than analyzing individual daily readings – which may occasionally stray from your "norm".

than it is during the second part of your cycle – after ovulation. If you're charting your BBT, you'll notice the bump up in temperature a day or two after ovulation day.

Keeping track of your BBT with a special basal body thermometer (which measures temperature in tenths of a degree instead of the standard two-tenth degree increments – a regular thermometer won't get the job done) can help you pinpoint ovulation – at least after the fact. Charting your BBT over a few months will help you to see a pattern to your cycles (once again, assuming your cycles are pretty consistent), enabling you to predict when ovulation will occur – and baby-making conditions are ripe – in future months.

On the horizon is a BBT monitor in the form of a skin patch worn daily under your arm that automatically collects temperature measurements and transmits the data to a digital reader. This promising development may eliminate the need for tedious temp taking and charting in the future.

Cervical Mucus

It's time to get up close and personal with your underwear – really. Because it's in your underwear that you'll discover the next – and one of the best – fertility clues.

Ever notice that sometimes your underwear is really wet and sticky, but other times you're quite dry down there? Ever wondered why (or even wondered if that occasional discharge was a sign that an infection was brewing)?

Actually, it's your cervical mucus at work – and it's one bodily substance you'll definitely want to get to know as you go about the business of baby making. That's because it reflects the normal hormonal ups and downs of your cycle, which you can use to help you pinpoint ovulation day.

Taking a closer look at your underwear – and keeping an eye on the cervical mucus you find down there – may not be the most appealing activity, but it's really one of the most effective ways of tracking your fertility. Here's what to look for as your cycle progresses (there's a cervical mucus change for every phase!):

- **Dry.** Right after your period ends, don't expect to notice any cervical mucus (CM). This dry spell – when your underwear will stay nice and fresh – usually lasts about 6 days to a week on average.

- **Sticky.** As your dry spell ends, things may start getting pretty sticky in your vaginal area (and your underwear) –

and generally stay sticky for a day or two. The texture and consistency of your CM during the sticky phase may be crumbly, tacky, rubbery, pasty, springy, similar to drying rubber cement (see how personal you're getting with it?). The colour of CM during this phase can be yellow or white.

- **Creamy.** For the next several days (beginning, on average, around day 8) your CM will take a turn for the creamy. It may have a lotion-like consistency, or a more milky one, but it'll most likely be white or pale yellow. This is where things can start getting pretty damp, too, or even pretty wet – often noticeably, and sometimes uncomfortably, so. In fact, you may be reaching for the panty liners at this point, to keep this creamy mess out of your underwear. If you try to stretch this CM between your fingers (how's that for fun in the bathroom?), it'll break apart.

- **Slippery.** Bingo! This is the sign you're looking for if you're TTC – CM that's slippery, stretchy (in fact, if you stretch it between two fingers, fertile CM may stretch up to a few inches),

Mucus Mysteries

Wonder exactly how you're going to obtain a sample of your CM-of-the-day, so you can properly assess it? For some women, the CM tap's always flowing – all they have to do to secure a CM sample is touch their vaginal opening (in fact, when they're fertile, these women might feel like they're swimming in egg whites). For those who produce CM on the scantier side, it may be necessary to insert a finger into the vagina and touch the cervix to cop a feel of

CM. But if you're like most women, paying attention when you wipe after peeing will tell you much of what you need to know about your CM. When you're fertile, the toilet paper will glide easily. During the unfertile times of the month, it'll feel drier when you wipe the toilet paper across. And of course, one of the easiest ways to keep track of your CM is to keep an eye on your underwear. When you're at your most fertile, your panties will likely spill the beans.

Did You Know?

Did you know that fertile CM tends to form a circle on your underwear, while CM during the nonfertile parts of your cycle is more likely to appear as a rectangle or line on your panties? So circle those circle days on your calendar!

clear in colour, with the consistency of egg white. This is the most fertile CM, and it indicates that ovulation is occurring (and that it's definitely time to schedule in sex, if you're already actively trying). There is usually more CM present during your most fertile time than there is during other parts of the cycle, but keep in mind that quality is more important than quantity when you're looking for the most fertile CM.

- Dry. Right after ovulation, the CM forecast is mainly dry – and it's likely to stay dry until your period arrives. Some women, though, notice a thicker, cloudier discharge during this time, and others feel a little wet-and-watery a day or two before their period begins (a result of the normal drop in progesterone that precedes menstruation).

Don't confuse fertile CM with that wet (and wild) slippery sensation you get when you're turned on. CM is something that you'll feel (or be able to detect) throughout the whole day – while arousal fluid (feeling "wet" when you're sexually aroused) is only noticeable when you're turned on, something you're not likely to be around the clock. Arousal fluid is also thinner and will dry on your fingers, while CM remains on your finger until you wipe it off.

If you're diligently checking CM each day to get to know your cycles, you'll also want to avoid confusing it with the semen that often dribbles out your vagina after sex. To stay out of that sticky situation, try to remember to do your CM check before you have sex. If you forget and have to run a check afterward, here's what to do: After sex – and before you try to obtain your CM sample – head off to the bathroom and pee. While you're peeing, try to push out as much of the semen as possible. Doing Kegel exercises (squeezing and releasing your pelvic floor muscles as you would to stop the flow of urine) can also help. Continue to squeeze and wipe away as much semen as you can with toilet paper. A quick rinse in the shower can get the job done as well. Once you've got the all-clear, you'll be able to test more easily for CM. (Don't try this if you're actively TTC, however, since you might push out the sperm you'd rather have reach your egg.) Another clue to consider: Seminal fluid is thinner than CM and, like

Action Plan

Now that you know everything you ever wanted to know about CM – or actually, probably a whole lot more than you ever wanted to know – it's time to start paying attention to it daily. Each day, take a look at your CM and note (on a chart such as the one on page 216) the consistency of CM you accumulate. Over the course of several months, you'll see a pattern, and you'll be able to pinpoint when your CM is at its most fertile (egg white slippery consistency, and most likely copious), so that you and your partner can hit the baby dance floor.

vaginal secretions, will dry on your finger quicker. CM, once again, sticks to your finger until you wipe it off.

Cervical Position

You're not done with your cervix yet. This tiny body part that you've probably never given a first thought to plays a pivotal role not only in pregnancy – but also in figuring out how to get pregnant. You've already explored the fertility clues your cervix leaves on your underwear or toilet paper, and now it's time to explore the cervix itself – that is, if you're game to. Feeling the shape and position of your cervix at different points in your cycle will fill in even more fertility blanks – and you don't have to be a gynaecologist to do it.

During most of your cycle, your cervix is firm (it's often described as feeling like the tip of your nose – go figure), closed, and low in your vagina. As ovulation draws near, your cervix rises, opens slightly (thanks to the increase in oestrogen) and becomes soft (described as feeling like your lips, which seems a little more like it). The reason for these changes? A soft, open cervix allows the sperm to pass through more easily on their quest for the egg.

Other Fertility Signs

Not all women notice the following other fertility signs, but if you experience any or all of them (and you may be more likely to if you know what you're looking for – many are easy to miss if you're not paying attention), you've got extra ammunition in your baby-making arsenal:

Crampy ache. Some women notice some sort of mild pain in their lower abdominal area around the time of ovulation. This pain, known in medicalese as mittelschmertz ("middle pain" in

Action Plan

Ready to get to know your cervix? It's easier than you'd think. No stirrups or speculums necessary – all you need is a clean finger with a short, smooth nail (you may want to skip the acrylic nails this month). To check the position and feel of your cervix, insert that finger into your vagina each day or every other day of your cycle, after your period ends. You may find it easier to find your target when you're checking in the squatting position, though you can also check while you're sitting on the toilet or with one foot up on the toilet seat. Relaxing your body will also help (if you clench those muscles, you'll have to fight your way in). For consistency's sake, use the same position (sitting, squatting) each time you check. Once your CM kicks into high gear, it'll be even easier to check because you'll be lubricated. It may take a few cycles for you to get used to your cervical position differences (practice makes perfect), but once you start making sense of them you can chart your findings on your fertility chart (see page 216).

If you've already had a vaginal delivery, your cervix will always feel slightly opened (no matter what time of month) and more oval than that of a woman who's never delivered a baby before, but you'll still be able to notice the subtle changes if you're consistent about checking.

English), can be felt near the ovaries (on one side or the other – likely the side that's about to release an egg) or in the lower abdominal area as a dull achiness, a cramp, or a sharp, fleeting pain. Experts hypothesize that the pain might be caused by the swelling of the maturing follicle or the bursting of the follicle at the actual moment of ovulation. Or the pain might be the result of contractions of the fallopian tubes around ovulation. The pain can last anywhere from a few minutes to a few hours.

Swollen vaginal lips. Just before ovulation, some women feel a fullness in their vulva and vaginal lips, usually on the side from which they ovulate.

Spotting. A few women notice light spotting midcycle, right around ovulation day. This so-called ovulatory spotting is thought to be caused by the sudden drop in oestrogen right before ovulation and the lack of sufficient progesterone at that moment to maintain the uterine lining. If that occurs, a little blood leaks out until progesterone kicks into higher gear and continues to build up the endometrium.

Ovulation Predictors

Don't want to mess around with mucus? You don't have to (unless you really want to). Visit the fertility aisle in your supermarket or pharmacy and stock up on any or all of the following (though be prepared to cough up a good chunk of change – technology doesn't come cheap). And keep in mind that no ovulation predictor tests can promise an accurate fertility forecast (or guarantee conception) – they can only indicate when ovulation may be occurring.

Ovulation predictor kits (OPKs) can help pinpoint your day of ovulation 12 to 36 hours in advance by looking at

TTC for You and Me

In the market for some TTC friends to share your baby-making adventure with – someone who can really relate? Someone who you can describe your cervical mucus to (without hearing, "Ewwww ... gross!"). Who you can swap baby dance tips with? Pass the time with while you're waiting for testing day to come (again!)? Someone to pump you up when a negative home pregnancy test result deflates you, or to share your excitement with when you finally see the readout of your dreams (and who won't think it's weird when you post that pee stick for all to see)? Check out the TTC boards at WhatToExpect.com. You'll make friends, find support, gain insights, and tap into an amazing community of hopeful, expecting, and new mums (and dads). Set up a profile page, blog, post, share video and photos, and more!

levels of LH, which is the last of the hormones to hit its peak before ovulation actually occurs. All you have to do is pee on a stick and wait for the indicator to tell you whether you're about to ovulate. (This way you'll be an expert at peeing on a stick by the time you're ready for your pregnancy tests.) Unlike pregnancy tests – where any line (faint or dark) indicates you're pregnant – the test line on an OPK has to appear the same or darker than the control line. Since there are always low levels of LH in your body, a sensitive OPK can detect it and show a faint line, but what you're looking for is the LH surge (therefore higher amounts of LH) – and a test line that reads bright and clear. You can bypass this confusing line reading detection by choosing those OPKs that have digital readouts (no squinting required!).

It's best to use an OPK between noon and 8 p.m. (though to make sure your urine is still concentrated enough, don't pee for an hour or two before you plan on testing) because most women experience their LH surge in the morning and LH won't be detected in the urine until at least 4 hours later. If you miss the LH surge when it actually happens (and only detect it on the way down), you may think you're ovulating a day after you truly are – throwing your baby dancing schedule off and possibly missing your monthly window of opportunity altogether. If you really want to make sure you catch your LH surge, consider testing twice a day (once between 11 a.m. and 3 p.m. and a second time between 5 p.m. and 10 p.m.). Whether you test once or twice a day, be consistent and test at the same time (or times) each day.

You'll want to start using the OPK tests a little before midway through your cycle (about 3 to 4 days earlier than your cycle midpoint). For a 28-day cycle, start using them on days 10 to 11. For a 31-day cycle, start on days 12 to 13. If your cycles are irregular, use the length of your shortest cycle in the last 6 months as a guide and begin testing 3 to 4 days sooner than the midpoint of your shortest cycle. The more irregular your cycles are, the more OPKs you'll likely use up (so figure that into your cost estimation). Most kits come with five to ten test sticks.

As soon as your LH surge is detected, begin having sex on that day and for 2 to 3 days after.

Fertility monitors take ovulation detection one step further. Instead of testing only for the LH surge, a fertility monitor will test for both LH and oestrogen in the urine, giving you a 6-day window of fertility opportunity. You use the monitor each day, beginning on day 1 of your cycle (the first day of your period), by turning on the device with the press of a button. The monitor keeps track of your cycle days – sort of like a fertility PDA – and the digital indicator reminds you when to start using the urine test strips that come in the package. When you get the heads-up signal from the monitor, you'll pee on the test strip, insert it into the monitor, and wait for the monitor to indicate whether your fertility status that day is low, high, or at its peak. When you see a high or peak readout, you're at your most fertile – which means it's time to get busy.

A saliva test allows you to monitor levels of oestrogen in your system, giving you a heads up that ovulation is near (oestrogen rises before ovulation – and before the LH surge – so by tracking oestrogen, you can get an even earlier indication of when you'll be ovulating). When oestrogen increases, so do the electrolytes (salt content) in your saliva. Testing your saliva can indicate when oestrogen is on the rise and when your fertile time is approaching (and you thought you were done with the bodily substance samples).

Each morning before brushing your teeth, eating, or drinking, put a dab of saliva onto the tip of your (clean) finger and gently smear it onto the lens of the saliva test. Some test brands suggest you put the saliva on the lens directly from your tongue. Wait about 5 minutes until the saliva is dry and then take a look under the test's eyepiece. When you're about to ovulate, a look at your saliva will reveal a microscopic pattern that resembles the leaves of a fern plant or frost on a windowpane (the rest of the time, you'll just see random dots). Once you see your fern, get ready to start baby dancing. Ovulation will likely occur within 24 to 72 hours.

The downside to this type of test is that not all women get a good "fern", and it can be very hard to interpret the test results.

A fertility "watch" is a biosensor worn on your wrist each day (or at night, if it's not your preferred fashion statement). The watch can detect the numerous salts (chloride, sodium, potassium) in yet another bodily substance, sweat – because the salt amounts change during different times of the month. Before ovulation (and even before the oestrogen and the LH surge), there is a surge in ion levels, called the chloride ion surge. Once the watch detects this surge, you've got a 4- to 6-day "warning" that ovulation is approaching, giving you plenty of time to schedule in some baby-making sex.

When You're Not Ovulating

What happens if you've been charting your BBT and checking for CM and even using OPKs, but for some reason, it seems that you're not ovulating every month – or maybe, not ovulating at all? You're not alone. About 6 to 15 percent of women have anovulatory cycles – in other words, they get their period but don't release an egg (and without that egg, conception can't occur). The most common reasons why otherwise healthy women may not ovulate in a particular month include illness, travelling, strenuous exercise, weight gain or weight loss, or extreme stress. Women who are chronically underweight or overweight plus those with a medical condition (such as polycystic ovarian syndrome or thyroid problems) may also have anovulatory cycles. If you think you might not be ovulating, check with your gynaecologist. He or she can turn to a host of low- and high-tech methods to help induce ovulation – and help you get closer to that baby of your dreams.

CHAPTER 6

Figuring Out Your Fertility

WONDERING HOW YOUR FER-tility stacks up on paper before you put it to the test in the bedroom? If you're the curious type, you'll probably want to dig into this chapter for clues about your fertility – how your cycles, your genetics, and your age (and your partner's age) might influence your reproductive profile. Keep in mind as you read, however, that no fertility forecast is a sure thing. Every woman's fertility is different, which means that certain fertility factors may never factor into your baby-making experience. And that also means you may end up making a baby a lot faster in the bedroom than you do on paper.

Rather just plunge into baby making without any fertility forecast? Skip this chapter, and get right to the action.

Am I Fertile?

Enquiring (and hopeful) minds want to know: Am I fertile? How eas-ily will I conceive once we start trying? There's no telling for sure how your fer-tility stacks up until you actually take it for a test-ride (or two, or three, or many more). Even if it's been tested in the past (and passed the test – in the form of a previous pregnancy), fertility can keep you guessing. Still, no need to be completely clueless about your fertil-ity – especially when there are so many clues that can reveal at least part of the baby-making picture.

Your Cycle and Your Fertility

"I'm about to start trying to conceive and I'm so excited. Is there any way to tell whether I'm fertile or not?"

There's really no way to know right out of the gate whether you can expect a smooth ride or a bumpy one to the baby finish line. It takes the aver-age, healthy couple 6 to 12 months of active trying to successfully make a baby. And short of either getting pregnant or undergoing a fertility screening (which you certainly don't need yet – and might never need), there is no way to find out definitively what your fertility prospects are at this early stage of the baby-making game.

Still, you can look to an old familiar (if not favourite) friend, your Aunt Flo, for some hints about what might lie ahead in your TTC future. In fact, tracking her monthly visits is one of the best ways to gauge your fertility and clue you in on the state of your reproductive health. So as you embark on your fledgling campaign to fill your nest, asking yourself some questions about your cycle can be a great place to start. (Keep in mind that you won't be able to get a good read on your cycle if you've been on oral contraceptives or another hormonal birth control method because such cycles are "artificial" and don't reflect what's normal for you. That's why it's a good idea to get back to cycling naturally after quitting birth control pills, before you start trying to conceive.)

How long are my cycles? A "normal" cycle is usually anywhere from 26 to 35 days between periods, with 28 to 30 days the average. If your cycles are much shorter or longer than what is considered "normal", it may be a clue to some fertility issues (though it may not be, too). Are your cycles all over the place? Occasional cycle-length irregularities aren't cause for concern. They're usually just the result of stress, weight loss or gain, or another temporary blip in your normal routine, and as long as they reregulate, they won't keep you from reaching your baby goal. But consistently irregular cycles can make conception slightly more elusive.

How much bleeding do I have? A normal period begins with light bleeding, builds to heavier bleeding, and then slowly tapers off, ending with light staining. *Excessive* bleeding (extremely heavy blood flow, blood clots, or large volumes of blood loss) or a flow that's watery or

---

It's Not Just Your Period, Period

Aunt Flo can tell you a lot when it comes to the state of your fertility, but she can't tell you the whole story. For the rest of the scoop, you'll need to keep an eye on ovulation, too – the most important component of fertility. If you don't ovulate, you can't get pregnant (without a little help from medical science, that is). And sometimes, even women who have seemingly "normal" periods may not be ovulating (this is called an anovulatory cycle). How can you tell if you're ovulating each month? See Chapter 5.

---

exceptionally light in colour could (but definitely doesn't always) signal a reproductive problem.

How long do I bleed? Most women have their period for 5 to 7 days, though usually they see heavy bleeding only on days 2 and 3. Bleeding should lessen by day 4 and continue with only light staining up to day 7. Heavy bleeding that lingers longer than 6 days or periods that last longer than 8 to 9 days may possibly (but by no means necessarily) be a sign that something is off reproductively. Ditto for periods that have very light blood flow for longer than 8 or 9 days or ones that end abruptly after 1 or 2 days.

Do I have pain or cramping? Some aches, pains, and cramps come with the time-of-the-month territory, though a few lucky women don't feel a thing. What's not normal is extremely severe cramping, nausea, vomiting, acute backache, dizziness, or headaches right before or during your period. Any of these could signal (though not necessarily) a reproductive problem.

Are my cycles erratic? If you go months without a period and then have a few periods in a row and then go months again without bleeding, it could signal fertility challenges ahead (unless, again, it's a sign of stress on your body – in which case the erratic cycles and the potential for fertility challenges should disappear when the stress does).

If there are any red flags in your period assessment – or if you have any other reason to believe you may be facing a fertility issue – talk over your concerns with your gynaecologist. Chances are, you'll get the reassurance you're looking for – and marching orders right onto the baby dance floor. If it turns out that your menstrual irregularities may signal a fertility issue, now's the time to have it checked out, diagnosed, and treated, so you can get back on the track to parenthood as quickly as possible.

Another Clue to Your Fertility

Interestingly, some women who do not ovulate regularly and/or have other fertility issues have a slightly increased amount of male hormones (and that's probably what's contributing to the irregular ovulation). How can you tell if that's the case with you? One sign is hirsutism (you're hairier than average on areas of the body normally not associated with hair on a woman, such as on the nipples, lower abdomen, face, even the big toe). Another clue? Acne that persists beyond the midteens can indicate increased male hormones. Check in with your doctor if you've noticed these symptoms.

Genetics and Fertility

"My mother had trouble conceiving me. Does that mean I'm going to have trouble conceiving, too?"

Like mother, like daughter? While it's not necessarily true that your mother's reproductive difficulties will be passed on to you (you may have a fertility walk in the park), there are genetic components to some fertility-related disorders and it's worth exploring your female family tree to see what may – or may not – be lurking beneath the leaves. Ask your sisters, mother, grandmother, aunts, and even female cousins about their TTC experiences and whether they had or have endometriosis, ovarian cysts, fibroids, thyroid disorders, or other potential fertility stumbling blocks. It may also be helpful to know how long it took each of them to conceive. Take all this information with you on your baby-making journey (being sure to let your practitioner know about it, too).

Baby Making After 35

"I'm 37 years old. Is it true that I should expect a harder time becoming pregnant?"

Thirty-five may be the new 25, and 40 the new 30 – but the question is, have your reproductive parts got the memo? Can baby making be on your calendar no matter how many calendars you've gone through?

Absolutely. Birthrates are currently soaring for women (and men) well into their 30s and 40s – proof positive that babies can come to those who wait (even if they sometimes come with a little help from a fertility specialist). If it's true that a woman's life begins at 30 (or even 40), it's also true that, more and more often these days, so does her active reproductive life. Fewer women are jumping on

Fertility and the Older Man

It's long been documented that a woman's biological clock eventually runs out, limiting her baby-making years. But what about men? Is your reproductive life also on a timer?

Actually, it might be, at least to some extent. Guys can – and do – continue their baby-making careers long after they've passed retirement age (and decades after a woman's fertility expires). And more and more are waiting longer to father that first child (there has been a 40 percent increase in first-time fathers aged over 35 in the last 30 years). But researchers have found that fertility does decline in men, too, albeit more gradually than it does in women – beginning at about age 30, and dropping more rapidly after age 45. In fact, it may take up to five times longer for a man to get a woman pregnant once he's 45 than it would have when he was 25.

And though a guy can continue producing viable sperm well into middle age, his age can affect the quantity of sperm (there may be fewer sperm in each ejaculate), the quality of sperm (aging sperm are more likely to be genetically damaged, and this is linked to a higher rate of miscarriage and possibly Down's syndrome and other chromosomal defects when a dad is older, independent of his partner's age), the motility of the sperm (if they can't move fast enough to reach the egg, conception can't happen), and the strength of the sperm (weak sperm will not be able to penetrate the egg's membrane to fertilize it).

Other facts of older life for guys: decreased potency (the force of a younger man's ejaculation is often more powerful than that of an older man, enabling the sperm to be ejected further into the vaginal canal) and problems with erectile dysfunction (which can definitely make fertility more challenging). And even those lucky older guys who notice no reduction in sexual function do experience a fertility drop-off. (By the way, taking Viagra could possibly lower your chances of conception – even as it makes the mechanics of the process possible – so before you pop that little blue pill, ask your doctor about the latest consensus in the research.)

That's not to say that your baby-making days are ever over when you're a guy. Far from it (just ask those who have fathered babies in their 80s) – only that there is a point of somewhat diminishing fertility returns for men as well as women. Though it's possible that you may have to wait a little longer to make that miracle happen, babies are always worth waiting for.

---

the baby train in their 20s, and a full 1 in 5 are opting to wait until they're well into their 30s and 40s to start a family.

Many of these mums are able to conceive within just a few months of trying (and have healthy pregnancies and healthy babies to show for it soon after). But for some "older" hopeful mums, the wait continues even after they've decided to take the baby plunge. They find it takes longer to conceive, or they find that they need a little help – or sometimes even a lot of help – from fertility treatments to make their baby dreams a cuddly reality.

That's because women are at their most fertile in their very early 20s, well before most are ready to tap into that fertility. By their early 30s, fertility has started to wane – the chances of getting pregnant goes from 20 to 25 percent per cycle for women 25 and under, gradually

How Fresh Are Your Eggs?

Since a woman is born with all the eggs she'll ever have – and they're gradually used up or break down as the months (and years) pass – she's left with fewer and fewer fertilizable eggs in reserve as she moves later into her reproductive life. But how do you know how many eggs you've still got left in your basket – and whether they're still functioning and healthy enough to make a baby?

When older women are trying to conceive for 3 to 6 months or more without success, doctors use a blood screening test to determine "ovarian reserve". This is done by measuring "day 3 FSH". Follicle-stimulating hormone – or FSH – is the all-important hormone that signals the ovary to release an egg. When lots of young and eager eggs are ready to burst out and get busy, a little FSH goes a long way – and less is needed to get the ovulation job done. But as the number of eggs dwindles, the brain senses that getting them ready to hatch won't be as easy as it used to be – and that it will take a little extra stimulating in the form of a lot of extra FSH. So the brain issues a signal to the pituitary gland to release more FSH. The fewer good eggs (and good follicles) left, the more FSH is released – the body's way of getting a productive egg up and running, and of compensating for the less-fertile conditions that come with aging. In fact, sometimes the body overcompensates by producing too much FSH, which explains why older women are more likely to drop two eggs at a time, upping their chances of conceiving twins (those follicles can get a little overstimulated from the flood of FSH). What's more, the body – never a quitter – keeps up its follicle-stimulating campaign long after there are no eggs or follicles left to stimulate. In fact, FSH levels are permanently elevated in menopausal women.

By measuring a baseline FSH on day 3 of a woman's cycle (through a simple blood test), doctors can get an indication of how close a woman is to menopause – and how close she is to having fewer and less viable eggs. The higher the baseline FSH, the lower her egg supply, or ovarian reserve. And most of the time, the lower the egg supply, the lower the quality of the remaining eggs will be, too. A normal FSH level is usually under 10. Measurements between 10 and 15 are borderline, and anything above 25 is considered abnormal. Once your FSH (and possibly oestradiol level) has been assessed, you and your doctor can discuss whether fertility treatments are a good next step.

An extension of the day 3 FSH test is the Clomiphene Challenge Test (CCT), which is more sensitive in detecting diminished ovarian reserve, especially for women closer to age 40. Like the day 3 FSH test, the CCT measures FSH and oestradiol on day 3, but it takes it another step: On days 5 to 9, you'll take 100 mg of Clomid (a fertility drug that encourages ovulation), and then on day 10, your FSH will be measured again. If FSH is abnormal on day 3 and/or day 10, it indicates poor ovarian reserve. The reason why this test is somewhat more useful is that some women have a normal day 3 FSH but an abnormal day 10 FSH, indicating diminished ovarian reserve.

Another hormone – AMH (antimüllerian hormone), detected via a blood test – may also be used to determine ovarian reserve in older women, though more study needs to be done before this test becomes widely available. AMH levels reflect the number of follicles present in the ovaries and can estimate how close a woman is to menopause.

down to about 15 percent per cycle for women in your age bracket, 35 to 39. Average chances of conceiving naturally at age 40 – about 5 percent per cycle. Still potentially doable, but clearly not as easy to do.

What causes this drop in fertility? Fewer eggs and less frequent ovulation, for one thing. For another, eggs that have been sitting on the shelf longer. As a woman ages, so do her eggs – and older eggs are less easily fertilized. Still another challenge: Older women don't make cervical mucus like they used to – the quantity and quality of this fertility-friendly fluid also tends to lessen as a woman ages. A woman in her 20s can expect 2 to 4 days of fertile (clear, thin, slippery, stretchy, egg white-like) cervical mucus per cycle, while a woman in her late 30s often has only 1 or 2 days of fertile CM. Less CM may spell more challenging swimming conditions for egg-seeking sperm. Gynaecological problems that can interfere with fertility – such as endometriosis or fibroids – are also more common as women get older, as are general health issues such as high blood pressure or diabetes that can make it harder to conceive. Those who do conceive have a somewhat higher rate of miscarriage, in large part due to those aging eggs.

Feeling daunted? Don't. The vast majority of women your age – 70 percent – conceive naturally and without a hitch. Even women who've passed their fortieth birthday have about a 40 percent chance of conceiving naturally. So don't bog yourself down with the numbers now. Instead, relax and go about your baby-making business (though you'll probably want to pay some extra attention to your cycles, so you can give yourself every fertility edge; see Chapter 5 for tips). If you're 35 to 38 and you haven't conceived within 3 to 6 months of active efforts, check in with your practitioner to see if it's time for a little

help in the fertility department. Check in sooner (after 3 months) if you're over 38, and check in right from the TTC start if you're over 40.

And, here's something else you may want to keep in mind. Being over 35 means conception can be a little trickier, but it can also make it more fruitful – meaning that when it rains babies, it can pour. Older mums have a greater chance of conceiving twins, even if they conceive naturally, without the benefit of fertility treatments. That's because older mums tend to ovulate irregularly, and because they produce more follicle-stimulating hormone (FSH), their ovaries are more likely to be stimulated into dropping two eggs at a time (see box, facing page, for more details). Two fertilized eggs – and presto, you've got two babies.

Action Plan

If you're over 35, you might want to put in a call to your doctor after 3 to 6 months of TTC with no luck. If you're over 38, consider making that call after 3 months of active efforts. If you're 40 or over, there's no reason to wait – check in right from the very beginning of your baby-making campaign. Why the earlier medical input for older mums? Not because you're definitely going to need help in the form of assisted reproduction (and, in fact, you may conceive naturally – and much sooner than you'd think). Just because taking a more time-sensitive approach to TTC makes sense when you're trying to conceive later in your reproductive years. If you do end up needing some help, it's a good idea to start the ball rolling sooner, so you're more likely to have time on your side.

Getting Busy Making a Baby

SO, SAY YOU'VE DONE YOUR PRE-conception prep. Your diet's on track, your weight's on target, you've traded in your 5-cup-a-day coffee habit for a 2-cupper and your tuna for salmon. Your nest egg is busy solidifying, and you've paid a visit to your doctor and dentist. You've got to know your cycle and your cervix, and you're an ovulation prediction pro. Or maybe you've opted to skip the prep phase altogether and cut straight to the good part – getting pregnant. Either way, all reproductive systems are go – and it's time to go make a baby. But how, exactly, do you go about doing that?

The logistics of sex you're pretty clear on – but how do you put that knowledge to its best baby-making use? Are there do's and don'ts to doing "it" now that your goal is conception? Should you let nature take its course, or help give nature a nudge? And what if nature takes her sweet time – how much doing it will you have to do? Are there ways to do it that speed conception or might make your pink or blue daydreams more likely to come true? Should you tap into the Complementary and Alternative Medicine (CAM) camp for a fertility boost? Read on for the answers to all your baby-making questions.

Making Love to Make a Baby

Before jumping into bed, you might want to give sex a second look. Sure, you've probably been doing it for years – and chances are you're pretty good at it by now. But will sex for procreation have to be different from sex for pleasure? In most cases, not at all (not surprisingly, egg and sperm typically meet up without any nudging nec-

essary). Still, a few minor adjustments here and there might be just the ticket you need to hop onto the baby express.

Stopping Birth Control

"We're ready to start trying for a baby. Do I just stop my pills and then get started?"

Ready to take the plunge into unprotected sex? Baby making might seem as easy as tossing the pills, pulling off the patch, or letting the condoms gather dust in your bedside drawer. But you'll need to look before you leap into the sack without that prophylactic parachute and give your birth control method a preconception assessment first. Here's the lowdown on how pregnancy protection can affect pregnancy planning:

Pills, patches, and rings. Because these contraceptives manipulate (make that, fool around with) your natural hormone levels, in effect creating artificial cycles, it's best to shelve the Pill, patch, or ring a few months before you want to start trying to conceive. That will allow your cycles to return to normal first, so that planning the pregnancy and dating the pregnancy will be easier. It'll also allow time for your uterine lining (the endometrium) to thicken, making it easier for an embryo to implant. Finish your Pill pack to avoid midcycle (breakthrough) bleeding before you ditch the package and use a barrier method (condoms are probably most convenient) while you're waiting for your cycles to get back up and running on schedule.

For some women, fertility returns as soon as they quit the hormones, but for others, it may take a month or so to resume ovulation – sometimes even longer, especially if you've been using the hormones for years. If you do get pregnant before your period becomes regular again, or if you get pregnant right after stopping a hormonal contraceptive, or even while using it, don't worry – there's no harm to the baby. The only tricky part if you get pregnant while you're transitioning might be figuring out exactly when you conceived. Early ultrasound can step in and solve that mystery.

Barrier methods (diaphragms, condoms). No need to plan way ahead with these types of contraception, so they're perfect for the spontaneous set. Just ditch the diaphragm or condom anytime (how happy are you about that?) and you're ready to get busy baby making. And

---

Hot to Trot

Feeling frisky? You might be about to drop that egg. Most women, in fact, report feeling their sexiest – and most in the mood for loving – right around the time they're ovulating. Convenient for baby making – and not surprising, either, given Mother Nature's master plan to keep all species, including humans, reproducing. Just as female animals go into heat when they're primed for procreation, females of the human race, too, have developed a heat of their own – biological responses to increase the odds that mating will occur when the chances for pregnancy are highest (at ovulation).

Both testosterone and oestrogen peak midcycle (just about the time you ovulate). Testosterone sends your libido into action (bringing out the sexual aggressor in you), and oestrogen hones your senses (and sensitive senses come in very handy when it comes to sex). What's more, these hormonally triggered friskiness factors (nature's answer to scented candles and mood music?) seem to increase as LH rises, peaking right before ovulation occurs – just in time for sperm to get in line for the egg's release. And leaving you wondering: Is it hot in here, or am I ovulating?

Your Voice Says It All

You may not hear it, but believe it: Your voice sounds sexier when you're most fertile. Think of it as a mating call to your mate, researchers say, a signal to him that you're ready to conceive. Even if he's not aware of the voice change, his reproductive parts apparently are, and they respond accordingly. All of this seems less random and more ingenious when you consider this fascinating fertility fact: The hormonal changes that result in egg release also change the shape and size of your larynx. These findings add fuel to the theory that women give off subtle signs (from scents to style) about their fertility – signs that can help put that fertility to good use. Now you're talking.

while you're ditching your diaphragm, you might as well toss it out, too. You'll need to be fitted for a new one after delivery since pregnancy and childbirth change the shape of your cervix (and ill-fitting diaphragms don't do their job).

Spermicides. Like barrier methods, spermicides don't need to be stopped until you're ready to roll. Don't worry if you accidentally conceive while using a spermicide – it won't hurt your baby.

Intrauterine device (IUD). Stop anytime by having your doctor remove the device. Once it's out, you may be able to start your baby-making efforts pronto (check with your doctor). Typically, your fertility will be the same as it was before the device was put in, with no or little downtime. Even an IUD that releases hormones shouldn't delay your baby-making efforts (the level of hormones is much lower than that in the Pill).

Depo-Provera. There's plenty of advance planning required here because it can take 6 months to a year for ovulation to resume after you stop getting these progesterone shots. Talk to your doctor about the best timing for you. And plan on using another method of nonhormonal birth control (condom, spermicides, or diaphragm) while you wait for your cycles to return to normal.

Natural family planning. As a practitioner of this method, you're ahead of the baby-making game, since you're likely an expert on your own fertility. Now that you're ready for a baby, just reverse your efforts. Instead of avoiding sex during fertile times, bring it on!

Sex Positions

"Is it true that some positions are better than others when it comes to conception?"

Is there a better way to do "it" (make a baby, that is)? Or will any way do? Will just getting it on get that baby on board – or will you have to get creative, too? Or even technical?

Though there's no need to pull out the old *Kama Sutra* book (unless you're in the mood for some spicy gymnastics), you also don't have to go back to on-your-back basics (as in the missionary position) either. The bottom (or top) line is that as long as sperm from your partner is deposited close to your cervix, you're in business. That's because healthy sperm are pretty good swimmers – even when they're swimming upstream, without the help of gravity – and they normally don't need any extra nudging along. Plus, though baby-making sex serves a brand new purpose, its other purpose still applies: having fun in bed (or wherever you choose to baby dance). After all, you're going to be doing it a lot while you're TTC, so you might as well relax and enjoy it. And don't get bent out of shape, literally, if you're happier in your same-old-same-old position. Medical studies haven't yet supported the theory that some positions are more effective for baby making than others.

Of course, there's no harm in doing a little research of your own, and trying a few of the positions often touted for optimum fertility success. After all, it can't hurt to head the little guys in the right direction – and it might even give sluggish sperm the mojo (or gravitational pull) they need to get the job done, or help them access that cervix of yours more easily. Because your vagina naturally tilts toward your back, lying on your back (with man on top) – and with a small pillow under your hips, if you'd like – can allow the sperm to pool right at the cervix. Too big a pillow, though, and you risk directing the sperm behind your cervix instead of up through it, so

elevate your hips only slightly to give gravity an edge (as opposed to a steep slope). If you have a tipped uterus (if your uterus tips toward the front; you can ask your practitioner if you're not sure), doggie-style (hands-and-knees position with penetration from behind) may give sperm that full-access pass to your cervix.

For now, you may want to avoid positions that allow the sperm to leak out (though it takes only one, there is strength in numbers when it comes to fertility odds), including any position in which you straddle your partner – sitting, standing, woman on top, and so on – though again, such a change isn't necessary for conception, and it could actually work against you if you find it doesn't float your love boat (if you're not having fun, you're going to start dreading your baby-making sessions – and that's not going to get you anywhere). Whichever position you choose, make sure your mate ejaculates deep within your vagina – and that he lingers in there as long as possible (you want to get every last drop of sperm).

Doing Headstands?

Wondering how to spend your post-coital time for best baby-making results? You've probably heard it all. Lie down for 20 to 30 minutes after sex to fast-track those sperm to your cervix. Or put your knees or legs up to enlist gravity. Or stand on your head – or twist yourself into some other kind of sperm-preserving pretzel position. And whatever you do, don't get up and pee.

But is there any truth to these tips? While they can't hurt – and potentially might help a little – don't get too hung up on them. Cuddling with your sweetie

for 20 minutes after lovemaking is satisfying for your relationship, and if it helps make a baby, all the better. But advanced yoga moves aren't called for. And neither is forcing yourself to stay prone after sex if you haven't got the time (you have to get to work after that early morning loving or back to work after that lunchtime quickie). Remember, healthy sperm are little men on a mission – and many of them will accomplish that mission without any help from you or gravity. After all, that's why a man's ejaculation is so forceful – to send those boys flying to their target.

Lubricants

"Now that we're timing sex so we can make a baby, the sexiness is gone – and I'm finding that I'm not as wet as I used to be. Is it okay for me to use lubrication?"

It's always easier (and much more comfortable) to get wild when you're wet – and vice versa, too. But when you're trying to conceive, you're better off sticking with nature's lube – your own vaginal secretions. Most experts agree that lubricants – particularly oil-based lubricants such as Vaseline or massage oils – not only meddle with your cervical mucus, preventing it from doing its job optimally, but can also alter the pH in your vaginal tract, causing it to be extra inhospitable to sperm. Some types of lubricants can even be toxic for sperm, killing them off before they can get started (and believe it or not, another natural lubricant – saliva – falls into the sperm-killer category). Water-based lubricants aren't green-lighted during preconception time either (even though they're the most doctor-recommended lubes at other times during a woman's sex life). Also off the bedside table: homemade or kitchen-found lubricants (such as olive oil or egg whites).

Some fertility specialists concede that a small amount of water-based lubricants (the size of a five-pence piece) won't hurt sperm or your conception chances. But if you can live (and make love) without it, it's probably best to lay off the K-Y until baby's on board (at which point you might not be needing any help in the lubrication department – pregnancy hormones typically turn on the secretions tap).

There are brands of lubricant that claim to be sperm friendly. According to the manufacturers, these lubricants mimic cervical mucus and have the same pH as sperm, helping them feel at home in the vagina. Anecdotally, many women who needed lubrication because of dryness say they conceived using these sperm-friendly lubricants.

If TTC has made lovemaking feel like a chore, try putting some pleasure back into the work of procreation. Spending more time (or at least some time) on foreplay before getting the deed done can pay off big time – and get your juices flowing again naturally. For tips on heating things up while trying to conceive, see page 112.

Take Your Sperm to a Movie

Did you know that watching a sexy movie with your mate right before you do the baby dance may actually help you conceive faster? Researchers (who apparently research everything) have found that when men watch a scene with sexual content (and it doesn't have to be X-rated) right before making love, the sperm they produce is higher quality. Why's that? You can chalk it up to good old-fashioned evolutionary male rivalry. When you see someone else getting it on, your innate sense of male competitiveness kicks in ("Hey, I can do that too, and I can do it better!") and your body revs up to produce superior sperm ("I'll show him!").

Orgasm

"Does my having an orgasm increase our changes of conception?"

It's no secret that for conception to have a shot (so to speak), the male partner has to reach orgasm – ejaculating, so that sperm-loaded semen can be

Winter, Spring, Summer, or Autumn

Flipping through the calendar, trying to figure out when to start pencilling in baby making? According to researchers, conception may be more seasonal than you'd think. With birthrates peaking in the summer and autumn (and counting 9 months back), they speculate that the best time to conceive is from October through to March – slow season on the beach, high season in bed. And there are more seasonal data you may want to factor in if you're thinking blue: More boys are conceived in October, researchers say, when there are 12 hours of daylight and an average outdoor temperature of 12°C. The possible explanation? An October conception results in an early summer birth instead of a harsh winter one – a good thing for boys, who tend to be less hardy at birth. Pining for pink? Girls are most often conceived in April, and born in the winter (the girls, it seems, can handle the chill better than the guys can).

The season you're less likely to conceive during, according to these studies? Early autumn. Just don't tell that to all the people whose birthdays are in late spring.

released and sent on its way. No male orgasm, no baby. But female orgasm, it appears, is optional. In other words, you don't have to climax to conceive.

Still, some experts maintain there's more to female orgasm than a good time. Here's why: When you have an orgasm, your uterus contracts, and these contractions may allow the cervix to dip into the semen pool to "suck up" more sperm. And once those sperm are in the uterus, the small contractions from a female orgasm can help move sperm toward the fallopian tubes. All these theoretical benefits are, of course, contingent on both of you climaxing at the same time (or relatively close in time).

So if you enjoy a good climax (and who doesn't?), go for it – that's at least half the fun of baby dancing. But don't get yourself all worked up trying to get all worked up in the name of conception (it'll probably only result in your missing the mark, anyway). And don't sweat it if you don't get it. Though sperm always appreciate a helping hand – or a little push from those uterine contractions – they can also swim exceptionally well on their own.

Frequency of Sex

"I've heard conflicting advice on how often to have sex when I'm ovulating. Every day? Every other day? Twice a day? Which is it?"

For men with a normal sperm count, more – the latest evidence seems to indicate – is more. If that description fits your guy (or you have no reason to believe it doesn't), once-a-day sex

Like What You See?

Is your mate looking extra, well, mate-able to you lately? Strange as it sounds, a woman's facial features are at their most attractive just as her ovary gets ready to drop its egg delivery. This monthly makeover (which is pretty subtle, yet scientifically identified by researchers) makes her more desirable to her partner – so that the couple's more likely to partner up for baby making.

during your fertile period is optimal for conception. For men with a low or marginal sperm count, however, sex every other day is probably best because it allows the troops to build up again in between deployments.

As for even more, that seems to be less. Making love more than once a day will not only wear out your man (and you, too, most likely), but it might actually decrease your chances of getting pregnant. That's because a guy needs time to regenerate his boys, and if he ejaculates more than once a day, he'll be doing so with depleted

The Smell of Love

Smell something? Smell everything? A baby – or at least an opportunity to make a baby – may be in the air. Your sense of smell, like your other senses, becomes heightened when you're in egg-release mode – thanks to stepped-up hormone production, particularly of oestrogen. You'll wake up and smell the coffee more keenly, the aftershave of a guy passing you on the street, the flowers in your boss's office, the hamburgers cooking two doors down. But what your nose knows also apparently allows you to sniff out a smell that no one else can: the musky pheromones of your male partner. This sensory response is instinctual and isn't something you're conscious of (so you won't be literally sniffing around your partner's armpits, which could be embarrassing in public). But before you know what hit you (the pheromones), your nose will lead you to your mate – and lead you both into the bedroom for a little baby making. Sweet!

sperm – which means those encore performances won't be packed, and they could be wasted.

Time of Day

"Is it better to make love in the morning if we're trying to conceive?"

Believe it or not, some research has shown that sperm levels are higher in the morning than later in the day. It could be related to your man's cooler testicles (body temperature is at its lowest after sleep, which explains why you take your BBT immediately upon waking), and you already know that cooler testicles make for happier – and more plentiful – sperm. What's more, a guy's hormones peak in the morning (and that may explain why he often wakes up with an erection). Which means that making hay when the rooster crows may possibly help you fill your coop faster.

Not a morning person – or just can't fit sex into the stressful get-to-work rush? Don't let the clock stop you from making love at a more convenient – or appealing – time. Sperm concentration may be higher in the A.M. (or may not be, since other evidence suggests it might be higher in the P.M., specifically during the 3 P.M. to 7 P.M. block) – but there are still plenty of sperm hanging around after hours, and definitely enough to get the job done 24/7. Besides, the best time to make a baby is when you're relaxed, ready to roll, and thoroughly in the mood – not when researchers say it's time to do it.

Oral Sex

"I heard saliva kills sperm. Is oral sex okay while TTC?"

You'd think that bodily fluids would all just get along – but it's true, saliva

Is Underwater Sex All Wet?

You already know that hanging around in hot tubs can land a guy in hot water, at least as far as his fertility is concerned. But did you know that underwater romance can also undermine your chances of conceiving – no matter what the water temperature? If you're fooling around in a pool, the chlorine can alter the pH in the vagina, making it extra inhospitable to sperm. But even plain water, the kind you'll be splashing in if you're doing it in the bathtub, can water down the cervical mucus that your partner's sperm count on as they try to hitch that ride to your waiting egg. For best results, save the water play for foreplay – and do your actual lovemaking on dry ground.

is a sperm killer. Which means that you'll probably want to limit the amount of saliva deposited in or near the vagina when you're trying to conceive (and that you'll definitely want to skip the saliva when you're looking for lubrication). But that doesn't mean oral sex is off the table (or the bed) for now. If you enjoy it, go for it – or tell your partner to go for it. Just keep the slobbering to a minimum. And don't worry about saliva you deposit on his penis when you offer him oral – there probably won't be enough left by the time he ejaculates inside you to hurt the sperm.

Vibrators

"Can using a vibrator hurt the chances of conception?"

Your good vibrations can continue even when you're trying for a baby. Having a good time with sex toys of any kind won't keep you from getting pregnant – and in fact, if a session with a vibrator puts you in the mood for the real thing, it can actually help you get pregnant, at least indirectly. As always, just practise proper sex-toy hygiene (clean them with soap and water after use, don't share them with others, and so on).

Douching

"Is it okay to keep douching while I'm trying to get pregnant?"

In trying to tidy up down there, you can actually mess up your fertility plans. The truth is, your body knows

Gee, You Smell Nice

The smell of love works both ways, it seems. Just as a woman can sniff out her mate's natural sexual scent, pheromones, when ovulation perks up her sense of smell – guys are more likely to respond sexually to a woman who smells like she's about to ovulate (Eau d'Egg?). Though you won't be aware that your partner smells differently or conscious of this animal-like response to her scent (you'll just know that you feel more like an animal) any more than she'll be aware of the pheromones that are attracting her to you, these subtle signals are among the many that nature transmits when the Egg Train is getting ready to pull out of the station (so your sperm can get ready to hop on board).

Dressing for Fertility Success

Looking for another sign that you're fertile? Take a look in the mirror. Researchers have found that women tend to dress (and primp) to impress when they're ovulating. This is probably nature's way of making sure you – like all the other females in the animal kingdom – attract your mate's attention and are more likely to mate (and make a baby). So next time you find yourself unexpectedly reaching for the tight red sweater with the plunging v-neck, or the stilettos that make your hubby weak in the knees – or if you're suddenly taking more pains with the blow dryer and painting on extra lipstick and eye shadow – consider that it might be just the time of the month to rip those clothes off, rumple your hair, and smudge your makeup.

how to clean itself naturally, and douching can upset the balance of good bacteria in your vagina, possibly setting you up for infections. But that's not the downside to douching when you're trying to conceive (though an infection isn't exactly an upside, especially when lots of sex is on the schedule). The drawback conception-wise is that douching can wash away that very important (and fertility-aiding) cervical mucus – something the sperm will miss, even if you don't know it's gone. Douching can also change the pH in the vagina, making it even less hospitable to sperm. What's more, if you douche after sex, you can be washing away the sperm – and washing away your odds of conceiving. And if that's not enough reason, women who douche regularly are at higher risk of developing pelvic inflammatory disease (PID), a leading cause of infertility.

The same drawbacks may apply to homemade douches designed for sex selection (they haven't been proven to work, anyway) or so-called natural douches. So bag the douching (and keep it bagged for good while you're at it).

Love that fresh feeling? Take a shower or bath – but skip the feminine hygiene sprays and wipes. These, too, can compromise your conception chances.

Action Plan

So what's the plan when you're looking for baby-making action? Here's a recap: Sex every day, man on top, on dry land, in the morning, stay put for 20 minutes, no lubricants or douching, simultaneous climaxes. Got it? Good. Now forget it. Though all these game plans may boost your chances of scoring that baby, they don't make it a slam dunk. You can do everything according to plan and not get pregnant. Or you can break all the make-a-baby rules (you have sex when you feel like it, how you feel like it) and still end up making a baby. So bottom line: Go for your bottom lines. Follow the how-tos if you want to; skip them if you don't. Approach procreational sex any which way that feels right for you, both physically and emotionally. Just do it!

Staying Connected While You're Making a Baby

Trying for a baby can be fun, it can be exciting – but it can also be trying. Though all those baby-making efforts may bring you and your partner together physically more often than ever, the emotional connection can sometimes take a hit in the process. But you can nurture your twosome even as you strive to become a threesome – and even fire up some of the romance that charts, ovulation predictor kits, and sex-on-demand may have left out in the cold. Just add a little TLC to your TTC.

Your Relationship

"We're so focused on trying to conceive that I'm afraid our relationship isn't what it used to be."

When you're baby making on all cylinders, it's understandable that you've both got less energy – and time – to put into romance. And while you're almost certainly having a lot of sex while you're trying to conceive, it's easy to lose sight of the other kind of intimacy that's needed to maintain a healthy twosome – the emotional kind.

But now, when you're striving to form that most perfect union (of sperm and egg), it's more important than ever to pay attention to the other significant union in your life – the one with your partner. These tips will keep your relationship on track – even when you're tracking your monthly cycle, tracking your BBT, tracking your cervical mucus, and tracking your sex life.

Is Her Stress Stressing You Out?

Planning a baby is exciting stuff – especially if it's a life event that you've looked forward to your whole lives. But it can also be stressful, particularly when it starts becoming an effort. Between the temperature taking, kits, and charts – and the monthly sex marathon that can make one of your favourite activities feel like a drag – it's no wonder anxiety is in the air. Though both of you are equally invested in baby making, it's often the woman who becomes a little (or sometimes a lot) more hyper about it. Females tend to excel at micromanaging, as you might have noticed, and sometimes to a fault. If your partner is driving you both a tad crazy these days – and is running Operation Conceive with more flowcharts than you've ever seen in a conference room and more preci-

sion than a military mission – maybe it's time for an intervention. Try explaining that though you both want this baby very much – and how, of course, you're willing to give this team effort your best efforts – the stress isn't good for either of you or for your fertility chances. And while all of those tools of the modern conception age may help you achieve your most adorable of goals, making them the focus of your daily lives – not to mention the ruler of your sex lives – can step up the stress unnecessarily (which can actually get in the way of that goal). For best results, suggest you both jump off that baby-planning roller coaster every now and again, and take a moment (or two or three) to appreciate each other – and the amazing ride that's about to begin.

Date Your Wife

Thought your dating days were over? You may want to think again. Dating your partner regularly is one of the best ways to make sure you stay partners for life – plus, it can help strengthen your twosome as it weathers the emotional (and physical) challenges of trying to become a threesome. A little rusty on the whole courtship thing? Here's a refresher course on romance:

Surprise her. Most women find surprises pleasant – and romantic. And if your partner has come not to expect any surprises, she'll be even more pleasantly surprised when you spring one on her – whether it's a bouquet of flowers or a reservation at her favourite restaurant or just a hand-drawn love note taped on the bathroom mirror (or tucked into her handbag, for her to discover later). An occasional surprise will keep her guessing – and keep her loving you more than ever. A little spontaneity will also be a welcome change of pace from all the scheduling you two have likely been doing lately – and that can quickly make even the most passionate relationship feel routine.

Notice her. When sex becomes procreational instead of recreational, it's easy for the mechanics to become the focus, for romance to leave the building (and the bedroom) – and for both of you to start taking each other for granted. So stop and smell her perfume. Take a second look when she curls her hair (and even when she doesn't have the time). Tell her how much you appreciate the view when she bends over to retrieve the keys she dropped. When you're having another session of scheduled sex, let her know how much you love her as your lover (and not just as the woman who you're making a mother,

and who's making you a father). Woo her as you do her (for the fifth time this week).

Date her. Re-create those early days of courtship (only this time you don't have to stress over that first kiss). Meet her for a latte at the coffee bar you two always sipped at after the movies. Make a reservation at the restaurant you lingered at over your first dinner – and impress her by remembering what she ordered (and if your memory's really good, what she was wearing). Take a drive to see the foliage, like you did that first autumn – and don't forget the picnic lunch. Hold hands at the movies, when you're out shopping – and whenever her hand is handy. Just because you've moved on to bigger and better things doesn't mean you can't go back to basics (which, by rekindling the romance in your relationship, may actually help heat up those bigger and better things).

Treat her. You already have her love, so you don't have to buy it. But that doesn't mean you can't occasionally do a little relationship reinvestment. Celebrate your baby-making adventure with a commemorative bracelet or necklace (one that you can add charms onto as you fill your nest). Or with a scrapbook that you can fill together with the memories you'll be making as you make a baby (ending, soon, with that positive pregnancy test!). Buy her a teddy bear that can one day reside in baby's room. And don't forget that some of the best treats don't cost a thing besides a little effort: Bring her breakfast in bed (or a bowl of ice cream with two spoons for an after-baby-dance nibble). Offer her a foot massage, complete with scented lotions. Or a neck rub while you watch TV.

Stay connected. Sure, your bodies may be connected now (as when the OPK says all systems go), but how about your minds? With all the sex you're having, don't forget about the other kind of intercourse – the talking kind. Stick around for some pillow talk after the baby dance. Snuggle on the sofa when sex isn't scheduled (and the TV isn't on), and share what's on your minds. Take a walk for the exercise, but also for the chance to talk, without interruptions. Your mate is the one person in the world who not only knows you best, but knows best what you're going through – because you're going through it together. And don't always stick with the baby talk. Healthy relationships are multidimensional – just like both of you are.

Get out of the bedroom. Maybe you haven't spent so much time in the bedroom since your honeymoon – but even back then you probably took a break in the action every once in a while and ventured out for a swim or a bike ride or a meal. So for a change of pace, schedule something else to do together besides sex – and rediscover the other side of romance. Splurge on a couples massage. Head out for a romantic dinner – or cook one together, and enjoy it with a side of mood music and without the TV. Take a nightly stroll around the neighbourhood at dusk. Plan a weekly movie night, complete with popcorn. Make a date for a game of miniature golf or bowling – or something else you can't help but have fun doing together (like paddleboating or ice-skating).

Get out of town. Treat yourselves to a prebaby holiday (once your conception mission is accomplished, travelling won't be quite as carefree). A week at a beach isn't feasible or financially possible? A night in a local hotel (with room service) can also take you away from all that baby-making stress – even if you'll be baby making during your stay – and remind you both why you're a couple in the first place. That's not in the (credit) cards, either? Improvise economically by staging a romantic stay-at-home weekend.

Take time away . . . alone. It seems counterintuitive, but it's true: Time apart can bring your twosome closer together. You both need time away to recharge and refresh – and to nurture yourselves. Take a Saturday afternoon break for a mani/pedi while your partner hangs out with his pals and watches the game. Catch a chick flick with your girlfriends while he sees the action movie you'd just as soon skip. Hit the gym while he takes a run. You'll find a little "me" time can make the "us" time even more satisfying.

Have a laugh. Making a baby is serious business – sometimes too serious. So loosen up a little. Rent that comedy that was too dumb to pay to see in a cinema – but is just dumb enough to keep you both rolling off the sofa at home. Play a silly board game that's sure to get you giggling (one where drawing is involved always gets a good laugh going). Challenge each other to a round of bad jokes – or watch some crazy YouTube videos together. And whenever you can, see the humour in the TTC process (there's plenty if you look objectively – like those comical mad dashes to the bedroom) and get a good laugh over it. Laughter isn't only the best medicine for your relationship, it's also one of the best ways to relax, which means it may help you with your baby-making efforts, too.

Making that love connection stronger isn't just important as you try to make a baby, it'll be important once

TTC Stress Cycle

Have you got yourself stuck in the TTC stress cycle? You chart, you baby dance, you wait, you test, and you stress. And you stress a little more each month your baby-making efforts end in a period instead of a positive pregnancy test. And then, if that's not stressful enough, you start stressing about whether all the stress over conceiving is making it even harder to conceive.

Many TTC mums who've been at it a while find themselves caught in the same stress cycle, and it's not surprising. After all, deciding to make a baby is exciting, but actually getting that baby on board, especially if the boarding process takes more than a few months, can be, well, stressful.

Though normal amounts of stress don't typically affect fertility, it makes sense to try to break the stress cycle before it starts spinning out of control (and increasing your stress to the kinds of excessive levels that may be implicated in lowered conception rates). For relaxation tips, see page 25.

that baby has arrived, too – and maybe more so. Remember, even when you're a couple of parents, you'll still be a couple.

Sex on Demand

"Sex seems like so much of a chore these days. How can we make it more fun?"

Take this little quiz: Which scenario best describes your love life these days?

A. Candlelight, back rubs, whispers of sweet nothings, leisurely foreplay, satisfying mutual climax.

B. Pee on a stick, shrieks of "it's time", missionary position with shirts still on, wham, bam, thank you ma'am, drive-through deposit made in under 3 minutes.

If you answered "B", chances are you've stumbled – or fallen head first – into the sex-on-demand rut that many hopeful parents-to-be find themselves stuck in when sex becomes a means toward an end (a baby) instead of a means toward a "happy ending". All work and no play makes any sexual relationship – even one that used to be all fun, all the time – dull. Yet it's not surprising that sex these days is more about getting it done than getting it on. After all, how sexy is temperature charting? How mood making is a beeping ovulation monitor? And who can get worked up over watching a fertility watch?

The good news is that trying to score (a baby) doesn't have to feel like a chore – even when OPKs line the bathroom counter and you're stretching cervical mucus between your fingertips. Here's how to keep the sparks flying even as you try to put a bun in the oven:

Get him thinking (of you). Leave love notes on his pillow or hide them in places he'll find throughout the day – in his car, his laptop, in his underwear drawer. Write him suggestive text messages or e-mail him alluring pictures on his mobile to whet his appetite for tonight's special (you). Tell him what you'll be wearing, and what you won't be wearing. Tell him what you'll be doing to him, and what you'll want him to do to you. Anticipation always adds sexual tension (the good kind of tension) to a lovemaking session – even if it's a fully scheduled one. And if you've never

You're Up ... Again

Feeling a little like a performing chimp lately (or maybe like a performing Chippendale?) That's not surprising if you've been TTC. After all, while the logistics of planning those baby-making sex sessions to coordinate with ovulation may be your partner's department, the sole responsibility for getting the deed done falls on your shoulders (or, let's just say, on another part of your body). Even if you're performing your favourite activity ever, being asked to perform it at a moment's notice, at inconvenient times (half an hour before you have to be at work), after an extra long day, and when you're not even remotely in the mood – can be a drag, and sometimes a stressful drag, one that can even make performance elusive.

You're not alone. Just about every dad who's in the thick of TTC experiences performance anxiety – or performance dread – at some point, and that's nothing if not understandable.

You're only human (as opposed to the studs in the rest of the animal kingdom, who don't give performance a second thought). But that doesn't mean you have to keep your feelings to yourself – and in fact, you shouldn't. Let your partner know that the sex scheduling is getting you down – and maybe, keeping you down when you'd rather not be. Suggest that you try adding a little spice to the sex-on-demand schedule, even if spontaneity isn't practical. You'll see plenty of tips on how to keep TTC sex exciting – and fun – on these pages. Thinking of giving that little blue pill a try, to give you a little extra boost on those down days? Ask your doctor for the lowdown on using Viagra when you're TTC.

Not having a hard time, so to speak, with all the sexual demands being placed on you these days (and nights)? Having the time of your life, actually? That's normal, too. So just sit back – or lie back – and enjoy the show.

tried naughty on for size, don't knock it until you've tried it.

Rev up the romance. You know the drill, but it's probably been a while since you practised those romantic moves that used to be lovemaking business as usual. Take a bath together, light scented candles, bring out the massage oil, play some soft music, dip some strawberries in chocolate (oh heck, just dip each other in chocolate) . . . you get the picture.

Turn up the heat. Debut a new piece of sexy lingerie each month. Play strip poker or nude Twister or an R18-rated board game. Pop in an erotic movie or unveil a sex toy. Bring on the whipped cream for a different kind of dessert. Get

kinky to your comfort level, of course, but if there were ever a time to push the sexual envelope, now would be it.

Don't just do it. Yes, you're goal orientated these days. But you can reach that goal and still have fun along the way. So don't just do it – take your time doing it (time permitting). Serve up some foreplay appetizers before you dive into the main course. Try for a slow build to increase tension and make the ultimate climax more explosive. Mind you, sometimes a quickie can be just as explosive – especially if plenty of clothes ripping is involved – and on a particularly busy day may be the only way to get the job done (you have 15 minutes to do it, change, and get to a client dinner). Just

TTC: To Tell or Not to Tell

Hoping to start a family soon, or add to it – but not quite sure when (or whether) to alert the media (as in, the mother and mother-in-law)? Do you tell as soon as you begin making the plans? Wait until your efforts are fully under way? Or keep your mission a secret until it's a mission accomplished?

If you're already being bombarded with questions about that baby-making barometer – at each and every family gathering, not to mention on each and every call from the parents (and your sister, and your great-aunt, and your friends) – then you may be tempted to tell all about your plans, just to get everyone (and your mother) off your back. You may be inclined to share the news, also, if you're feeling like you need a little TTC support or cheerleading – or if you're just too excited to stay mum about your plans to become a mum (and a dad).

You might want to think it through before you spill the TTC beans too soon. That cheerleading squad may be nice – as can having mum on speed dial when you need a preconception pep talk – but will you really want to deal with that monthly deluge of questions from friends and family? And all that advice? Those comments you could definitely do without ("you're just trying too hard" or "you're not getting any younger!")? The added pressure of offering up pregnancy test results to a long list of well-wishers anxious to hear the monthly update?

Don't feel obliged to tell if you're afraid that spilling those beans will open up too many cans of worms. In the meantime, try to field those inevitable questions about your future plans to start your family with a sense of humour. "You'll be the first to know" is sure to get you off the hook (who can argue with that?).

On the other hand, if you decide you're happy to make the whole gang part of your pregnancy planning, go right ahead – after all, you know yourself and your family better than anyone. And if the barrage of unsolicited advice you'll inevitably receive on how to become pregnant makes you second-guess your decision, you may want to arm yourself with this one-size-fits-all comeback: "Thanks, but we actually know how to make a baby."

---

try, as you go about reaching that all-important goal you're so understandably focused on, not to forget the other goal in all this: mutually satisfying sex and intimacy.

Change the scenery. You've likely been spending a whole lot of time in bed these days. But guess what – babies can be made in other locales, too. In a car. On the kitchen table. Even in the laundry room (talk about a spin cycle). And don't just assume your positions, either, without some thought to the pleasure component. Nothing says rut like the same-old, same-old – so spice things up with a brand-new *Cosmo*-worthy move or two. (And if you're concerned that pretzel positions won't get the baby-making job done as efficiently, start off with the creative stuff, then finish off in a more conception-friendly pose; see page 102.)

Talk him up. So you, at times, may be feeling like a sperm receptacle, which is understandable. But keep in mind that he may be feeling like nothing more than a sperm provider, which is also understandable. Remember, too, that he's the one who's under all that performance pressure, to rise to the occasion at the beep of a fertility monitor. So make sure you let him know how much you love him and appreciate him (and find him studlike when he's not performing those services, also), even as you're asking him to hop-to and hop into bed for yet another round of fertilize-my-egg.

Get physical. Even when it's not ovulation time, stay in tune by touching each other often, swooping down for unexpected kisses, catching each other for hugs, cuddling whenever you can, and yes – making love at other times of the month, too . . . just for the fun of it.

Take a break. Not from the pleasures of lovemaking, but from the stress of baby making. Remember that sex isn't only about getting pregnant (though it may seem that way these days) – there's also an important emotional connec-tion that's involved, one that often gets neglected when the mechanics of conception get in the way. If you're finding the CM stretching and BBT charting is taking its toll on your relationship (and on your quality of life), ditch it and let nature take its course. Not only can taking a break from all those gadgets and charts help you reconnect as a couple, but it can help you relax about conceiving (and remember, the more relaxed you are about it, the more likely it is to happen).

Consider this: Studies show that the average unstressed couple has sex 2 to 3 times per week. If you're on that type of schedule, chances are nature will work pretty well on its own and you'll likely get pregnant within 6 to 12 months (and maybe a whole lot sooner) even without "working" at it. So take a break from TTC, and who knows – you might find you've conceived without even trying!

Making a Baby with CAM

There's nothing more natural than making a baby – so what could be a more natural way to boost your fertility than tapping into the CAM camp? Complementary and alternative therapies – from acupuncture to hypnosis to herbal medicine – are being used more and more often to give Mother Nature (and sometimes medical science) a needed nudge. Whether that nudge works or not hasn't been demonstrated consistently through research, and a lot more research will have to be done before any conclusions can be made. Still, here's what's known so far about so-called natural fertility boosters.

CAM for Fertility

"My friend says using acupuncture helped her conceive when she was undergoing IVF. Is there any truth to that?"

Can a little bit of CAM go a long way in your fertility quest? It's possible. Though the modern study of these therapies – which are rooted in ancient practices – is still in its infancy, more and more research seems to be showing that they do have applications to successful baby making. And though the jury's still out, adding acupuncture

CAM for Men

CAM isn't just for women looking to get a leg up on fertility. Acupuncture appears to reduce the number of abnormal sperm and increase the number of healthy sperm in men with a low sperm count. It can also be used to pump up blood flow, which may definitely help pump up something else. Mind-body strategies, including hypnosis, massage, relaxation, yoga, and visualization, can reduce stress and promote healthy blood flow – important components of a healthy libido, which in turn is an important component of making a baby.

and/or other mind-body techniques to infertility treatments may, some studies suggest, increase your chances of getting pregnant. By extension, it's speculated, such therapies may also help speed the conception process in a woman without known fertility issues.

This may be news to practitioners of traditional Western medicine, who've scoffed at such once-fringe therapies, but CAM experts aren't surprised at all. Long respected in Eastern medicine, alternative treatments have gained increasing popularity in the West for a variety of illnesses and conditions. More and more often, these treatments are being integrated into traditional medical care, in the form of CAM.

East is meeting West, as well, when it comes to fertility – and the preliminary feedback has been promising. A few published studies have shown that acupuncture may help a variety of fertility issues at almost every age and promotes reproductive health in general (though, again, there's no scientific consensus on how much – or even whether – acupuncture really helps). Acupuncturists contend that the technique increases nerve stimulation and blood flow to the ovaries and uterus, improving reproductive function. What's more, acupuncture may increase the production of feel-good endorphins that also play a role in regulating your menstrual cycle and, therefore, your fertility. Acupuncture may bust stress, too, which can interfere with fertility.

Some evidence indicates that chiropractic techniques, too, can help the fertility cause in certain women. Chiropractors hold that if the nerves going to your reproductive organs are impaired, fertility can be impaired as well. Manipulation of the spinal column and nerves to those areas may restore balance, and possibly with it, fertility.

Hypnosis and hypnotherapy may also boost fertility, particularly in cases when the mind (often a stressed one) is interfering with the body's normal reproductive functions. Some CAM practitioners say that the reduction in stress and the relaxing benefit of hypnosis can even aid in embryo implantation, resulting in an increased rate of pregnancies among women who practiced hypnosis while undergoing fertility treatments. A few less obvious examples of mind-body techniques are proving to be effective as well. For example, emotionally connecting with others is a powerful component when it comes to getting pregnant, and researchers have found an increase in pregnancy rates for infertile women who take part in support groups (another reason to check out those TTC boards). Other mind-body strategies include diet changes, movement, relaxation, yoga, and visualization.

It's as yet unclear if these documented fertility improvements are the result of the actual CAM technique being used or the result of a placebo effect (and if they work, does it really matter why?).

Cough It Up to Some Medicine

Could cough syrup actually be good medicine for fertility? While no scientific studies have backed up (or hacked up) the anecdotal evidence, some women aren't sneezing at it. Here's how an expectorant can theoretically help you expect:

The active ingredient in cough medicines like Lemsip Cough Chesty is guaifenesin, a substance that helps thin the mucus in your lungs – helping to decrease coughing. But it doesn't differentiate between the mucus in one part of your body (in your lungs) and another. Which means that guaifenesin also thins cervical mucus, possibly allowing sperm to move through it faster and better, and potentially making it easier to hit their target on time.

Willing to do your own clinical trial? Take 1 to 2 teaspoons of cough syrup once a day beginning a few days before ovulation. One major caveat: Read labels carefully before purchasing your cough syrup or before pulling it out of your medicine cabinet. Not all cough medicines are alike – and some contain antihistamines, which can actually have an anti-fertility effect by drying up that sperm-friendly mucus.

Still, most experts agree that as long as the CAM techniques do no harm, there's no harm in trying them – and there could be many benefits, especially if the therapies make you feel less stressed and more empowered. If you do decide to incorporate these and other alternative techniques in your baby-making mission, take the safe route. First, make sure any CAM practitioner you engage is qualified and experienced and specializes in women's health and fertility. You can visit the British Acupuncture Council (www.acupuncture.org.uk) to find an acupuncturist in your area. Other resources include the NHS Directory of Complementary and Alternative Practitioners (www.nhsdirectory.org), the British Holistic Medical Association (www.bhma.org) and the Institute for Complementary and Natural Medicine (www.i-c-m.org.uk).

Second, be sure to remember the "C" in CAM – complementary. For CAM to be a valuable part of any medical care, it needs to be integrated into your traditional care. So let your traditional doctor know about any CAM techniques you might be using or considering because some therapies could interact with each other (and not in a good way), making your goal of conception more elusive. And if you're having fertility issues, don't rely on CAM alone to find your way out of them – also seek the help of a doctor who can diagnose and treat any reproductive problem.

Mind Over Matter

"I've heard that it's possible to boost fertility just by thinking positive. Is there any truth to that?"

The power of positive thinking may be more powerful than you think when it comes to fertility. It's true – your ability to conceive could actually be impacted by your thoughts and feelings. Not directly, of course (as in "if I just wish it hard enough, I'll get pregnant"), but indirectly. It is now becoming more recognized that physical health (including your reproductive health) is related

Say Good-Bye to Your Tighty Whities

Hey guys: Looking for another way to enhance your fertility? It could be as simple as raiding your underwear drawer. Though scientists have yet to rule definitively on the boxers versus briefs debate, it can't hurt to push those tighty whities (and those lycra shorts you work out in) to the back of the closet for the TTC duration to give those vital testes some breathing room and a cooler environment in which to hang out.

to emotional health. A negative state of mind (as is common with excessive stress, depression, and pessimism) can have a negative effect on hormone levels and fertility. Experts well versed in this mind-body theory suggest that you can boost your fertility by boosting your emotional well-being (and you may benefit from an emotional boost even if your fertility issues have a clearly physical cause – in fact, it may make other forms of treatment more effective). Managing stress, depression, anxiety, and other emotional challenges through yoga, meditation, acupuncture, visualization, and relaxation exercises, according to these researchers, may indeed help give your fertility a boost – and bring you one step closer to the baby you're hoping for.

As powerful as positive thinking can be, it's also important to be mindful of the mind's limitations. If stress is interfering with your fertility, thinking happy baby thoughts may be just what the doctor ordered – without the doctor. But if it's another fertility issue that's standing between you and conception, seeking medical help – while continuing

to think those happy baby thoughts – is always a smart strategy. For more on the stress–conception connection and stress relief, see page 24.

Herbs and Fertility

"I take herbs daily, just for overall health. Are any unsafe now that I'm trying to conceive? And are there any herbs I can take to increase my chances of getting pregnant?"

That depends on who you listen to. According to some holistic practitioners, certain herbs can give your reproductive efforts an edge. For example, black cohosh is touted as a way to establish regular ovulation. Siberian ginseng and dong quai are said to help regulate the menstrual cycle. Chaste tree berry is said to stimulate the release of LH and regulates the levels of progesterone and oestrogen. Red clover blossom is rich in oestrogen-like isoflavones and might be helpful in regulating hormones. Fish oil (or other omega-3 supplements) is said to boost your fertility and your mood (and an emotional lift may further boost fertility).

Sounds promising, huh? The only problem is, when it comes to most herbal supplements, it's hard to know how effective, or how safe, they are – especially when it comes to fertility. Some supplements – that echinacea you pop to ward off a winter cold, or the gingko biloba you swallow to give your brain a boost, or that St. John's wort you take to turn your frown upside down, among many others – may interfere with conception in both hopeful mums and hopeful dads. Others may be dangerous to your pregnancy if you do conceive (and that includes some of the so-called conception-promoting herbs).

So before you buy out the supplement section of your local health food market or stock up online – or continue taking supplements you've been taking for years – think twice, once for you and once for your baby-to-be. Here's why: First, herbal supplements are not evaluated, so the safety and risks associated with them are, for the most part, unknown. Second, no regulations govern the manufacturing and selling of herbal products, so there's no way of knowing whether you're actually getting what you think you're getting – or what you're paying top dollar for (though products from Germany, where regulations are tighter, may be more reliable). Finally, there's still a significant shortage of clinical studies on these supplements – especially when it comes to reproductive matters. Even the few that seem promising are still preliminary. Which means that in the case of many herbs, it's not clear whether they help with fertility or compromise fertility. Further complicating the supplement equation: If you're TTC, there's always the possibility that you've succeeded – and no

large reliable studies have been done on pregnant women to assess the effect of herbals on developing babies.

The bottom line when you're trying to create that very cute bottom line: Though herbs are natural, natural doesn't always mean safe. As with any medicine, herbs should be taken only under the supervision of your doctor and/or an alternative medicine practitioner who knows you're trying to become pregnant. Not only to find out if they're safe, but also because some herbals may interfere with other medications or fertility boosters (or treatments) you're currently using. Also keep in mind that herbs can react very differently in different people, so even though your sister-in-law swears her herbal concoction got her pregnant, it might not offer you the same happy result. So ask before you pop. And until more is known, you'll probably want to be cautious with supplements – just to stay on the safe side.

One CAM supplement – albeit not technically a herbal – you can feel good

Can Popping Make You a Pop?

It seems as if everyone's hopping on the supplement bandwagon these days – including those who are hoping that hopping will help make them a pop. But what can herbals and other supplements really do for your fertility? That scientific debate (like most scientific debates) is still ongoing. A small study showed that Pycnogenol can boost male fertility. L-carnitine and arginine are said to promote good sperm motility and sperm count. Ginseng is a classic Chinese aphrodisiac and, according to classic Chinese medicine practitioners, also a fertility booster, upping testosterone levels and increasing sperm count.

Astragalus may increase sperm motility, and lycopene may increase sperm count.

On the fertility flip side, however, large amounts of St. John's wort can negatively affect the genetic makeup of sperm, echinacea can change the composition of the sperm head (making it less able to penetrate an egg), and ginkgo biloba can have a detrimental effect on sperm health. Ditto, possibly, for other herbs. Which means that before you pop a supplement, ask your doctor (one who knows you're trying to get your significant other pregnant) whether it's safe and what the risks may be.

Baby Help from a Box?

Been trying for a few months to hit baby bingo, but without success? Remember that the average couple conceives within 6 to 12 months. If you're not a very patient waiter – but you're still nowhere near ready to head down the fertility treatment route, there may be a happy compromise in a box. On the market in the US (it is available online) is a kit that claims it can help bring you one step closer to a baby without going that extra mile to the fertility specialist's office.

The product premise is pretty basic: If you concentrate your partner's sperm pool and deposit it closer to your cervix, there's a greater chance you'll conceive. Here's how it works: The kit contains a nonlatex condom (one that doesn't contain spermicide, for obvious reasons) that's used to collect semen from an ejaculation (during intercourse) and a cervical cap into which the collected semen is transferred. The cervical cap is then placed into the vagina and onto the cervix for 6 to 8 hours – allowing the sperm to bypass the vagina and head right into the cervix sooner and in a more concentrated form. Which isn't easier than it sounds – getting that cervical cap into position without spilling those seeds can be tricky, especially if the silliness factor of the process has given you the giggles.

The kit isn't cheap, and though there's no harm in using it, it's probably not necessary for most fertile couples, who can conceive the time-honoured way (though it can definitely give you something entertaining to do while you're waiting for nature to take its course). It also isn't helpful for couples who have more complex fertility challenges. Those with the most potentially to gain from spoon-feeding sperm into the cervix would be those who are dealing with a diagnosed low sperm count, since it gets the boys closer to where they need to go.

about taking: omega-3s. Whether these phenomenal fatty acids can boost your fertility is still open to debate (and further scientific investigation), but there is evidence they can lift your mood – a lift that may give your fertility a leg up after all.

Making a Baby Boy – or a Baby Girl

These days, not only are some couples trying to pick the perfect time to conceive a baby (after I get a raise . . . so that the baby's born in the spring . . . once we're able to afford a bigger home), they're also trying to select the baby's sex – or, at least, to influence those time-honoured odds of 50-50 in the favour of their preferred gender. But can gender selection methods deliver the bundle of pink (or blue) that you've been dreaming of? Maybe . . . but probably not. Still, in most cases there's no harm in giving them a shot – as long as you don't count on the results, and just have fun trying.

Choosing the Baby's Gender

"Is it possible to choose the sex of my baby? We already have two boys and we'd love a baby girl."

Thinking pink? Eat lots of veggies and pile on the chocolate (and perhaps the pounds?). Make sure the moon is full when you conceive and take the sexual lead. Have sex only on a certain day of the month based on calculations involving the calendar and your birthday. Rooting for the blue team? Have sex lying on your right side, be sure there's a quarter moon, and eat lots of red meat.

There's no shortage of far-fetched methods promising to deliver you the baby of your gender dreams – and you can access dozens without consulting a single old wife (the Internet's loaded with them). The only thing is, they work just 50 percent of the time – giving you the same 50-50 odds of having a girl (or a boy) that you'd have if you left the selection of your baby's sex up to nature (and your partner's sperm).

Not thrilled with those odds? Hoping to give sex selection an edge, even if it's just a slight nudge in the direction of your choice? Old wives' tales and Internet legends aside, a number of low-tech techniques claim to up the odds of conceiving one or the other gender, but have no scientific evidence to back up their claims. A few high-tech (and expensive) sex selection methods are more likely to work but involve assisted reproduction, and are consequently not available to every couple.

First, the do-it-yourself techniques. Try these at home, if you're so inclined, keeping in mind that all three recommend completely different approaches, often conflicting – and none has been proven to work the way it claims:

The Shettles Method. This theory holds that the Y-sperm (boys) are faster swimmers yet don't live as long and are not as strong as the X-sperm (girls). Because of the resiliency of X-sperm, female babies are more often conceived in less ideal conditions, such as when there is a lower sperm count or when the sperm are kept waiting a long time for the egg to be released (and only the fittest – and most resilient – still survive when the egg finally shows up). On the other hand, males are more often conceived when conditions for fertilization are ideal because, as the faster swimmers, they will win the race to the finish faster.

To up the odds you'll conceive a girl, according to the Shettles method:

- Have lots of sex starting 3 days before ovulation (more frequent ejaculations means fewer Y-sperm, and the longer sperm wait for the egg, the better the odds that the stronger female sperm will be the last woman standing).

- Use the missionary position.

- Avoid female orgasm, which will only help the weaker male sperm along. (Clearly, this involves some sacrifice on the part of the female partner – how's that for a touch of irony?)

If you're trying for a boy, take the opposite approach:

- Avoid intercourse until the day of ovulation (this way the faster-swimming boy sperm won't be kept waiting for the egg – and will, hopefully, race their way to the finish line faster).

- Achieve female orgasm (to help propel those less hardy boys to the egg and to improve the alkalinity of the vagina).

- Use the rear-entry position.

- Have the male partner drink something caffeinated an hour before sex (to speed up his boy-making boys).

Pick Your Food, Pick Your Baby's Gender?

Can the food you eat affect the gender of your soon-to-be-conceived baby? There's plenty of conjecture (and a fair share of message board rumours) to answer that question. You may have heard, for instance, that eating a diet rich in calcium and magnesium and cutting back on red meat and salty food will increase the odds of conceiving a girl. Or that eating foods rich in sodium and potassium will up your chances of making a boy. Some salt with that banana?

But is there any grain of truth to these theories? That's still unclear. Some scientists theorize that a baby's sex may possibly be linked (somewhat) to mum's diet around the time of conception. One controversial study even suggests that eating your corn flakes (or your Cheerios, or any other cereal) may increase your chances of conceiving a boy. Ditto for a diet high in energy foods (aka high-calorie foods) and in such nutrients as potassium, calcium, and vitamins C, E, and B_{12}.

Does that mean you should switch from yogurt to Special K if you'd especially like a boy (or quit cold cereal cold turkey if it's a girl you're hoping for)? Should you increase your calorie consumption around conception time if your heart's set on a baby boy, or cut back if sugar and spice would be nice? Not so fast. First, it's not smart to increase or decrease your calorie intake when you're trying to conceive (unless your practitioner has advised that you do, to gain or lose weight preconception), or to restrict nutrients by eating only certain foods and avoiding others. Second, this research is definitely not conclusive – and in no way promises that a change in diet can help you choose your baby's sex. In fact, the boy-to-girl proportion of babies born in the overall sample studied by these researchers was 50-50 – pretty much the same as would be expected without any diet modifications. Food for thought, but not necessarily for breakfast.

The Whelan Method. This method contradicts the Shettles method completely (go figure). According to this theory, the closer to ovulation you have sex, the more likely you are to conceive a girl. That's because of certain biochemical changes that could favour Y-sperm the earlier you are in your cycle. Therefore, if you want a boy, have sex 4 to 6 days before ovulation, and if you want a girl, only have sex when you're ovulating.

The O + 12 Method. This method claims to up the chances for conceiving a girl by having sex 12 hours after ovulation (hence the name of the method: ovulation plus 12 hours). Contrary to the Shettles technique, this method requires the father to abstain completely from ejaculation until 8 to 12 hours after ovulation – and then to have sex only once.

Getting a lot more high tech, pricey, and invasive (and leaving it up to the pros) are these options:

The Ericsson Method. This in-the-lab technique separates the faster swimming boy sperm from the slower swimming girl sperm. The method relies on the theory that the faster Y-sperm will be able to swim through a solution and reach the bottom of a test tube faster than the X-sperm, allowing the two types of sperm to be separated. Once the X- and Y-sperm are separated, the desired gender is introduced via intrauterine insemination. There is no guarantee of success (the odds of conceiving the gender of choice using this method range from 50 to 80 percent), and many say this technique has not been shown to work reliably at all.

The Microsort Method. This high-tech (and costly) method also separates the X and Y sperm in the lab. Though not foolproof, the technique seems to work because Y-sperm contain less DNA than X-sperm, making them a bit smaller and lighter, and allowing the male-producers and female-producers to be sorted. It appears to be more successful in producing a girl than a boy.

Preimplantation Genetic Diagnosis (PGD). This procedure, which is also used to screen embryos for genetic defects, is an effective sex selection method – but one that's always reserved for couples who have a medical reason to

choose their baby's sex (when there's a genetic condition that's X-linked recessive, for instance, such as haemophilia or fragile X syndrome, that is inherited by sons, but not daughters). Using embryos conceived in vitro, doctors determine the sex of each, implanting only the embryos with the gender of choice.

Sex Selection Kits

"I already have a girl and would really like a boy. A friend of mine mentioned something about sex selection kits. What's the deal with them?"

You've seen them advertised, you've heard other TTC couples chatting them up, and you've probably wondered: Do these do-it-yourself sex selection kits really work? Do those gender vendors have any scientific leg to stand on – or are they just peddling false hope – at inflated prices – to those thinking pink or blue?

Some kits claim to determine the sex of your already-conceived baby – as early as 5 weeks of gestation – using just a drop of maternal blood to detect the baby's DNA. If you do opt to try one of these kits, keep in mind that the accuracy rate claimed by the manufacturers is questionable (so it's probably not a good idea to base your nursery colour scheme on the results).

Other kits claim to improve your odds of conceiving the gender of your choice by using nutritional supplements that allegedly alter the conditions around the egg and sperm and douches that supposedly make the vaginal tract receptive to one or the other gender-specific sperm. Again, many experts consider these claims to be scientifically suspect, especially since there's a 50 percent chance that you'll get the gender of your choice without doing anything at all.

As always: Buyer beware – or at least be aware.

And They Say Girls Keep You Waiting

Laugh all you want at the irony – but interestingly, the longer it takes you to conceive, the greater your chances that a baby boy will show up. How do researchers explain these late-breaking boys? They speculate that two factors are at play: First, women with thick cervical mucus have a harder time conceiving in general, so it takes them longer to get pregnant. Second, the Y-sperm (male) swim faster through that thick mucus – while the X-sperm (female) swim faster in thinner mucus. Put these two factors together, and you're somewhat more likely to end up playing on Team Blue – that is, if you wait long enough.

CHAPTER 8

Are You Pregnant?

Y OU'VE CHARTED, YOU'VE CHECKED your cervical mucus, you had sex at all the appropriate times – and in all the recommended ways. And now you're wondering: Were those baby-making efforts successful? Has our conception mission been accomplished?

Did we score that fertilized egg? Hit the baby jackpot? Could I be pregnant? Sure, you can just wait until your period's expected to take a home pregnancy test and find out for sure. But what if you're not the waiting type? Read on for the very early pregnancy scoop.

Early Pregnancy Signs - or Are They?

I s this month *the* month? Or is it just that time of the month – again? Are those early pregnancy signs – or early PMS signs? Or just your imagination gone baby wild? Hard to know for sure, but it doesn't hurt to wonder . . . does it?

Tender Breasts

"My breasts feel achy on the sides. It's sort of what I feel right before I start my period. Could I be pregnant – or is it just PMS?"

B reasts are often the first body part to get the memo when sperm meets egg, at least the first part noticeable to you. Their response to the big news varies from woman to woman, but newly

pregnant breasts can be tender, full, achy, swollen, tingly, sensitive, and even painful to the touch. Sometimes these signs show up within a few days of conception; sometimes they hold off until weeks later. Sometimes the changes are over the top (and have you quickly coming out of your tops), and sometimes they're more subtle (especially if they come on gradually instead of seemingly overnight).

There's just one little catch. As you're already surmising, early pregnancy breasts are not all that different from PMS breasts – except that breast changes due to pregnancy hormones stick around instead of disappearing with the arrival of Aunt Flo. Problem for you – and lots of other hopeful TTC mums – is that until AF arrives (or doesn't), it's really tough to tell these two types of breast changes apart. The puzzle is even harder still to solve in women whose breasts normally change a lot premenstrually – since these same women are more likely to experience pronounced breast changes with pregnancy.

Confused? Frustrated? Anxious for a sign that you can actually take to the baby bank? Well, here's one to look out for: changes in your areolas (the circles around your nipples). Pregnancy hormones (even those really early ones) can cause the areola to darken in colour and increase in diameter somewhat in the weeks after conception – though, again, that timetable can vary a great deal. You may also notice, as those hormones kick in, an increase and enlargement in the tiny bumps on the areola (they'll resemble goose bumps). These bumps are actually glands that produce oils to lubricate your nipples and areolas in preparation for lactation (talk about planning ahead!). These areola alterations will appear only if you're pregnant, not if you're PMS-ing. However, because every mum-to-be experiences these changes to a different extent and also at different times (some will notice obvious changes almost immediately, others won't notice any at all until much later), not seeing these differences in your areolas now doesn't mean baby isn't already on board – just that you might have to wait until that passenger list is officially confirmed by a pregnancy test.

Implantation Spotting

"I'm TTC and though it's a week before I'm due to get my period, I'm noticing some pinkish discharge when I wipe. Is my cycle messed up?"

The spotting you're noticing could actually be the positive sign you're looking for – or, at least, a prelude to the positive sign you're hoping to see on that as yet unopened pregnancy test. A significant minority of newly expectant mums (around 20 percent) notice scant spotting when an embryo burrows its way into the uterine wall. Such so-called implantation bleeding will likely arrive earlier than your expected monthly flow – usually around 5 to 10 days after conception. Much lighter than your period (it'll be spotty, not continuous bleeding) and lasting anywhere from a few hours to a few days, implantation bleeding is usually pale to medium pink or light brown in colour – sometimes merely pink-tinged mucus. It's rarely red, like a period.

Don't have any spotting at all? Remember, implantation bleeding is the exception, rather than the rule. The majority of mums-to-be (80 percent) do not have any spotting when an embryo implants – which means you definitely don't have to spot to be expecting.

On the other hand, not all pre-period spotting is related to implantation, or a sign that you're expecting – and this can lead to frustration. Women with irregular cycles (or cycles that are disrupted in a particular month for whatever reason) may assume that the pink they're seeing on their panties or on the toilet paper is implantation bleeding, only to find later that it's a midcycle blip or a harbinger of that monthly visitor coming a little earlier than expected. Adding to the frustration is the fact that home pregnancy tests may not be able to produce a reliable result this early (though if the result is positive, you can be positive, too; if it's negative, you can't consider it definitive yet). If your spotting does end up being implantation bleeding and a pregnancy test confirms your happy news – congratulations. If the spotting turns to bleeding, and ultimately ends up being your period, don't give up. Next month might be the one that's marked for success – so try, try again.

Urinary Frequency

"All of a sudden, I feel like I have to pee all the time. Could it mean I'm pregnant?"

Feel like you're peeing for two? It's possible you are. The need to pee with annoying frequency can appear on the pregnancy scene fairly early – usually about 2 to 3 weeks after conception. That's because pregnant kidneys must work overtime (keeping mums-to-be on the toilet overtime) to filter waste from the blood once there's an extra waste producer on board. What's more, even a just-pregnant uterus has begun to grow, and because it's still low in the pelvic cavity, it presses squarely on the bladder, triggering that gotta-go feeling. Also sending an expectant mum to the bathroom more often: those pregnancy hormones (most predominantly, progesterone) step up urinary frequency.

The best way to find out if all this peeing is a sign of pregnancy is to pee – on a home pregnancy test (HPT). Since this symptom typically appears right about the same time reliable results can be expected on an HPT, this purposeful peeing should give you your answer. And weren't you on the way to the bathroom again, anyway?

If it turns out you aren't pregnant – and retesting confirms this – the need to pee frequently could be a sign that either you've been increasing your fluid intake (which is fine) or that you may have a urinary tract infection (which isn't so fine – and needs to be treated). To find out for sure (and especially if it burns when you're urinating), put in a call to your doctor.

Not peeing up a storm? That doesn't mean there isn't a baby brewing. It could just mean this particular symptom hasn't kicked in yet or won't be kicking in at all (first rule of pregnancy: Every pregnant woman is different – so no pregnancy symptom is experienced universally by all pregnant women). Test – when the time is right and you have to pee – to find out for sure.

Elevated BBT

"I've been tracking my BBT and noticed the expected temperature rise right after ovulation (luckily we had sex right before) – but it hasn't come down, like it usually does. What's going on?"

If you've been tracking your first morning temperature for a few months, you're probably pretty familiar with your BBT ups and downs. As you've noticed, your BBT shifts upward right after ovulation, thanks to the increase in progesterone. As soon as progesterone falls (right around the time you'd expect your period), your temps will drop back down again – if AF is on her way, that is. But if you've conceived, there is no drop in progesterone (in fact, elevated progesterone is what keeps a new pregnancy going) – and that means there is no drop in your BBT. So if you notice 18 or more consecutive days of elevated BBT, there's a pretty good chance – make that a very good one – that you're already hosting a baby. And if for some reason you continue to take your BBT each morning during your pregnancy (though there's definitely no need to do that, unless you've become really attached to that thermometer), you'd see those increased progesterone levels keeping your temperature up throughout your pregnancy.

Does a persistently elevated temperature provide proof positive that you're expecting? Not exactly – you'll also need a positive pregnancy test to positively confirm your happy news. There are other, far less common explanations for a continued elevated temperature (such as an ovarian cyst), so if you don't see a drop in your temps, and if you don't get your period, yet all your pregnancy tests come out negative, put in a call to your gynaecologist to find out what's going on. It's definitely still possible that you're pregnant (sometimes it's just too early to call on an HPT, especially if you've been testing before your period was expected), but it's always a good idea to check out the situation.

Other Pregnancy Symptoms

"I'm TTC and I'm wondering if I'm pregnant, but it's too early to take a pregnancy test. Are there any other symptoms – besides breast and temperature changes – I can look for to know for sure?"

The only way to be positively sure that you're positively pregnant this early on is to get a positive result on a pregnancy test – and that may be impossible to secure just yet (depending on how early you're testing and how sensitive the test is). While you're waiting for testing day to dawn – and that waiting can be tough – you can be on the lookout for any early pregnancy clues your body may be sending (such as those tender breasts or that perpetual peeing). Unfortunately, those clues (plus the ones listed here) can also point to unrelated conditions (most notably PMS, but stress or a stomach bug are among the other possibilities). Still, experiencing any of these symptoms may be just the excuse you need to run to the store for an HPT (the pricier, more

sensitive models will be more accurate earlier; see page 132).

Fatigue. Too pooped to pop? You may be on your way to becoming a mum. Early pregnancy – actually the first 4 months – is typically exhausting, leaving you feeling sluggish, sleepy, sofa-loving. That's because your body is beginning to crank up its baby-making machine (particularly the placenta manufacturing), and that takes a lot of energy – just about all the energy you have on hand. Those newbie hormones surging through your body also do a number on your energy levels (would you believe that surging progesterone can actually put you to sleep?). Lower blood sugar, lower blood pressure, and increasing metabolism can also zap you of energy. Does an attack of the sleepies guarantee that you're providing bed and board for a baby? No – it can also indicate that you're PMS-ing, fighting off an infection, working (or playing) too hard, stressing too much, or not sleeping enough.

Nausea. Here's a symptom that can sign on early – in some cases, just days after conception, though it's more likely to show up 4 weeks later, at about 6 weeks of pregnancy – and hopefully, check out by the end of the first trimester. Though pregnancy hormones are responsible for so-called morning sickness, not every mum-to-be gets the queasies, and far from all experience vomiting, since hormones affect every woman differently. Not feeling green? That morning sickness could be just around the corner, but you may dodge it altogether. Still, nausea – or even a bout of vomiting – isn't a definite sign of pregnancy. It can also be caused by PMS, by a stomach bug or food poisoning, or even by mind games (it's possible to talk yourself into feeling queasy if you're really anxious to be expecting).

Smell sensitivity. Does your nose know something you don't know (but are hoping for)? Some newly pregnant women report a heightened sense of smell early on – and that could be owing to the increasing amount of oestrogen in your system during early pregnancy. If your sniffer's suddenly more sensitive (and easily offended), pregnancy might be in the air. But (and there is a but), some women also experience this smell surge during PMS.

Bloating. That bloated feeling can creep up (and out) on you very early in a pregnancy – though it may be difficult to differentiate between a pre-period bloat and a pregnancy bloat. While it's too soon to attribute bloating and swelling to your baby's growth (remember, your baby's not much bigger than the size of the full stop at the end of this sentence), it's likely due to early pregnancy hormones (in particular progesterone).

These hormones slow down your digestive tract (to better allow what you eat to feed baby), allowing gas to hang out in your intestines. Of course, as every woman knows from months and months of experience, bloat doesn't always spell baby – it can also spell P-M-S.

Cervical mucus. If you've become a student of your CM (maybe a graduate student if you've been at it a while), then take this test: Check your CM. If it becomes creamy and stays creamy after ovulation, that's a good sign that you'll pass the next test (the pregnancy one).

Missed period. In the stating-the-obvious department, if your 2-week wait doesn't end with a period (especially if your periods generally run like clockwork), it may be time to celebrate. Break out the pregnancy test, and hopefully, the sparkling apple juice!

Diagnosing Pregnancy

Maybe boxes of pregnancy tests are stacked up in your bathroom waiting for the right moment to be ripped open and peed upon. Or maybe you're waiting until the last minute (as in the day you miss your period) for a mad dash to the pharmacy to pick one – or seven – up. Wherever you fall in the waiting-to-take-a-home-pregnancy-test spectrum, you're sure to have questions about taking that pregnancy test (when? how? how often?). Keep in mind, though, that even though pregnancy tests may answer one question, they often leave you with lots more.

Pregnancy Tests

"How soon can I use a home pregnancy test to find out if I'm pregnant?"

Soon . . . but definitely not soon enough for most hopeful mums. Though it would be nice (note to Mother Nature and manufacturers of home pregnancy tests) to get the heads up – or thumbs down – as soon as the last baby dance of the month is over, that's not the way it works, at least not yet. There's an average of 2 weeks of waiting from the time you ovulate until

Who Needs a Blood Test?

With HPTs as easy as one-two-pee, why bother with a blood test anymore – especially if you're not fond of needles? Actually, there are a couple of good reasons. First, less waiting time. While you can't rely on an HPT to provide reliably accurate results until approximately 2 weeks post ovulation (3 weeks for a 97 percent accuracy rate), the more sophisticated blood pregnancy test can pick up those pregnancy hormones with virtually 100 percent accuracy as early as 1 week after conception. Second, the blood test offers more information than those pee-on-a-stick tests can. Since it measures the exact amount of hCG (an at-home test only lets you know whether it's there or not), and those values change as pregnancy progresses, a blood test can also help to date the pregnancy – a very good thing if your cycles are irregular, but actually valuable even if you run like clockwork. That's why many doctors will follow up with blood tests even if you've had a positive HPT, but also if your HPT was negative but your period hasn't shown up or if you're not sure when you conceived. Blood tests are routine, too, if you've been undergoing fertility treatments (so the pregnancy can be detected as early as possible). Either way, a blood test can give you a heads-up on your pregnancy status and a head start on your pregnancy care – and who doesn't need that?

the time you have (or miss) your period. And that's a lot of waiting, especially if you already feel like you've been waiting forever for that happy news.

Luckily, HPTs are quick, accurate, and reliable – and most important of all, they can keep the waiting to a minimum. You can start using many of them even before your period is scheduled to arrive, though the closer to P-day, the more reliable your results.

So how exactly can peeing on a stick give you the pregnancy scoop, and what's the earliest it can issue that baby bulletin? It's actually pretty simple. All those HPTs lined up on the shelves of the pharmacy work by measuring the levels of human chorionic gonadotropin (hCG) in your urine. HCG, a developing placenta-produced hormone of pregnancy, finds its way into your bloodstream and urine almost immediately after an embryo begins implanting in your uterus, between 6 and 12 days after fertilization. As soon as hCG can be detected in your urine, you can get the positive result you're looking for – that is, theoretically. But HPTs aren't always sensitive to hCG until levels begin building up, which they do as the days pass. Though some hCG is in your urine a week after conception, it's not likely to be enough to register on the HPT – which means that if you test 7 days before your expected period, you're likely to get a negative result even if you're pregnant. A good reason to hold off until your period's expected to break open that HPT.

Waiting's not your thing? Some tests promise 60 percent accuracy 4 days before your expected period. Not crazy about those odds? You'll have a 90 percent chance of netting the correct result if you sit tight until your expected period. Test a week later, and the accuracy rate jumps to 97 percent (so if at first you don't succeed, or get your

HPTs, Circa 1350 BCE

So you thought peeing on a stick to find out if you're pregnant was an invention of the modern era? Well, the stick may be – but the peeing, apparently not. An Egyptian papyrus from 1350 BCE describes a home pregnancy test that definitely predates EPT. To test for pregnancy – and her future baby's gender – a woman would urinate on a pile of wheat and barley seeds. If barley grew, it meant she was pregnant with a boy. If wheat grew, it meant she was expecting a girl. No sprouts at all? Then there was no little sprout growing in her, either.

Were those ancients onto something? Believe it or not, there's some grain of truth (both barley and wheat) to this wisdom from the ages. When replicated in our times, it's been found that this test is 70 percent accurate for predicting pregnancy (not gender), probably because the elevated levels of oestrogen in a pregnant woman's urine cause those seeds to sprout. Farmers, take note?

---

period, try that test again). Whether you test early or late (or every 12 hours for 2 weeks straight), the good news is that false positives are much less common than false negatives – which means if your test is positive, you can be, too.

HPTs offer a very accurate diagnosis very early in pregnancy – all in the privacy of your own bathroom. Still, you'll have to leave the bathroom and follow up with a professional. If the result is positive, you should have it confirmed by a blood test and a complete prenatal checkup. If repeated tests are negative, but your period still doesn't show up, check in with your practitioner to see if there's another reason why you're so late.

Can't test on the day your period's expected because you never know for sure when that day will come? Your best testing strategy if your periods are irregular is to wait the number of days equal to the longest cycle you've had in the last 6 months – and then test. If the result is negative and you still haven't got your period, repeat the test after a week (or after a few days if you're not the patient type).

Best Way to Test

"I heard it's better to take a pregnancy test in the morning. Is that right?"

Any time is a good time for a home pregnancy test, but first thing in the morning is the best time of all – especially if you're testing early, before your period's expected. That's because the longer you've gone without peeing (and drinking), the more concentrated your urine will be. The more concentrated

Action Plan

Though you might not want to hear it, the truth is, it's best to wait until the day your period is expected (or a day or two before depending on the brand of test) to whip out the HPT. Sure, the waiting is tough to take, but the results will be more accurate and you'll save yourself a lot of uncertainty – not to mention all the money you'd be spending on retests.

your urine, the more likely those still low levels of hCG will show up – and the more likely you are to get an accurate (and hopefully positive) result. Can't wait for the morning? You definitely don't have to – just keep in mind that you might not score that result as easily early on.

As for other test prep tips, start by reading the package directions thoroughly, and then following them. No, it's not rocket science, but since each pregnancy test has a slightly different protocol, it pays to look before you pee. Depending on the brand, you'll either hold the test stick in your stream of urine for a few seconds, or collect your urine in a cup, and then dip the stick into it. Midstream urine is usually preferred for any urine test because it serves up the cleanest sample (and you might as well master the midstream now, if you haven't already; if your test is positive, you'll be spending a lot of time provid-ing these samples to your practitioner at your prenatal appointments). To pee just right, urinate for a second or two, stop, hold it, and then put either the stick or the cup in position to catch the rest of the stream.

Once you have a properly peed-on stick, take a deep breath and get ready to read the result. Make sure you follow the recommended waiting period; not waiting long enough – or waiting too long – can affect that result. In fact, it's possible for a test that originally came out negative (using the timing indicated on the packaging and directions) to turn into a positive result hours or days after it was done, even if you're not really pregnant. The test result that's accurate – and the one you should count on – is the one that appears after the recommended waiting time. If you see a different result hours later, take another test before jumping to any conclusions.

Stress Tests

Is it that time of month again – testing time? If you've been TTC for a while, you know the drill, and maybe you've come to look forward to it – and at the same time, dread it a little bit. That's understandable. All of those efforts you're both putting in to your baby-making mission each month, all the anticipation, all the excitement, all the hopes and dreams – all come down to a trickle of urine, a stick, and a knot-in-the-stomach wait for a sign (or a line, or a readout).

If the monthly testing – and her monthly second-guessing of symptoms – is stressing you both out, hang in there. Baby making can take longer than you'd think (ironic, considering how much effort you may have made over the years trying *not* to get your partner pregnant), but most often, it does happen – and it's always worth waiting for. In the meantime, try taking some of the stress out of the monthly testing (remember, stress isn't good for baby making). Plan a little something special each month – a dinner out, a bouquet of her favourite flowers, a cupcake from her favourite bakery, even a card that lets her know how happy you are to be working on making a baby with her. Whether you end up celebrating a baby-to-be or toasting next month's efforts, it'll remind you both not only how lucky you are to be starting a family together, but how lucky you are to have each other.

Faintly Positive

"When I took a home pregnancy test, it showed a really faint line. Am I pregnant?"

Get ready to faint – from excitement. Any positive line (or readout) is a positive sign – and a sign that you're positively pregnant. That's because the only way a home pregnancy test can produce that positive result is if there's hCG circulating in your system and making an appearance in your urine. And the only way that hCG can show up is if you're pregnant (only pregnant bodies can manufacture this pregnancy-centric hormone). Bottom line on that line (or that digital readout), no matter how faint: It means that you're officially expecting.

Not the dark, emphatic, no-doubt-about-it line you were looking for – the one you were going to snap a picture of and send to everyone in your e-mail address book? That's probably because the test you used wasn't as sensitive as others (some are more sensitive than others; see box, below), or because you're testing so early that there isn't enough hCG to generate that loud-and-clear message you hoped to see (those levels rise each day, so if you test early there's only a little hCG to tap into). Also possible: you're not as far along as you thought.

If you feel you need a more definitive result before you start celebrating (or if you're just determined to get that photo op), wait until at least the first day of your missed period and test again. Chances are you'll see the line that will delete your doubts, and convince you that you've conceived after all.

The Sensitive Type

Sensitivity is always a plus in a partner – but it's also a plus when you're looking for a positive home pregnancy test. The more sensitive the HPT, the more likely it is to give you an accurate result sooner. To figure out just how sensitive your pregnancy test is, check out the packaging. Look for the milli-international units per litre (mIU/L) measurement. The lower the number, the better (20 mIU/L will tell you you're pregnant sooner than a test with a 50 mIU/L sensitivity). Not surprisingly, the more expensive tests usually have greater sensitivity, and more reliable results – though a less sensitive test can still tell you if you're pregnant, just maybe not as early on.

Positive Result... Then Negative

"My first pregnancy test was positive, but a few days later I took two more and they were both negative. And then I got my period. What's going on?"

Early testing does come with a downside, and unfortunately, it sounds like you may have experienced it: the diagnosis of a chemical pregnancy. Because an HPT can diagnose a pregnancy so very early in the process, it can sometimes also diagnose one that isn't meant to continue – one that isn't capable of developing or surviving, and ends practically before it begins. In a chemical pregnancy, the egg is fertilized and starts to implant in the uterus, but for some reason it never completes implantation. Instead of turning into a viable pregnancy, it ends very quickly in a period. Though experts estimate

I'm Pregnant. Now What?

Maybe it was your first time at the baby-making plate, or maybe you've been swinging away for months. Either way, sperm and egg have made contact – and you and your partner have made a baby. Congrats on a job well done! But guess what? Your work is just beginning. If you thought that making a baby was demanding, wait until you start growing that baby. That's why you're going to need all the help you can get, not just from the daddy-to-be in your life, but from your pre-natal practitioner. Don't know where to begin with anything pregnancy related (what to do, what not to do, what to eat, what not to eat, what to make of all those crazy, seemingly random symptoms you may already be experiencing)? You'll get lots of help from *What to Expect When You're Expecting,* as well as *Eating Well When You're Expecting*, and get all the support you need from fellow mums-to-be on WhatToExpect.com. Hey, look at that – you've graduated to expecting!

that up to 70 percent of all conceptions are chemical, the vast majority end before a woman even realizes that she's conceived (certainly in the days before home pregnancy tests, women didn't know they were pregnant until much later, so chemical pregnancies weren't diagnosed at all). Often a very early positive pregnancy test, followed by negative testing and then a late period (a few days to a week late) are the only signs of a chemical pregnancy. Unless you tested early, you never would have known about it.

Technically, a chemical pregnancy is more like a cycle in which a pregnancy never actually occurred than it is a true miscarriage – it's a random event that requires no medical treatment or follow-up, and is no cause for concern. Emotionally, it can be a very different story. The loss of the promise of a pregnancy, no matter how early it happens, can also be upsetting for both you and your partner – especially if you've been trying to conceive for some time. Talking to other women who've gone through the same thing may help you work through your feelings – and also help you realize that you're far from alone (you will probably find plenty of these women on TTC and pregnancy message boards; as more and more women are testing earlier, more and more are encountering chemical pregnancies).

Here's the good news: There's no medical reason to wait if you'd like to TTC again on your next cycle, and experiencing one chemical pregnancy usually doesn't increase the chances of having another one. Keep in mind, too, that having conceived once makes it more likely that you'll conceive again soon (though you may want to wait a little longer to test next time) – with the much happier result of a healthy pregnancy.

Pregnancy Symptoms Without the Positive Test

"I have all kinds of early pregnancy symptoms, but I must have taken six tests in the last week and all have been negative. What should I do?"

Having spent your whole life living in it, you know your body well – possibly even better than a pee-on-a-stick test does. If you're experiencing multiple symptoms of early pregnancy, but can't get those HPTs to corroborate, wait a week, give your body a chance to accumulate some more hCG, then test again. Your pregnancy may be too early to call with an HPT (after all, pinpointing conception isn't a precise science). In the meantime, take optimum pregnancy care of yourself (you know the drill, and you're probably already practising it: take your prenatal vitamins, don't drink or smoke, eat well). Or, if waiting's not your game, call your practitioner and ask for a blood test, which can diagnose a pregnancy more accurately sooner.

If your hunch isn't confirmed by follow-up testing (especially if a blood test also comes back negative), it becomes much more likely that you aren't pregnant after all. Because just about every early pregnancy symptom – including a missed period – can have other triggers, it's possible to feel pregnant and not be pregnant. To screen out physical causes for your symptoms, check in with your practitioner, especially if your period is uncharacteristically late. Testing again is probably also a good idea – just in case your cycle was out of whack this month and you may have conceived much later than the calendar suggests.

If your pregnancy tests are consistently negative, but your practitioner can't find a physical explanation for your symptoms, it's possible that they could have emotional roots. The mind-body connection is strong, but it can be especially strong when your mind is so anxious for your body to become pregnant – and that is completely understandable, especially if you've been waiting for that happy result for a while. As many TTC mums have found, even the power of suggestion – reading about pregnancy symptoms, hearing about them from friends – can summon up everything from nausea to food cravings to fatigue when you very much want to be pregnant. Being so keenly tuned into your body, which many TTC mums are, can also make you hypersensitive to every little possible change – which can make you see symptoms where they might not actually be. And what wishful thinking can't summon up, PMS symptoms very easily can (including bloating, breast pain, crampiness, moodiness, headache, and fatigue). What's more, being stressed out about being in pregnancy limbo (am I? am I not?) can actually keep your period from arriving, which can keep the limbo going longer – and even exacerbate those pseudo-pregnancy symptoms.

This isn't to say that you're imagining your pregnancy symptoms – or that they're all in your head (emotionally triggered symptoms can be surprisingly convincing) – only that your mind and body may be collaborating to play tricks on you. It isn't fair, but it's very common. Most hopeful mums find themselves second-guessing symptoms, even when those pregnancy tests won't back them up – and some find themselves doing that with each and every cycle. Bring the topic up with others who are TTC and you'll likely get an earful of empathy.

So if it turns out that the miracle didn't happen this month, realize that accepting this reality doesn't mean you're giving up on those baby hopes – just that you're giving up on this month's and moving on to the next, which will be here before you know it!

There's Always Next Month

So another round of testing has arrived, along with the waiting, and hoping, and wishing, and seemingly endless anticipation. Will you be? Won't you be? You head for the toilet, heart in your stomach, emotions on your sleeve, HPT in your hand. You pee, you wait some more, you steel yourself, and you peek at the results (eyes half closed at first because you're almost afraid to look).

Negative, again, even after you retest, and retest – and wait and retest? There's no denying it – it's disappointing, whether it's the first month you've tried, or the tenth, or more. Frustrating, too, especially if you've been meticulous in your fertility charting, precise in your sex scheduling – and fully expected your efforts to pay off in the form of a positive HPT.

It's definitely hard to put a positive spin on a negative pregnancy test when you were so hoping this would be your lucky month – the one when all the efforts you and your partner have been putting into your conception mission would finally provide the ultimate pay-off. But here's one way to try. Instead of lingering over what didn't happen this month, try to think about what might just happen next month. Instead of looking back at this month's negative result, think ahead to next month's possibly positive one. Remind yourself that successful baby making, like most of life's best rewards, often takes time. But it's time that's well worth it – even if it sometimes feels that all those efforts are getting you nowhere. If you can, and if it seems to help you stay positive, try to find just one way you can improve on this month's efforts (unless you're already doing everything so by the book that there's no room for improvement) – whether it's cutting back on caffeine or stepping up your fruits and veggies, or hey, learning to love oysters. Taking another positive step can always make you feel a little better about that negative test – and can help you summon up the motivation you'll need for next month's challenge.

Most of all, in your quest for a baby, don't forget about the guy you're on the quest with. Though he may not be showing it – probably for fear of stressing you out – he's probably also feeling a little drained over all the emotional ups and downs of TTC, too. So as you look forward to next month's baby making, remember to look next to you, too.

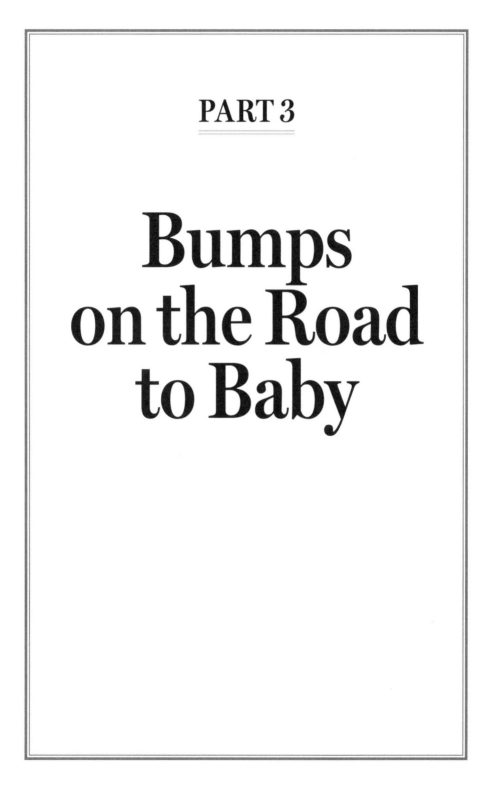

PART 3

Bumps on the Road to Baby

CHAPTER 9

Challenges to Fertility

DID YOU ALWAYS SORT OF ASSUME that getting pregnant was going to be as easy as chucking the birth control and getting busy? Sometimes it is, but often it isn't. Making a baby can take more time than you'd expect – even when everything's in working order on both sides of the bed, but especially when something (or someone) needs a reproductive tune-up, or more. For almost a quarter of couples, it's not just a matter of time, it's a matter of fertility challenges. A number of bumps along the road to baby can slow the way, or even make a detour or two necessary. Fortunately, in most cases fertility challenges don't have to signal the end of your hopes of starting (or adding to) a family. The right treatment for these conditions can get you right back on the baby-making path and pave the way for conception.

Fertility Challenges

Often, overcoming infertility is as easy as finding out what's blocking your path to pregnancy, and clearing it up. Sometimes, it's a condition you already knew about – but maybe didn't realize would affect your fertility. Other times, it's a condition that you didn't have a clue about until a fertility workup uncovered it. Either way, treatment is almost always possible, and usually successful. Here are some of the more common fertility challenges and what can be done to overcome them.

Fibroids

What is it? Uterine fibroids are almost always benign (in other words, non-cancerous) tumours that grow inside or around the wall of the uterus. Fibroids can grow individually or in clusters and each can be as small as a grain of sand or as large as a melon.

As many as 25 percent of women in the UK have fibroids, and nearly a quarter of these women have symptoms ranging from painful, extremely heavy,

The Good News

Research shows that treating and/or removing fibroids can increase fertility in those women who are having trouble conceiving because of their fibroids.

longer-than-normal periods and pressure in the pelvic area, to constipation, urinary incontinence, and backache. Some women don't have any symptoms at all.

Though it is not completely clear what causes them, fibroids are more common among overweight women (it's believed that high levels of fat-derived oestrogen contribute to the growth of fibroids). Women of African descent are 9 times more likely than Caucasian women to develop fibroids. There's also a genetic component: If your mother had fibroids, you may be at higher risk for getting them.

How is fertility affected? Most fibroids do not affect fertility and can safely be left alone. Around 2 to 3 percent are thought to interfere with conception by causing blockages in the reproductive tract and by changing the shape of the uterus, making it harder for an egg to be fertilized or for a fertilized egg to implant. Fibroids can also cause inflammation of the blood vessels of the uterus, which in turn can complicate implantation.

What are the treatment options? A number of treatment options for fibroids are available, but only one is appropriate for women who'd like to conceive. That treatment is a surgical procedure called a myomectomy, during which numerous or large fibroids are removed from the uterus. A myomectomy is generally done laparoscopically in an outpatient setting.

Pelvic Inflammatory Disease (PID)

What is it? Any time an infection causes inflammation in your pelvic organs, the condition is known in medical-speak as pelvic inflammatory disease (PID). PID can result from a wide range of pelvic infections, including an infection of the uterus (endometritis), of the fallopian tubes (salpingitis), or of the ovaries (oophoritis). PID can occasionally be caused by a ruptured appendix, but most often it's triggered by untreated sexually transmitted diseases (STDs) such as chlamydia or gonorrhoea. In fact, up to 40 percent of women with untreated chlamydia or gonorrhoea develop PID.

The symptoms of PID include pelvic pain (which can come on suddenly or build up over time), smelly vaginal discharge, excessive bleeding during your period, fever, chills, painful urination, backache, nausea, and/or vomiting.

How is fertility affected? Twenty percent of women with PID become infertile. That's because if PID is left untreated, the inflammation can cause scar tissue to form in the fallopian tubes, making it difficult both for an egg to travel through them after ovulation and for the sperm to reach the egg. If fertilization does occur, the scar tissue in the fallopian tube can stop the fertilized egg from reaching the uterus, increasing the risk for an ectopic pregnancy (when a

The Good News

Early and aggressive treatment of infections and STDs can decrease the chances that PID will prevent you from becoming pregnant.

STDs and Male Infertility

Men with STDs usually exhibit symptoms soon after they are infected, which means many seek treatment right away – and that's a good thing. Untreated STDs can damage a man's fertility by causing epididymitis, an inflammation of the vessels that transport sperm from the testicles. In severe cases, the inflammation can cause the vessels to be completely blocked – and blocked vessels won't allow sperm to get through at all, resulting in infertility.

Getting tested and treated for STDs early, as well as practising safe sex with infected partners, can help men protect their fertility.

fertilized egg remains in the fallopian tube and grows there instead of implanting in the uterus). If the uterine lining is affected by PID, it could be difficult for a fertilized egg to implant normally.

What are the treatment options? If you notice any of the symptoms of PID, visit your doctor for a diagnosis. If PID is diagnosed, antibiotics can get rid of the infection and may protect your fertility. Getting treated right away for STDs and following safe sex practices with partners who have STDs will decrease your risk not only for an STD, but also for PID. If the PID leads to scarring, surgery may be recommended (see facing page). Unfortunately, antibiotics can't reverse damage that is already done, so if PID is not treated, and even in some cases when it is, it's possible to suffer infertility that can't be treated with surgery. In such a case, IVF will be necessary in order to conceive.

Endometriosis

What is it? Endometriosis, a condition that affects approximately 2 million women between the ages of 25 and 40 in the UK, occurs when tissue from the uterine lining (the endometrium) gets deposited during menstruation on other parts of the pelvic area (such as the fallopian tubes, ovaries, bladder, appendix, or even intestines) and grows. Because this tissue acts the same way as it does inside the uterus no matter where it ends up, each month when oestrogen levels rise as part of a normal menstrual cycle, the endometrial tissue will grow and then bleed if there's no pregnancy. This results in extreme pelvic pain, severe cramps during your period, painful intercourse, lower back pain, and nausea and vomiting.

Endometriosis is thought to be caused by a combination of factors, including a malfunction of the immune system; a backup of endometrial tissue during menstruation (instead of all the tissue flowing out in the form of a period, some tissue backs up the wrong way and into the abdominal cavity); and genetic factors (if your mum or another close female relative had endometriosis, your chances of developing the condition are increased).

How is fertility affected? Fortunately, endometriosis can be treated. But if left undiagnosed or untreated, the endometrial tissue can continue to grow and block the fallopian tubes, or impede implantation of a fertilized egg in the uterus (if the growths invade uterine muscles, and not just the uterine lining). It is estimated that 6 percent of European women with untreated endometriosis are infertile.

What are the treatment options? Though there is no cure for endometriosis, there are ways to treat the condition and protect (or recover) your fertility. Such therapies include:

The Good News

Treating endometriosis and removing or shrinking the endometrial lesions can give you an excellent window of opportunity in which to become pregnant. And there's even more good news ahead once you successfully conceive. The pain associated with endometriosis is often diminished during pregnancy, plus pregnancy provides a reprieve from new growth.

- Surgery (usually laparoscopic) to remove the endometrial lesions.

- Possibly, diet modifications – including avoiding high-fat dairy and stepping up intake of complex carbs, as well as essential fatty acids found in sesame seeds, salmon, flax, walnuts, or walnut oil – may help ease symptoms, though there isn't any conclusive evidence to support their effectiveness. Since all of these foods are fertility- and baby-friendly anyway, there certainly isn't any downside to adding them to your eating plan, and there could definitely be some benefits.

- Hormonal treatments to reduce the level of oestrogen can shrink some of the lesions. Your doctor may suggest a specific course of birth control pills as part of a hormone therapy, though clearly this is not the best treatment if you're trying to conceive.

Scar Tissue/ Surgical Adhesions

What is it? Scar tissues are bands of fibrous material that can develop in and around your uterus as a result of inflammation from PID or endometriosis, or after a gynaecological procedure such as a dilation and curettage (D & C). Scar tissue can grow in any part of your body after it's wounded (like in your finger – the one you sliced along with the tomatoes that time). If your uterus feels wounded because of a D & C or because of PID or other infections, protective layers of tissue (known, not surprisingly, as scar tissue) form in the areas of inflammation as healing takes place. Sometimes, layer upon layer of scar tissue (or adhesions) can grow. An overgrowth of scar tissue in the uterus, called Asherman's syndrome, may cause symptoms, including pain and light or absent periods.

How is fertility affected? Most scarring in the uterus doesn't lead to fertility problems, but in some cases it can stop the endometrium (the uterine lining) from forming properly. Without a robust and healthy endometrium, it's difficult for a fertilized egg to implant and grow properly. Rarely, scar tissue can also form on the cervix, and if it blocks the cervical opening completely, it can impede fertility.

What are the treatment options? If you have lots of adhesions, if you have pain, or if you have trouble conceiving, your doctor may recommend surgery to remove scar tissue. Often, the surgery is performed with a hysteroscope, an instrument inserted through the cervix and into the uterus that is used to visualize the uterine cavity. If any adhesions

The Good News

For women with mild to moderate adhesions, there is a 70 to 80 percent chance of getting pregnant (and having a successful pregnancy) once the adhesions are removed.

Cervical Stenosis

Sometimes, women may develop small amounts of scar tissue on the cervix after undergoing surgical procedures on their cervixes – such as a LEEP procedure or a cone biopsy. In some cases, the scar tissue can grow thick enough to cause cervical stenosis, or a narrowing of the cervical canal. Since sperm needs only a tiny opening to swim through, most of the time cervical stenosis doesn't negatively impact your ability to conceive. In rare cases, however, scar tissue completely blocks sperm from entering the uterus through the cervix. And in those cases, fertility may be impeded. Luckily, intrauterine insemination (IUI; see page 167) with cervical dilation can get the sperm where they need to go – so you can get on with your plans for having a baby.

are found, additional instruments can be inserted through the hysteroscope to remove the scar tissue.

Ovarian Cyst

What is it? A cyst is a soft, fluid-filled sac that grows on the ovary or in one (or more) of the egg follicles. For most women who get ovarian cysts, these blister-like growths come and go with a normal menstrual cycle and are completely harmless. But for others, ovarian cysts can linger, grow large, and even cause symptoms, including pain localized on one side of your abdomen when you ovulate (not to be confused with the small normal twinges sometimes felt midcycle). They can also cause irregular periods.

The Good News

The vast majority of ovarian cysts have absolutely no effect on fertility. For those that do impact your ability to conceive, treatment almost always makes it possible to have a baby.

How is fertility affected? If too many cysts cover the ovary, eggs could fail to develop or be released.

What are the treatment options? Often, cysts resolve on their own, but if a cyst persists or gets larger, or if your symptoms get worse, you may need laparoscopic surgery to remove the cyst.

Polycystic Ovarian Syndrome (PCOS)

What is it? About 1 in 15 women have polycystic ovarian syndrome (also known as PCOS), and the condition is the most common cause of infertility. PCOS occurs when the body starts producing too much LH and the ovaries start producing too much testosterone (they usually produce only a small amount). Excess amounts of these two hormones disrupt ovarian function and a normal menstrual period (because without ovulation, the body doesn't produce progesterone, the hormone responsible for normal periods).

PCOS can be marked by irregular periods, extra long menstrual cycles, excess body hair, acne, and obesity. While it's not known for certain what causes PCOS, experts speculate there is a genetic component (if your mother or a close female relative had it, your risk is higher), and that it might also have something to do with the body's inability to use insulin properly (not only does insulin control blood sugar, but it also controls ovarian function). Women with PCOS generally have other out-of-sync hormones (including thyroid hormones) as well as elevated levels of other male hormones – and that might also be a contributing factor.

How is fertility affected? When the ovary can't perform as it should because of the hormone irregularity characteristic of PCOS, the developing follicles (eggs) can't mature properly, and instead of one egg dominating each month and eventually bursting out in normal ovulation, the developing follicles stay trapped inside. After time, so many follicles collect in the ovary that cysts begin to form. Eventually, a shell also forms around the outside of the ovary, causing further disruptions to ovulation.

What are the treatment options? Weight loss, regular exercise, and medications (such as metformin) may all help the body better use insulin. With less insulin around to stimulate ovarian production of testosterone, the ovaries function more normally. Eating a healthy, well-balanced diet (one that's rich in complex carbs, such as whole grains and fresh vegetables, and low in refined carbs and sugar),

---

PCOS and Thyroid Disorders

Some women who suffer from PCOS also have thyroid disease – and often, they don't know it. If you've been diagnosed with PCOS, be sure to ask your doctor to test for a thyroid condition and thyroid antibodies. For more on thyroid disease, see page 147.

---

plus ensuring an adequate intake of vitamin D and the B vitamins, may also help. Losing weight is key to restoring normal hormone function and cycles, however, and for some women weight loss alone can regulate ovulation.

Irregular Menstrual Periods

What is it? Irregular periods (cycles lasting longer than 35 to 40 days), no periods, or abnormal bleeding are usually signs that you're not ovulating. Called anovulation, this condition can be caused by many factors, including stress, an eating disorder, too much exercise, illness, and/or hormonal imbalance (such as a thyroid condition or PCOS).

How is fertility affected? Irregular or abnormal ovulation and menstruation is responsible for up to 35 percent of all cases of infertility. If you don't ovulate, you can't get pregnant.

What are the treatment options? First, take a good look at your weight and your lifestyle. If you're overweight or underweight, getting your weight close to where it should be (see Chapter 2) may reregulate your cycles (but don't do any extreme dieting, which can also

---

The Good News

Treating PCOS and then (for some women) using fertility drugs, such as Clomid, to stimulate ovulation can often solve associated fertility problems.

Secondary Infertility

Getting pregnant with number one was a piece of cake, but getting a second bun in the oven has been a surprising struggle? You have a lot of company. Actually, more couples experience secondary infertility (in other words, infertility that shows up after you've already had at least one baby) than primary infertility (infertility the first time around). In fact, secondary infertility accounts for 25 to 30 percent of infertility cases. Yet those stats don't seem to be reflected in attitudes about secondary infertility. Far more attention is focused on first-timers who are having a hard time getting pregnant than those who are getting nowhere on round two. Friends and family may feel a couple's pain less keenly when they already have a pride and joy to enjoy. Doctors may downplay secondary infertility, urging a couple to "just keep on trying" – reassuring them that getting pregnant once means it'll happen again. And a couple who's having trouble conceiving baby number 2 may be less likely to seek help – after all, who has time for fertility screenings and treatments when you've got a little one to run after? For that matter, who has time to devote to complicated baby-planning activities – to charting, to testing, to carefully choreographed sex . . . or any sex for that matter – when you're busy scheduling an older child's activities?

Occasionally, secondary fertility problems are triggered by a situation that's related to a previous pregnancy or delivery, such as an infection or a difficult childbirth that damaged the uterus. Most often, however, secondary infertility is caused by the very same kinds of conditions that cause primary infertility.

First, try to find the time to do your own assessment of your preconception prep (unless you've already been on top of that game). Have you been keeping track of your fertility – and baby dancing at all the appropriate times? Have you noticed any changes in your cycles that might be keeping you from conceiving? How's your diet and caffeine consumption been lately (nobody needs an IV coffee drip more than a mum does, but too much caffeine can interfere with fertility)? Is there any room for improvement when it comes to your lifestyle? Have there been any changes in your health – or medications you've been taking – since your first baby was born? How about your weight – has that been relatively stable, or have you put on some pounds since your first baby boarded? Or, maybe, lost a few too many since your first baby was born – because you no longer have time to eat? You're obviously older than you were when you conceived the first time, but has enough time passed that your age might now be an factor when trying to conceive? Your partner should ask himself the same questions about his health, lifestyle, weight, diet, and age, too, because his fertility can also be impacted by any or all of the above. Read over Chapters 1, 2, and 3 to see if a few modifications in how you're living could help you live the pregnant life again sooner.

Then, check in with your doctor for a more professional assessment. A year of trying to conceive (or much less if you're older) definitely qualifies you for a fertility workup, so there's no reason to hold off. In many cases, treatment for anything that's discovered can be quick and easy (as with the treatment of a thyroid condition, something that's fairly common after the birth of a baby), so you can finally get that second passenger on board. In some cases, treatment may take longer, but either way, moving those fertility bumps off your path to pregnancy can get that bump on your belly once again.

Of course, if you're having trouble conceiving baby number 2 (or 3, or 4), you're not only dealing with all those typical TTC ups and downs – you may also be dealing with emotional issues that are unique to those experiencing secondary infertility. First, the surprise ("I got pregnant right away last time – why not this time?") and the denial ("How can I have a fertility problem, when I've been fertile before?"). Then the guilt ("Why aren't I happy with just one child?"). And the jealousy ("Everyone else can have two kids – why can't I?"). You may feel, strangely, more alone than other hopeful parents who are facing fertility challenges in round one – you're not a member of the primary infertility group since you have a child already, but you're not fully at home with fertile friends, since you're having trouble conceiving again. This may make it harder to find the support every struggling-to-conceive couple needs. Those around you may imply that you should be grateful for what you've got – or may seem not to get what you're going through, or summon up much sympathy for your child-making frustrations because you're not childless.

Just because you already have a child doesn't mean you aren't entitled to feeling discouraged when you're having trouble making another. Nor does it mean you're not entitled to all the empathy and support you need as you go about facing this challenge. So seek it out. If your friends and family just don't understand, talk to those who do – those who are experiencing or have experienced secondary fertility problems. You can find them on online message boards and in support groups (you'll be surprised how many you'll find, since secondary infertility is so common).

Remember, too, you're not facing secondary infertility completely alone – you have each other to face it with. Staying connected as a twosome always takes more effort when you're also a threesome, but it's especially important, particularly as you try to become a foursome (or more). Chances are you're both feeling the same frustrations, and the same disappointment, and the same guilt, and you'll both feel better if you share those feelings with each other. But also try to make time for the kind of romance that will keep your baby-making campaign – and your relationship – going strong.

One other person may be feeling the effects of your fertility struggles, even if he or she doesn't know about them: your child. Kids, even very young ones, have keen mood radar – so though your child almost certainly isn't in the loop about your conception efforts, he or she may be riding that emotional roller coaster right alongside you. To make sure those ups and downs don't leave your child feeling off balance, try to keep family life as normal as possible – even as you push forward with your efforts to add to that precious family.

Clomid to the Rescue?

Clomiphene citrate, the drug found in fertility treatments like Clomid or Serophene, is often the first line of defence when a woman has trouble conceiving and the suspected culprit is ovulation issues. Your doctor will likely start you off with 50 mg per day for 5 days, beginning on the second, third, fourth, or fifth day after your period begins. Most women can expect to start ovulating about 7 days after the last dose of clomiphene. For those who don't begin to ovulate right away, the dose can be increased by 50 mg per day each month up to 150 mg. Once the drug is working and you've begun to ovulate, you'll likely only be kept on Clomid 3 to 6 months. If you haven't conceived by the sixth month on Clomid, more medications and/or other assisted fertility techniques could be used (see page 161).

One thing to keep in mind about Clomid: Since it's a medication that induces ovulation, there's a chance that it'll work so well, you may ovulate more than one egg. If you conceive during a cycle where more than one egg is released, there's a 5 to 10 percent chance you'll be seeing double in the future – as in a twin (or more) pregnancy. As far as other side effects when you're on Clomid, some women experience breast tenderness, mood swings, hot flashes, vision changes, and night sweats.

---

throw your cycles off). A regular exercise programme can boost your general health – and possibly, your fertility – but overexercising can prevent you from ovulating (and getting pregnant), so try cutting down if you've been hitting the gym too hard. Eating disorders (anorexia, bulimia, or even just periodic bingeing) can also throw off your cycles, so if you – or anyone around you – think you might need help overcoming such a problem, don't hesitate to seek it. Extreme stress can also derail your cycles, so try to relax, too (see page 24 for some tips on how). If none of these tactics seems to work – and screenings for a thyroid condition or PCOS have come up negative – your doctor may prescribe fertility drugs like Clomid to induce ovulation and normal periods.

Premature Ovarian Failure

What is it? Premature ovarian failure (POF) occurs when the ovarian folli-

cles are depleted before age 40 or when the ovaries stop working properly long before they should have. POF can be caused by type 1 diabetes; genetic factors such as metabolic disorders, Turner's syndrome, or fragile X syndrome; autoimmune diseases; or cancer treatments.

How is fertility affected? If the egg reserves are nearly depleted, it becomes

The Good News

Though POF causes a woman's egg supply to be depleted much faster than it would normally, many women with POF may still have some eggs left with which to conceive. Depending on how many eggs are still viable, fertility treatments like ovarian stimulation and retrieval to get those last few eggs may be useful and promising for women with POF.

Is It You . . . or Is It Me?

When a couple has trouble conceiving right away, it's typically assumed the woman is responsible for the fertility glitch. That's a long-held assumption. After all, for centuries it was believed that women were always the weak reproductive link when a couple came up empty-handed (and empty-nested).

It turns out, though, that men and women can both contribute to infertility – and actually at about the same rates. Statistics show that 35 to 40 percent of the time, the problem lies with the man, in another 35 to 40 percent of cases it's with the woman, and the rest of the time both partners have contributing factors or the cause is unknown.

While either partner can contribute to a conception standstill, it's almost always easier to diagnose and treat infertility in a man than it is in a woman. So if you're finding the baby making is slow going (keeping in mind, once again, that conception can take an average of 6 to 12 months for healthy couples), it's always a good idea to start fertility testing with him. Then if he aces his tests, you can proceed with testing for you. See page 154 for more on the fertility workup.

extremely difficult to conceive (and if the egg reserves are completely depleted, as is sometimes the case with POF, conception becomes impossible).

What are the treatment options? The most common treatment for women with POF who want to get pregnant is cyclic hormone replacement therapy (HRT) or cyclic progesterone to provide a regular period without suppressing ovarian function. If that doesn't work to induce ovulation (because there are too few eggs), fertility treatments using egg retrieval or possibly a donor egg would be the next step.

Thyroid Disorder

What is it? Thyroid disorder affects about 15 percent of women of childbearing age. Thyroid disorder can show up as hyperthyroidism, when too much thyroid hormone is produced, or more commonly, hypothyroidism, when too

The Good News

Thyroid condition is one of the easiest chronic health problems to control and to treat – and one of the easiest fertility challenges to overcome. Women with properly managed thyroid disorders routinely have perfectly safe and uneventful pregnancies. Taking your medications (though your dosing may have to be adjusted once you become pregnant), keeping your thyroid levels under control (by having regular blood tests), and getting regular medical monitoring are the keys to your fertility success. Though your regular physician or gynaecologist may be able to treat your thyroid condition successfully, it's sometimes best if an endocrinologist supervises your care, too.

Male Infertility

When a couple has difficulty conceiving, approximately 35 to 40 percent of the time the issue can be traced back to the man – usually in the form of a sperm disorder. Low sperm quality (such as sperm with chromosomal defects) can cause fertility problems and/or lead to miscarriage. Any deficiency in sperm count (the number of sperm), sperm motility (ability to move), forward progression (quality of movement), and/or sperm size and shape can also cause fertility difficulties. The ability of sperm to move and the quality of that movement are more important to overall fertility than sperm count. In fact, many men with low sperm count are still fertile.

What are some of the causes of sperm disorders?

- Anatomical problems, such as scrotal varicocele (in which varicose veins around a testicle hinder sperm production – about 15 percent of men have varicoceles, and most can be repaired with surgery); retrograde ejaculation (in which the ejaculate flows backward into the bladder instead of out through the penis); undescended testicle (in which the testicle failed to complete its descent into the scrotum by infancy and therefore doesn't function normally); or erectile dysfunction (ED, the inability to get or maintain an erection, essential for ejaculation). Sometimes medications and/or surgery can correct these problems so that fertility is restored. Assisted reproduction techniques (such as IVF) can also get around these problems.

- Age. While men can be fertile well into their 80s, sperm quality and mobility gradually start to decline at age 40. Sometimes this downward trend begins to affect fertility, sometimes it doesn't.

- Immune problems. In rare cases, a man may produce antibodies that treat sperm as foreign invaders. These antibodies attack the sperm, adversely affecting sperm motility and sometimes its ability to fertilize an egg. Corticosteroids can be used to decrease the production of anti-sperm antibodies. If that fails, fertility treatments (such as IVF or ICSI; see pages 169 to 171) can help bypass the antibody problem.

- Underweight. Very low weight in men can be linked to lower sperm count and decreased sperm function. Once an underweight man gains weight, this fertility issue can disappear.

- Obesity. Men who are obese or even overweight may have infertility prob-

little thyroid hormone is produced. Signs of an underactive thyroid (hypothyroid) can include a goiter (a ball-like swelling in the neck), unexplained weight gain (or trouble losing weight), thinning hair, dry skin, low energy, depression, constipation, irregular or otherwise abnormal periods, and problems getting pregnant. Those who have an overactive thyroid (hyperthyroid) can have such symptoms as fatigue, hair loss, shortness of breath, constant hunger, weight loss, sweating, weakness, and irregular periods.

Thyroid condition often runs in families (the association between female family members is particularly strong), so if anyone in your family has it, you lems. That's because excess fat converts the male hormone testosterone into the female hormone oestrogen, possibly suppressing sperm production and lowering overall sperm quality. Weight loss can reverse this type of infertility.

- STDs. Untreated sexually transmitted diseases could damage the male reproductive tract, making it hard or impossible for sperm to be transported properly. Treatment of STDs can restore fertility in most cases.

- Uncontrolled chronic diseases such as diabetes can cause ED. Some medications can also impact sexual function, as well as affect sperm (see page 10). Getting chronic conditions under control can increase your chances of conception.

- Mumps (if it was contracted after puberty) can sometimes adversely affect testicular function, as can some other childhood infections and diseases.

- Cancer treatments. Chemotherapy and radiation targeting certain areas of the body may contribute to fertility issues in men (see box, next page).

Lifestyle and environmental factors can also play a role in male fertility problems – in these cases, eliminating the factor can eliminate the problem:

- Prolonged exposure of the testicles to high temperatures (in hot tubs, hot baths, from laptops, or with electric blankets, for instance) can damage sperm.

- Extreme bicycling, sports trauma to the penis and/or testicles, or extremely intense exercise routines may lower sperm production.

- Exposure to toxic substances (such as pesticides, X-rays, or other environmental or occupational hazards) may affect sperm production and quality.

- Use of illegal drugs, including pot, excessive use of alcohol, and smoking can also impact male fertility and sperm production, as can some medications.

- Lubricants can affect sperm quality (see page 104 for more on lubes).

- Extreme emotional stress can also depress testosterone levels and thus sperm production.

- While the jury is still out, there is some preliminary data that excessive mobile phone radiation may possibly alter sperm cells (see page 35).

If you have concerns about the quality or health of your sperm or if you suspect any kind of sperm disorder or testicular dysfunction, be sure to schedule an appointment with a doctor to check it out.

---

may want to be tested for it. Even if there's no one in your family with the condition, some experts recommend you get tested during the preconception period anyway – particularly if you're having trouble getting pregnant. Testing for abnormal thyroid antibodies may also be recommended. Even women who test normal for thyroid levels sometimes have abnormal thyroid antibody levels, a sign of a related autoimmune dysfunction.

How is fertility affected? Many women with a thyroid condition have no problems getting pregnant, but for some, thyroid dysfunction can prevent ovulation by disrupting the balance of reproductive hormones, leading to irregular periods and problems becoming pregnant.

What are the treatment options?
Normalizing thyroid function is usually as easy as popping a daily pill and having regular blood tests to keep an eye on your levels. Once any imbalance is corrected, a thyroid condition shouldn't interfere with your fertility.

Cancer and Fertility

Cancer diagnoses are always heartbreaking, but they can be especially devastating to men and women who plan to have children one day. Happily, thanks to advanced treatment options, cancer survival rates for young people are at an all-time high. Though these treatments are life saving, some of them can also lead to infertility. Educating yourself about the fertility risks and options for becoming a parent after cancer is important so you can make the choices that are best for you.

So what are your options for saving your fertility before cancer treatments?

- Egg freezing. In this procedure, your eggs are retrieved following hormonal stimulation and then frozen until needed.

- Embryo freezing. Once your eggs are retrieved, they are fertilized with sperm (from a donor or your partner) and the resulting embryos are frozen until needed.

- Ovarian tissue freezing. If you don't want to (or can't) have hormonal stimulation to retrieve eggs, ovarian tissue freezing is an experimental surgical procedure in which ovarian tissue is removed, frozen, and then reimplanted after treatment with the hope that it will resume normal functioning.

- Ovarian shielding, or moving the ovaries outside the radiation field, is a method that minimizes the dangers of radiation to your ovaries and eggs and may be an option depending on the type of cancer you have and the treatments that are necessary.

Sometimes, fertility returns after treatment, making a natural conception possible. If it turns out that your fertility has been permanently affected and you're unable to conceive naturally, you can use assisted reproductive techniques with the frozen eggs or embryos. Donor eggs can also be considered as an option. You'll need to talk to your doctor and oncologist to make sure pregnancy will be safe. Most of the time, it will be.

For men, cancer and its treatment can damage fertility, too. Sperm banking before treatment can preserve the ability to father a baby. Testicular tissue freezing is an experimental option that may be available for you, too.

For more information and help for cancer patients regarding fertility, go to www.cancerhelp.org.uk.

When You Need a Little Help

YOU'VE BEEN WORKING HARD AT TTC. You can pinpoint ovulation with your eyes closed, you've got your sex timing and positioning down to a science. But things (as in sperm and egg) are just not clicking yet and you're still not pregnant. Maybe you (and your doctor) have found a reason for your fertility frustrations. Maybe there's no known cause. Whatever the case, you're probably wondering: How long should we keep trying on our own? Is it time to consider seeing an infertility specialist? And if we do need a little help, what are our options?

Do You Need Help?

If your plans to start a family are going nowhere fast, you might be thinking about seeing a fertility specialist. But are you getting worried too soon? Should you just continue trying for a few more months? Or should you get started with a fertility workup just in case? Read on for answers to these (and other) questions.

When to Get Help

"We've been trying to conceive for 6 months already. Is it time to find a fertility specialist?"

Considering how fundamental a human function it is (there couldn't be humans without it), conception isn't as easy to achieve as you'd think. Sure, it can happen overnight – or even after one early morning quickie – but it usually takes much longer. In fact, under the best of circumstances, a couple with no known fertility issues has only a 20 to 25 percent chance of conceiving in a given menstrual cycle – which means they have a 75 to 80 percent chance of coming up empty at the end of any given month. So no need to jump to any conclusions about your fertility – or to jump in your car and head for the nearest

Fertility Treatment and the NHS

When you're feeling those fertility frustrations, help is at hand. Make an appointment with your GP, who can tell you about the fertility treatments available on the NHS in your area – options vary depending where you live. The criteria for treatment may differ from region to region, too, so your doctor can advise whether you are already eligible for a referral, or how you can go about qualifying for one. Sometimes there are waiting lists, which can understandably add to frustration. If you are keen to get that baby on board sooner rather than later, treatment at a private clinic may be an alternative to explore – that is, if it's financially feasible (private treatment can be very pricey).

Three main types of treatment are available on the NHS:

■ Fertility drugs. For those women who ovulate irregularly or not at all, fertility drugs such as Clomid or Metformin may be given to encourage the monthly release of an egg (see page 160).

■ Surgical procedures. If your fallopian tubes are scarred or blocked, a surgical procedure to repair the tubes may be suggested. For women with endometriosis, laparoscopic surgery is often used (see page 140).

■ Assisted conception. The option for assisted conception is in vitro fertilization (better known as IVF; see page 169), which in some cases may include intra-cytoplasmic sperm injection (ICSI; see page 171). Donor eggs or sperm may also be used in IVF. The number of cycles of IVF and ICSI the NHS will cover varies from region to region so, depending on your situation, you could be eligible for between 1 and 3 funded cycles.

fertility clinic – if sperm and egg don't meet up right away.

That said, if you've reached the 6-month mark of active trying (following all the recommended baby-making guidelines) without accomplishing your mission, you might want to start thinking about next steps – though it might be too early to actually start taking those steps right now. Here's the usual fertility rule of thumb when it comes to when to seek help: If you and your partner have no known reproductive problems and you're under 35, consider trying on your own for a year. If you're older than 35 and don't have any known fertility issues, help is usually suggested after 3 to 6 months of trying without success, though you can seek it earlier if you're concerned about running out of time. If you are 38 or older, many doctors recommend beginning those workups after just 3 months. And if you're over 40 or have a history of medical problems or a family history of infertility or any other factors that might impede fertility, it makes sense to arm yourself with the right help right from the start, to give your more challenging campaign the best chance for success.

But before you start Googling fertility specialists in your area, pick up the phone and make an appointment to see your regular doctor. Find out if he or she can handle your fertility needs (at least any initial workup) or whether you'll likely need a specialist on board, too. Even if your regular practitioner would be out of his or her league with your particular fertility scenario – and suggests that a fertility specialist be called in to consult or take over your diagnosis and treatment – he or she should still be on your team.

Keep in mind that you may not nab an appointment with your doctor right away, and that you'll almost certainly have a wait before getting on the books with a fertility specialist, so plan ahead (in other words, call for that appointment a month or two before your "cut-off" date). The worst (or rather the best) that can happen? You make the appointment, and then have to cancel – and schedule a prenatal visit instead – because you're pregnant!

Which Specialist Is Best?

"I don't know the first place to start with finding a fertility specialist – all I know is we're having trouble conceiving and we have no clue why."

If sperm and egg aren't meeting on their own, which type of practitioner would be the best matchmaker? Your doctor is a good place to start because he or she can begin a basic fertility workup and either treat your fertility issues on his or her own or send you for a more complete workup and more advanced

treatment with a reproductive endocrinologist (RE) – a fancy way of saying "fertility specialist".

The good news is that in most cases, fertility difficulties can be resolved by a doctor without an extensive fertility evaluation or treatment by an infertility specialist. And even if you're sent to an RE, it doesn't mean you're starting down the path of high-tech (and expensive) fertility treatments. In fact, most couples can be treated with simple medications and/or minor surgery and possibly intra-uterine insemination (IUI) and never even have to attempt the more involved in vitro fertilization (IVF).

Whichever type of doctor you're seeing (or even if you're seeing more than one), come prepared with a list of questions. Knowledge is power, and the more you know about tests and treatment options you might be facing, the easier they'll be to face. Here are some suggestions for questions you may want to ask your doctor or RE:

- What tests and workups would you recommend to figure out why I haven't conceived yet?

- Should my partner be tested? Should he be tested first or at the same time?

- What are the tests for male fertility?

Finding a Reproductive Endocrinologist

How do you go about finding a fertility specialist if you end up needing one? Your best lead will probably come from your doctor, who will likely refer you to one who he or she recommends and works with often. You can also ask friends who have had fertility challenges. Or go to the Human Fertilisation and

Embryology Authority (www.hfea.gov.uk), which regulates all UK fertility clinics. You'll definitely want a specialist you feel comfortable with – one who comes with a stellar success rate and unbeatable credentials, but also an exam-side manner that puts you at ease – so consider a consult before you sign up for care.

- How much will the test cost, if I'll be paying out of pocket?

- How long will it take to diagnose a problem if there is one?

- Based on the results of those tests, what are my treatment options?

- How much will the treatments cost, if I'll be paying out of pocket?

- How long do we try one treatment option before we move on to another?

- What is your success rate with fertility treatments?

- Are there any side effects to the fertility treatments you're suggesting?

The Fertility Workup

"What's involved in a fertility workup? And do we both get worked up at the same time?"

Trying to find out why the seemingly simple process of reproduction isn't working can be a little complicated – especially for women (sorry). In fact, the workup for men is so much easier (as is the treatment of any diagnosed fertility issue), that it's sometimes recommended that workups start with him. Talk to your practitioner about the best way to proceed, and whether you should be worked up one at a time or in tandem.

At-Home Fertility Screening

Anxious to access the state of your fertility, but not so anxious to head off to the doctor's office for all that poking, prodding, and testing – at least not yet? Is your partner not especially enthusiastic about doing his business and providing a sperm sample in such a public setting (even with the door locked)? There are some his-and-her screening tests that both of you can try at home, at least to get you started.

For him, the test can measure the concentration of motile sperm using a special test device that gives results using a test line (like a pregnancy test). One line indicates a low level of motile sperm; two lines indicate a normal concentration of motile sperm. Some brands measure sperm count (but not whether they are motile) with colour-changing solutions to show the results or with a microscope (provided with the kit).

For her, the at-home screening test measures the level of FSH on the third day of a period using a urine test similar to a pregnancy test. An abnormally high level indicates a low ovarian reserve (see page 98).

Though this at-home screening isn't a substitute for a thorough exam and evaluation by your doctor or fertility specialist (the results, while more than 90 percent accurate, are not definitive), it does give you a heads-up on what you might – or might not – find if you do eventually go for the full fertility workup. It's also far from comprehensive in what it can look for and find (you'll only be able to test for the very basics, not for such fertility-related issues as blocked tubes, cysts, varicoceles, and so on).

Finally, though an at-home screening is definitely cheaper than a full-on fertility screening, it's still pricey – so you may want to decide if you'll be getting what you pay for before putting in your order.

Just You and a Cup

Not convinced you want to perform *the* activity at a doctor's office – with medical personnel waiting outside to retrieve your sperm sample? Not to worry. First of all, you may be able to take care of this business at home, depending on how far from the doctor's office or lab you live (though you will have to deliver it pretty promptly after producing it, and keep it at room temperature en route). So ask if at-home masturbation is a possibility for you. If it isn't, keep in mind that the staff at the facility will be nothing if not professional and discreet. They'll also give you all the time and privacy you need – as well as an impressive stack of visual aids (magazines and/or DVDs) to get your mind off your sterile surroundings (and the fact that you're romancing a cup). Plus, you'll be more than ready to produce since you'll have been instructed to avoid ejaculation for anywhere from 48 to 72 hours in advance of generating your sample.

Either way, here's what you can typically expect from your fertility workups.

For him. The male fertility exam includes:

- A general physical, as well as a thorough examination (while standing) of the testes, scrotum, and penis, and perhaps a culture from the opening of the penis to rule out infection (don't worry – it's quick, easy, and usually painless). Since one possible cause of fertility difficulties is varicoceles in the scrotal sac (see page 148), the doctor will carefully examine the testicles to make sure everything checks out fine in that department. Believe it or not, the doctor may also want to do an underwear check (since overly tight briefs may have fertility implications).

- A semen analysis. While it's inherently unfair that the female workup involves (as you'll read later) needles and ultrasounds, and the male workup involves a stack of porn and one of his favourite pastimes since school, a semen analysis is still a crucial first step in figuring out where the fertility problem might be coming from. A sperm analysis checks the quantity and quality of sperm in the ejaculate (there should be more than 20 million sperm per millilitre of semen and more than 50 percent of them should be moving). The sperm analysis may also look at sperm DNA fragmentation (in other words, sperm that is "broken"). For optimum fertility, no more than 30 percent of sperm DNA should be fragmented. If the numbers come back low, the test is repeated (sperm count varies from ejaculate to ejaculate).

He'll likely be told to avoid ejaculation for 2 to 3 days before the semen analysis so that his sperm count will be at its highest. If multiple samples will be necessary, it's best to obtain them using the same spacing (in other words, if his first sample was produced 3 days after his last ejaculation, the next should also be produced after a 3-day wait). To produce the semen sample, he'll be asked to ejaculate into a clean sample cup – either in a private room in the doctor's office or, if you live close enough to the office, at home just before bringing it to the office for

Taking the Emotional Leap

You've put your all, and then some, into making a baby – devoting months to exhaustive fertility charting, exhausting baby dancing, and emotionally draining ups (it's time to test again!) and downs (it's negative again!). You and your partner have done absolutely everything you physically can to conceive on your own – but emotionally, you're not sure whether you're ready to look for help.

Beginning the fertility treatment process is an emotional leap. Making a baby is supposed to be a natural process, and a beautiful one – one that brings two people in love together in the most intimate of physical acts, so they can create a child who will forever be a symbol of that love. Taking that process out of the bedroom and into sterile exam rooms and treatment centres, making it a clinical experience instead of a personal one, can seem to rob it of its wonder and its innocence. It's also, once and for all, an admission that you have a fertility problem, and no amount of trying and waiting is likely to change that. And that can be tough for you both to accept.

Not only aren't you alone in your situation (about 1 in 6 to 1 in 8 couples have problems with infertility), you're not alone in feeling this way. Just about every couple experiences a wide range of conflicting emotions – from sadness to anticipation to guilt to ambivalence to jealousy of those who conceive with ease – as they contemplate ending one path to conception and beginning another. But the truth is, the sooner you overcome this emotional hurdle, the sooner you can begin the treatment that can make your baby dreams come true, finally.

Which isn't to say getting the help you need will bring you the results you're hoping for right away (depending on the cause of your infertility, treatment may be quicker than you'd imagine or take even longer than you feared). There may be plenty of ups and downs ahead of you – just as there were when you were trying to conceive naturally. And considering the even higher stakes (especially if you're paying a premium for the treatments), any downs may be harder to handle. But the first step, deciding to take the leap and make that first round of appointments, is the most important one. You're on your way – and you're on your way together.

The more support you gather for your journey, the better. Look to each other, of course (open communication will not only help you both get through the experience, but it will also help strengthen your bond), but turn, too, to those who know exactly what you're going through. Join a support group online or in your neighbourhood for insights, reassurance, validation of your feelings, and the pep talks you'll sometimes need.

---

testing. If it's possible to produce the sample at home, be sure to get it to the office within an hour, carrying it in a bag or coat pocket (it shouldn't get too hot or cold – room temperature is best). If the thought of masturbating into a cup isn't appealing to your guy, ask the doctor if you can use a special condom during intercourse to collect the sample instead. That sample, too, would have to be rushed to the lab (so much for the post-coital cuddling).

For her. The female fertility workup is a little more involved than the man's. It can include:

- A physical exam and a comprehensive pelvic exam if one was not done recently (during a preconception visit). A Pap smear will also be done to rule out abnormal cervical cells or infections.

- A blood test to determine levels of reproductive hormones. Usually taken on day 3 of your cycle, the test will check FSH levels to gauge ovarian reserve (see page 98) and oestrogen (abnormally high levels on day 3 may indicate ovarian cysts or diminished ovarian reserve). Another blood test taken after ovulation will test for pro-

gesterone to confirm that ovulation has taken place. Other hormone levels (such as thyroid and prolactin) may also be checked.

- Pelvic ultrasound (usually performed vaginally) to determine the number of egg follicles in the ovaries and how they are growing, as well as to visualize the uterus and cervix.

- A post-coital test (the name says it all) performed a few hours after intercourse. The test, which uses a cervical mucus swab to look at how his sperm swims in your cervical fluid, is done 1 to 2 days before ovulation (you'll need to be keeping track of your cycles to time it right). Within 2

Getting Help Doesn't Hurt

Maybe going to the doctor is not your favourite thing. Maybe you even have a long list of reasons why you've spent your entire adult life avoiding medical treatment (unless it's the kind you can buy yourself in the pharmacy, preferably in a box that doesn't call a lot of attention to itself). Maybe the last thing you feel like doing is sharing your most personal bodily functions – and your most private body parts – with a stranger wearing a white coat and latex gloves. Or even worse, sharing with that stranger the trouble you and your partner have had making the baby you both want.

Completely understandable. Completely normal. But getting the help you and your partner need to conceive can help you achieve that happiest outcome you've been hoping for and trying for – and help you achieve it sooner. Yes, there will be exams and tests involved – and a lot

of waiting (waiting for appointments, waiting for test results). Yes, it may be financially draining – if you decide to go private. Yes, it'll often be emotionally draining, too. But it will all be for the ultimate payoff: that beautiful bundle of baby you've been longing for so long.

Read up on fertility screenings, as well as on the most common fertility treatments, so you'll start the process with some idea of what you can expect. Talk over your fears and anxieties, if you have any, with your partner (she's probably feeling the same ambivalence – even if she's been the one who's been actively lobbying for seeking fertility help). It's a big step, but it's a step you'll be taking together. Remember, although you're bringing on another team member or two, and you're considering a major change of strategy, the game plan is the same – go out there and make a baby.

to 8 hours after you have sex with your partner (in private at home), you'll go to the doctor's office where the test (similar to a Pap smear) will be done.

■ A hysterosalpingogram (HSG) – an assessment of the uterus and fallopian tubes using X-ray imaging and dye (for contrast) to make sure there are no blockages in the fallopian tubes or scarring in the fallopian tubes or uterus that might be preventing conception. Alternatively, your doctor may perform a sonohystogram, an essentially painless test where saline is infused into the uterus through the cervix while the uterus is visualized on ultrasound.

Sound like you (and your doctor) have your work cut out for you? You definitely do. Be prepared for the workup to take 6 to 8 weeks before all the tests are completed and the results compiled and evaluated. Once the results are back in, your doctor will discuss with you the best plan of action to help you conceive.

Treatment Options

So you've both been worked over, maybe more than once. You've done plenty of waiting – and more waiting – for the results. But it's all worth it, you figure, because finally, you'll have the diagnosis that will solve the mystery of your infertility, and with it, the treatment that will bring you one step closer to filling your belly – and, ultimately, your arms – with the baby you've been hoping for.

Sometimes, it is as simple as that – diagnosing is easy and treatment an easy fix. A correctable condition is discovered, and all that's needed is minor surgery to remove some scarring or a cyst, or some thyroid replacement therapy to jump-start your cycles.

But that discovery isn't always easy, or even possible to make. Often, not even that exhaustive – and exhausting – full battery of tests and screenings (and needle pokes and embarrassing sperm collections) uncovers the exact cause of a fertility problem. Many couples end up with the finding "unexplained infertility" – and isn't that where you started in the first place, before all the testing began?

Fortunately, in most cases you don't need a definitive diagnosis to treat a fertility issue. No matter what the cause – and even if there is no known cause – there's usually at least one treatment option for every couple that's facing a fertility challenge. The following is an overview of the most common treatments – including, fertility fingers crossed and double-crossed, the one with your beautiful baby-to-be's name on it.

Surgery

While surgery to correct fertility problems used to be the first line of defence in treating infertile couples, doctors today are depending more and more on assisted reproductive techniques (ART; see more in this chapter) instead of surgery. Still, depending on what's causing your infertility, your doctor might suggest certain surgical procedures to help get you closer to conception.

Surgery for Male Infertility

For men struggling with infertility due to a sperm flow problem, a number of surgical procedures may offer some help depending on the type of problem:

- If you are among the 15 percent of men who have a varicocele (a condition in which sperm production is compromised due to abnormal blood flow to the area and varicose veins around a testicle, elevated scrotal temperature, and a reflux of toxins back into the testicle) your doctor may recommend a varicocelectomy to treat the problem, and hopefully restore fertility. The surgery is relatively simple, involving one or two small incisions in the lower abdomen that allow the doctor access to repair the abnormal veins. Once the repair is made, sperm production should return to normal. Whether the surgery helps resolve infertility problems is still being debated. Critics of the surgery say that there is little improvement in pregnancy rates after the surgery, while experts who favour varicocele repair say it's an easy – and proven – treatment for male infertility.

- If you've had a vasectomy but now want to have it reversed so your partner can conceive, surgery can help. Your doctor will perform a vasovasostomy (or, depending on how many blockages you may have, a less common procedure called an epididymostomy). In a vasovasostomy procedure, the doctor restores sperm flow simply by reconnecting the ends of your previously cut vas deferens. In an epididymostomy, the doctor connects the vas deferens directly to the epididymis to allow the sperm to flow through. Nearly all men who have a vasovasostomy produce sperm following the surgery. As many as 90 percent of men who have had an epididymostomy will produce sperm – but since the procedure may affect sperm quality, conception success rates are lower than with vasovasostomy.

- If tests have found you have blockages in the vas deferens or the epididymis (often caused by STDs, infections, or trauma) or in the ejaculatory duct (usually the result of cysts in the prostate or scarring), surgery (either a type similar to a vasovasostomy or sperm duct microsurgery) can help the sperm bypass the blockages and get to where they need to go for conception. These types of rare blockages can also be bypassed by removing sperm directly from the epididymis (in a procedure called microsurgical epididymal sperm aspiration, or MESA) or directly from the testicle (called testicular sperm extraction, or TESE) and then turning to assisted reproduction techniques to attempt conception.

For instance, if tests find that you have anatomical problems in your uterus, cervix, or vagina (and these problems are preventing you from conceiving or maintaining a pregnancy), surgery can be a quick way to fix the problem and enable you to conceive a baby on your own. If you have scar tissue in your uterus or fallopian tubes, surgery can clear the path for sperm and egg to meet. Tumours, cysts, fibroids, and endometrial lesions can also be removed surgically.

Often, surgery is performed with a hysteroscope, an instrument inserted through the cervix and into the uterus that visualizes the uterine cavity. If any abnormalities are found (such as fibroids, scar tissue, or a septum – when tissue divides the uterus in two), additional instruments can be inserted through the hysteroscope to remove or repair the problems. Another procedure, known as laparoscopy, is used to view all the pelvic organs and, if necessary, to remove endometrial lesions, ovarian cysts, scar tissue, or fibroids. Your doctor inserts a long viewing tube (or laparoscope) through an incision in your belly button. To perform the surgery, he or she inserts the necessary surgical tools through small incisions near your bikini line. Laparotomy microsurgery (in which the surgeon looks through magnifying glasses while removing scar tissue or endometrial lesions) is another option, but is used less often. For women suffering with fibroids, the surgery of choice is often a myomectomy using laparoscopy (see page 139). Most of the time, surgery is done as an outpatient procedure (you'll be able to go home only a few hours after the surgery is complete) and the recovery is usually quick.

Tubal Reversal Surgery

What if your tubes are tied – but now you're wishing they weren't (so you could pick up your nest filling where you last left off)? Luckily, those tied tubes won't likely stand between you and your renewed baby dreams. One option is to bypass the tubes altogether, and go directly to IVF. Because fertilization takes place outside of your body with IVF, and the resulting embryo (or embryos) is placed directly into destination uterus, the fallopian tubes (the tubes that are "tied") aren't needed.

If you'd like to try to conceive the old-fashioned way, you may be able to have surgery to reverse your tubal ligation (depending on whether your fallopian tubes were cut, tied, cauterized, or nonsurgically blocked). Tubal reversal surgery is most commonly performed through an incision in the abdomen (though some doctors perform it laparoscopically). The surgery is not a walk in the park, unfortunately (you'll need to stay in the hospital for a few days) and recovery can take a few weeks. Still, it could definitely prove worthwhile – there is a 70 to 80 percent pregnancy success rate (for women under 35 with no other fertility problems) within a year post-surgery (though the procedure slightly elevates the risk of ectopic pregnancy).

Before you go the surgery route, however, you'll want to make sure your partner's sperm is top notch (it would be a waste to have the tubal reversal only to find out later that his sperm count is low and IVF is your only conception option). Your doctor will also want to verify (through a hysterosalpingogram) that your remaining tubes are long enough to be reattached successfully (the shorter they are, the lower the chances for a pregnancy), and that you have no other fertility issues.

Clomid

If your fertility workup shows you're not ovulating regularly, you've got a lot of company. About a third of all women struggling to get pregnant have ovulation issues, sometimes explained, often not. But for many, there's an easy fix in a little pill. Clomiphene citrate, aka Clomid or Serophene, stimulates your ovaries to release eggs and corrects irregular ovulation. You'll begin by taking 50 mg of Clomid on the second or third (or sometimes fifth) day of your period for 5 days. If you don't begin to ovulate right away, the dose will be increased by 50 mg per day each month up to 150 mg. Once the drug is working and you've begun to ovulate, you'll likely be kept on Clomid for 3 to 6 months. If you haven't conceived by the sixth month on Clomid, you'll move on to other medications and/or assisted fertility techniques.

Clomid works by making your body think oestrogen levels are low (who said you can't fool Mother Nature?). When your body finds itself low on oestrogen, it compensates by producing more FSH and LH, stimulating the development of the follicle (and egg) and causing ovulation to occur. After that, it's a sort of domino effect – but the good kind (the kind that's meant to knock you up, not knock you down). The development of the eggs kicks up your oestrogen, which in turn helps produce better quality cervical mucus (for most, but not all, women; some women find their CM becomes dry and sticky while on Clomid), making it easier for those sperm to hitch a ride toward the egg or eggs now being released. Higher levels of oestrogen also beef up your uterine lining, and a thicker lining makes a much more hospitable implantation site for a fertilized egg – and one in which it'll be easier to stay implanted. And there's more to this chain of happy events: More eggs means more progesterone (produced by the corpus luteum that's left behind after an egg is released). More progesterone also helps build a strong lining for that egg to latch on to, plus helps maintain a new pregnancy. Best of all, by the time fertilization occurs, Clomid is out of your system, meaning it won't harm your newly conceived baby (or babies).

Happily, there are few side effects with Clomid, at least as far as hormone treatments go, and if you do experience them (bloating, nausea, headache, hot flashes, breast pain, mood swings, and in rare cases, ovarian cysts), don't worry – they're only temporary. Some women also experience vaginal dryness. Though there's an increased chance that more than one follicle and egg will be stimulated (you'll have a 10 percent chance of conceiving twins), your doctor will keep you on the lowest dose possible to keep those chances down. While you're taking your first round of Clomid, you'll have to see your doctor or RE often for ultrasounds and blood tests to make sure the drug's working the way it's supposed to.

While Clomid is the most common fertility drug, it's far from the only one. There are other drugs that your doctor or RE might prescribe instead of or in addition to Clomid, all with about the same side effects. Whatever the drug, its mission is the same: to encourage the maturation of eggs. And ready-to-roll eggs are good news when you're trying to fill your nest.

Hormone Shots

If Clomid doesn't do the trick, your doctor might kick it up a notch to hormone injections, which pack a more powerful fertility punch. Your doctor or fertility specialist will put together a cocktail of hormones that you'll learn to inject yourself with (see box, next page), or your partner will learn to inject you with if you're too squeamish. These injectable hormones work directly on the ovaries to help mature the follicles and eggs and stimulate ovulation – basically triggering the same reproductive chain reaction as Clomid, but with much more bang. You'll use injectable hormones in conjuction with intrauterine insemination (IUI) or, if that doesn't work, with in vitro fertilization (IVF).

Some possible side effects to hormone injections – though you may not

Shots: A Pain in the . . . Thigh?

So, chances are you've been on the receiving end of your fair share of needles over the years – but unless you're a medical professional or a diabetic, it's not likely you've ever given an injection, particularly not to yourself. Yet, if hormone injections are going to be a part of your fertility treatment plan, inject you must (that is unless you can talk your partner into wielding the needle – if so, have him read over this tutorial, too).

Needle-phobic by nature? Afraid to take the plunge (into your soft, delicate skin)? Some needle novices find it helps to start with some fruit – not for a snack, but for practice. Using an empty syringe (no need to shoot up a plum with hormones), stab away until you're feeling like a pro – at least when it comes to produce.

Don't try your first stab at real injections at home, though. You'll feel more comfortable if you (or your partner) tackle your first shot attempt at your doctor's office, under close supervision and with supportive guidance. You'll be given specific instructions on when, where (in the muscle or under the skin), and how to give the injections. It's best to follow doctor's orders, of course, but just in case you've forgotten the basics by the time you get home (or you blank on everything that the doctor or nurse showed you yesterday), here's a step-by-step guide. Keep in mind that the first few times may be stressful (especially for the squeamish), but before you know it, you'll be injecting with ease.

1. Pick a spot in your home. Ideally, you'll want to find a quiet area where there will be minimal distractions (and away from any clamouring kids or curious pets). Also important is that the area is clean, for obvious reasons. The bathroom or kitchen are good choices because of the countertop space, and because they're easy to sanitize (compared to the living room sofa).

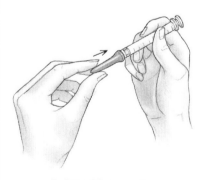

A. Attaching needle to syringe

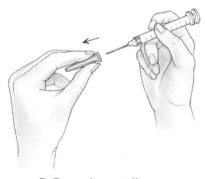

B. Removing needle cap

2. Set up. Wash your hands and set up a clean zone on a countertop to spread out your injection supplies (medication, syringes, alcohol swabs, needles, and disposal container). If you're going to want to numb your skin first, you'll need some ice handy, too. Make sure the needles do not touch anything other than the medication containers or the injection site – otherwise they'll become contaminated and unusable (in other words, keep the cap on the needle until you're ready to use it – just like the professionals do).

3. Choose the right syringe and needle (as directed by your doctor). If you're injecting the drug into your muscle (intramuscular), you've probably been told to use a 1-mL or 2-mL syringe. If you're injecting the drug under your skin (subcutaneous), you'll probably use a 1-mL syringe. Needles for subcutaneous injections are shorter (usually only 1¼ centimetres long) than ones for intramuscular injections (2½ to 5 centimetres long). If you need to mix the solution, you'll have to attach the large "mixing needle" firmly to the syringe first (illustration A). Continue with step 4.

4. Prepare the medication. Depending on the type of medication, you may need to dissolve powder into a solvent (liquid) before you inject. (Note: If your syringe comes prefilled, or if your medication comes in a prefilled "pen", skip ahead to step 6.) First remove the cap (illustration B) and pierce the rubber-stoppered cap of the solvent container with the larger mixing needle (illustration C). Draw up the solvent to the prescribed amount (you'll see the measurements on the side of the syringe; illustration D). You might have been instructed to turn the syringe so the needle is facing upward and then to tap out the air bubbles (illustration E). Then squirt the solvent into the container containing the powdered medication by piercing the rubber-stoppered cap with the same needle. Repeat until the proper dose of solvent is in the powdered solution. The powder, by the way, should dissolve

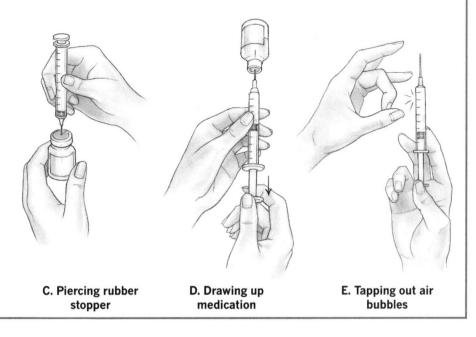

C. Piercing rubber stopper   **D. Drawing up medication**   **E. Tapping out air bubbles**

on contact with the fluid and the solution should look clear; if it doesn't, you can gently roll the vial between your hands to mix. (If the medication comes in glass vials – or ampules – you'll have to break off the tops and then prepare the medication as described.)

5. Replace the large needle that you used to prepare the medication with the finer needle necessary for the injection and load the prescribed amount of medication into the syringe by drawing up on the plunger.

6. It's shot time. You can do this!

For intramuscular injections:

■ First, identify your location. The best place to inject the medication is in the upper outer quadrant of your buttocks (just below the hip bone) or on the middle of the outside of the thigh (alternate sides for each injection so your muscles won't get sore).

■ Lie down, sit, or stand with your weight off the side you'll be injecting.

■ If you'd like, numb the targeted area with an ice cube.

■ Give the area to be injected a swab of alcohol and then let it air dry.

■ Remove the needle cap (illustration B, page 162), hold the syringe straight up, tap the sides of the syringe so no air bubbles remain (illustration E, previous page), and push the plunger slowly until you see a drop of the medication come out.

■ Take a big pinch of the area to be injected – taking both the skin and muscle – with your fingers. (Some doctors recommend pulling the skin taut instead of pinching; ask which is preferred in your case.)

■ Holding the syringe as shown in the illustrations below, quickly insert the needle at a 90-degree angle completely into the pinched skin and muscles, making sure none of the needle is exposed.

■ Draw back on the plunger. (In the unlikely case blood appears in the syringe, remove the needle, replace it

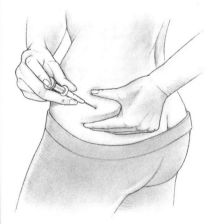

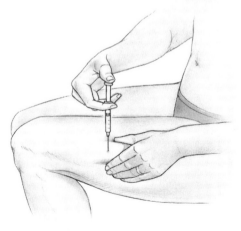

Injecting in the upper outer quadrant of the buttocks.

Injecting on the outside of the thigh

with a new needle, and repeat the process.) Then *slowly* push the plunger all the way to inject the medication.

- When you're done, quickly (but gently) pull the needle straight out.

- Gently massage the injection site for 30 seconds afterward to spread the medication. Ice can help minimize the pain.

- Dispose of the syringe in a biohazard container or another container that you can seal. Never reuse needles or syringes.

For subcutaneous injections:

- Identify your location. The best place to inject the medication is a few inches below and to the side of your belly button. You can also inject it on the top of your thigh or in the back of your upper arm.

- If you like, numb the area with an ice cube.

- Sterilize the area with the alcohol swab and let it air dry.

- Remove the needle cap (illustration B, page 162), hold the syringe straight up, tap the sides of the syringe so no air bubbles remain (illustration E, page 163), and push the plunger slowly until you see a drop of the medication come out.

- Pinch the area you'll be injecting with your fingers.

- Holding the syringe as shown in the illustration below, quickly insert the needle at a 45-degree angle until it's completely submerged, then release the fingers doing the pinching.

- Slowly depress the plunger, and when all the medication is injected, quickly (but gently) pull the needle straight out.

- Apply pressure to the injection site to stem any bleeding.

- Dispose of the syringe in a biohazard container or another container that you can seal. Never reuse needles or syringes.

7. Give yourself a pat on the back (after you've disposed of the syringe, that is).

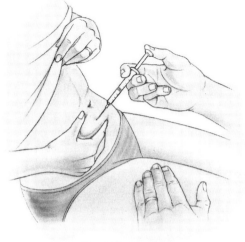

**Injecting below and
to the side of the belly button**

get any – include breast tenderness, mood swings, headache, abdominal pain, nausea, and, in rare cases, ovarian hyperstimulation (in which too many eggs are stimulated, causing pain and possible problems down the line). In most cases, women on these inject-able fertility drugs notice more cervical mucus – and that might aid in your con-ception quest (if you'll still be trying for a baby the natural way). While on fertil-ity drugs, you'll have to see your doctor or RE often for ultrasounds and blood tests to make sure everything's working the way it should be.

Here's the lowdown on some of the hormone shots you might be needing, but keep in mind that depending on your situation and the preferences of your doctor, you may be prescribed only one or two of these medications:

- Follicle-stimulating hormone (FSH). These injections (brand names include Fertinex, Fostimon, Puregon, Gonal-f, and Metrodin) act like your own natu-ral FSH to stimulate the development of egg follicles. You'll need to inject FSH daily, usually starting on days 2 to 4 of your cycle. Your doctor will use blood tests and ultrasounds to monitor the ovarian response, and if necessary, fine-tune the FSH dosage.

- Human menopausal gonadotropin (hMG). While "menopausal" doesn't sound promising when you're trying to make a baby, these hormones can deliver. The injections (brand names include Merional and Menopur) con-tain both FSH and LH – two impor-tant hormones necessary to stimulate the development of the follicles and the maturation of the eggs. You'll take the injection daily beginning at the start of your cycle for about 12 days. Blood tests and regular ultrasounds will allow your doctor to monitor how your ovaries are responding to the hormones

and whether or not the dosing needs to be tweaked.

- Human chorionic gonadotropin (hCG). This sounds more like it (after all, hCG is *the* pregnancy hormone). The brand names of this type of hormone injection include Ovidrel, Pregnyl, and Choragon, and they are used in conjunction with FSH or hMG injections, or even in conjunc-tion with Clomid. When one or more follicles reach the point of no return (ready to release a mature egg), you'll inject the hormone hCG. HCG is considered the pregnancy hormone because it shows up in your blood and urine once the embryo implants, but in this case, hCG will help trigger ovu-lation. Another bonus from the hCG: It improves the quality of the uterine lining, effectively plumping and fluff-ing it for the arrival of an embryo.

- Gonadotropin-releasing hormone, or GnRH agonist. Sometimes FSH or hMG injections can stimulate the release of eggs before they are mature. Enter a GnRH agonist (fortunately you don't have to spell it, you just have to inject it; brand names include Zoladex and Goserelin). GnRH agonist works on the pituitary gland to help prevent immature eggs from being released too soon. It does so by first increasing and then suppressing FSH and LH, pre-venting the LH surge (which triggers ovulation) and allowing additional time for more quality eggs to develop. It also helps produce a higher number of quality eggs. You'll probably start injecting Goserelin just before FSH and hMG shots are started if you're doing an IVF cycle.

- Gonadotropin-releasing hormone (GnRH) antagonist. Like GnRH ago-nists, this hormone injection (its brand names include Orgalutran, Ganirelix, and Cetrotide) is used in IVF cycles before FSH and hMG injections are started to prevent a too-soon LH surge – ensuring that eggs are released when they are mature and not before. GnRH antagonists work much faster than GnRH agonists, making this the drug of choice when premature ovulation needs to be prevented right away.

- Progesterone. In some cases, your doctor might tell you to inject progesterone daily, beginning 2 days after egg retrieval (if you're attempting IVF) and ending when the placenta is producing appropriate amounts of progesterone. Progesterone isn't always given as an injection. You might be able to use a vaginal gel, suppository, or even a pill.

Keep in mind that it may take several cycles and adjustments in your medication cocktail before you hit your optimal fertility prescription. Since every woman's fertility needs are different, every woman's fertility treatment plan will be different. To save yourself some stress and confusion, try not to compare your hormone injections to those of other hopeful mums you know (or hang out with on your TTC message board) who are undergoing treatment.

Intrauterine Insemination (IUI)

Sometimes, overcoming fertility challenges isn't just a matter of adjusting your hormones – sometimes either partner (or both) needs a little extra help in making the miracle of conception happen, for a variety of possible reasons. Intrauterine insemination (IUI) is performed when sperm count is low, when sperm have poor motility, when cervical fluid is found to be inhospitable

to sperm (as detected in a post-coital test), or when there is just no known infertility cause. IUI can be employed alone – without the use of fertility drugs or injections – or it can be used in conjunction with Clomid if ovulation issues have been identified as well. (IUI isn't often combined with hormone injections – most often injections go hand in hand with IVF or other assisted reproductive technology). The procedure gives the sperm a better chance of reaching their target by bypassing the initial hurdles they would encounter in the vagina – sort of a running (or swimming) head start.

The ART of Conception

For as long as there have been men and women, sperm and egg have been meeting up the old-fashioned way: through sex. And more often than not, they still do. But sometimes, physiological factors intervene to make that amazing meeting impossible, or at least, highly improbable. And that's when conception is turned over to science, and becomes an ART. Assisted reproductive technologies (ART) is the umbrella term for fertility treatments that bring sperm and egg together without intercourse. The objective of ART? To create an embryo in the lab, instead of in bed, thereby bypassing those fertility obstacles altogether. The most common ART procedure is in vitro fertilization (IVF). There are currently around 700 treatment cycles of IVF per million of the population in the UK, resulting in 10,000 babies born each year – that's a whole lot of ART!

A Look at IUI

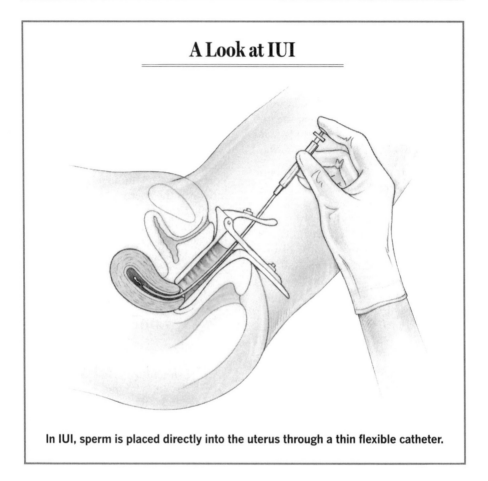

In IUI, sperm is placed directly into the uterus through a thin flexible catheter.

How does IUI work? Think turkey baster – only a little more sophisticated and a lot more precise. Around the time you're ovulating (either on your own or with the help of Clomid) and using a sperm sample from your partner that has been "washed" (the sperm is separated from the semen and the nonmotile sperm are separated from the motile sperm in a centrifuge), your doctor or nurse will insert a thin flexible catheter through your cervix and inject the healthy sperm directly into the uterus close to the fallopian tubes. The same process would occur if you are using donor sperm. In intracervical insemination, the sperm will be placed right at the cervix, and with FAST (fallopian sperm transfer) insemination, the sperm is placed directly in the fallopian tubes. The whole process takes only a few minutes and there isn't much discomfort (about as much as you'd have during a Pap smear).

Once the insemination is complete, the doctor places a cervical cap into your vagina and on your cervix to make sure the sperm doesn't drip out. You'll be able to remove it after a few hours (there's a string like on a tampon for easy removal). If after trying IUI for 3 to 6 cycles you still haven't achieved conception success, you'll likely be advised to move to the next step – IVF.

Ranking Your Clinic

How can you tell if the ART clinic you're about to visit has a good track record? Most reputable IVF clinics are licensed by the Human Fertilisation Embryology Authority (HFEA) – see www.hfea.gov.uk. You'll want to focus on the number of live births per retrieval as opposed to pregnancies (which doesn't factor in the miscarriage rate) when researching your clinic. Equally important: the clinic's multiples rate. Multiples come with the potential for multiplied risks. Triplet and higher-order multiples are associated with high rates of very preterm birth and other complications. Some centres achieve their high success rate by transferring more embryos, despite the possible risks, and that's a red flag.

If your clinic doesn't show up on the database, it could mean its success rate is so low that they're not reporting their numbers at all (and that's not a good sign). It could also mean the clinic you're visiting is too new to show up on the database (there's about a year or two delay with the reporting to allow for the pregnancies to conclude and to compile all the data). Still, you might want to think twice about going to a clinic without a proven track record. The HFEA website contains information on how to research clinics and what to expect in terms of treatment.

In Vitro Fertilization (IVF)

In vitro fertilization (IVF), considered the most effective of the ART techniques, is a good choice when there are blockages in the fallopian tubes, ovulation disorders, or a lot of sperm deficiencies. Here's how it works: Hormone injections (see page 161) are used over the course of a cycle to help stimulate your ovaries to produce eggs. Around days 12 to 14 of your cycle, the stimulated eggs will be mature and ready for retrieval. But instead of letting them "ovulate" on their own, your doctor will remove them for fertilization in the lab.

The eggs are retrieved transvaginally with a needle that reaches your ovaries and aspirates the egg from the follicle. The egg retrieval takes 20 to 40 minutes on average, and since you might feel some discomfort, your doctor may give you a light anaesthetic or pain reliever. While you're busy with the egg retrieval, your partner is busy producing a sperm sample. The healthiest eggs (as determined by an embryologist who examines and grades each egg immediately after retrieval) are placed together with "washed" sperm (the sperm is separated from the semen and the non-motile sperm are separated from the motile sperm in a centrifuge) in a laboratory dish for fertilization. Estimates are that at least 50 percent of mature eggs become fertilized during IVF.

Approximately 3 to 5 days after the eggs are successfully fertilized (though it could be shorter or longer than that depending on your doctor's preference), the embryos (usually more than one, though the number will depend on your choice and that of your doctor, your age, cause of infertility, and other factors) are slowly and carefully transferred into your uterus. Under ultrasound guidance, your doctor will insert a thin flexible catheter through your vagina and cervix into the uterus, and then gently

A Look at IVF

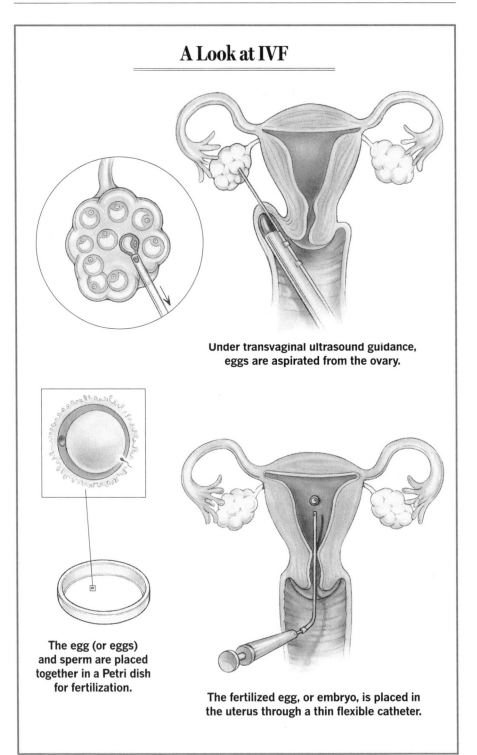

Under transvaginal ultrasound guidance,
eggs are aspirated from the ovary.

The egg (or eggs)
and sperm are placed
together in a Petri dish
for fertilization.

The fertilized egg, or embryo, is placed in
the uterus through a thin flexible catheter.

depress the attached syringe containing the embryos, placing them in your uterus with the hope that they will implant and continue to grow just as they would with unassisted conception. You'll likely rest for a short time (about half an hour) in the recovery room and then be advised to take it easy for a few days post-transfer. Then it's a 2-week wait from your egg retrieval until the blood test that will confirm whether or not the procedure was successful.

Intracytoplasmic Sperm Injection (ICSI)

ICSI, pronounced ICK-see, takes IVF one step further, focusing on a solution for male infertility. ICSI is used when the male partner has a very low sperm count, low sperm motility, or poor quality sperm. Instead of merely mixing your eggs and your partner's sperm in a Petri dish and hoping they get together, seal the deal, and make an embryo, the doctor actually injects a single sperm directly into an egg to assist with fertilization – basically eliminating all of the challenges that the little guy would otherwise have had to face (see illustration, this page).

Here's how it works: Egg retrieval is the same as it is for a regular IVF cycle. Once the eggs are retrieved, they are "washed" to loosen their protective outer coating. Then the sperm is slowed down with a chemical solution so it's easier for the technician to "catch" one. Then its tail is immobilized so it can safely puncture the egg's membrane and be injected deep inside the egg. Once the sperm is injected into the egg, fertilization (hopefully) occurs. As with IVF, if fertilization occurs, the embryo (or embryos) is transferred into the uterus – and less than 2 weeks later, you discover whether mission conception has

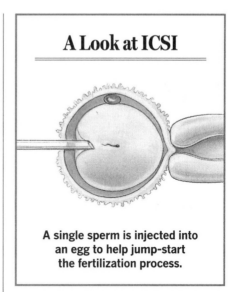

A Look at ICSI

A single sperm is injected into an egg to help jump-start the fertilization process.

been accomplished. For couples who undergo ICSI because of male factor infertility, when the woman is under 35 years old, the procedure is successful about 43 percent of the time. Women ages 35 to 37 can expect an almost 33 percent success rate; women 40 and over will have around an 8 percent chance of conceiving.

Assisted Hatching

Though assisted hatching sounds like something you'd find going on in a chicken coop, it's actually a highly specialized ART technique designed to make the implantation process less challenging for a fledgling lab-grown embryo. For an embryo to implant inside the uterus, it must "hatch" out of its protective shell (called the zona pellucida). When you conceive naturally, the trip the embryo takes down the fallopian tube enables the shell to thin, making it easier for the embryo to implant successfully in the endometrium. Embryos grown in a lab, however, don't have the benefit of that trip down fallopian lane, so some – though certainly not all – embryos created in vitro have a thicker than normal shell and may need an extra push to break out of it. In some women, this extra-thick shell may be the reason previous IVF attempts have failed. Enter assisted hatching – a procedure in which a laser is used to make a microscopic hole in the zona pellucida right before the embryo is transferred to the uterus. This tiny opening enables the cells of the embryo to escape the shell and attach more easily to the uterine wall. What will reproductive science come up with next?

Gamete Intrafallopian Transfer (GIFT)

There's no greater gift than a baby – and gamete intrafallopian transfer (GIFT) is a procedure that can help deliver that gift to some hopeful couples. GIFT is a more expensive and more invasive ART treatment than IVF, which is why it's used much less frequently, but it allows fertilization to occur naturally inside your fallopian tube instead of in a Petri dish. Eggs are stimulated and retrieved and sperm is collected as with IVF, but instead of having them meet up in the lab for their fertilization

The Agony of the Two-Week Wait

If you've been trying to conceive for a while (and if you've turned to ART, it's probably been a pretty long while), you've already done more than your share of waiting. Waiting for ovulation. Waiting to do an HPT – and then waiting to retest. Waiting for medications to work. Waiting for test results. Waiting for appointments with specialists and treatment centres. But probably the toughest wait is the one you have ahead of you after a round of IVF. Though you might feel hopefully pregnant the moment your embryos are transferred into your uterus, you'll have to wait 2 weeks from the day your eggs were retrieved for confirmation of a pregnancy.

Just because you've become a pro at waiting doesn't mean those two weeks won't be hard to handle. They can pass agonizingly slowly, and the mounting anticipation and anxiety can make it difficult to focus on anything else (work, romance, relationships, eating, sleep-

ing). As always, relaxation techniques may help you stress less while you're waiting. Eating well, as hard as it might be when you're so nervous, may also help reduce stress (and at the same time, reducing stress will help you eat well – which is so important if you do turn out to be expecting). Keeping a journal – writing down all of those conflicting feelings (excitement that you might be pregnant, dread that you might not be) – can help pass the time, and also help contain the emotional mayhem (you can use the journal starting on page 256). Venting in a blog will accomplish the same goal, and opening up a dialogue with others confronting fertility challenges can be enormously helpful all around. And speaking of dialogues, if you haven't already found an online support group (or a place to blog), check out the fertility treatments message board at WhatToExpect.com. No one knows what the waiting's like better than others playing the same waiting game.

How Many Embryos?

Since not every fertilized egg (whether it was fertilized inside a woman's body or inside a lab) turns into a baby, and because the process of egg retrieval, IVF, and embryo transfer is arduous (and costly) – not to mention emotionally draining – many doctors and their eager patients choose to implant more than one embryo when undergoing ART. The more the better when trying to up the odds of a successful pregnancy – right? Well, not always. Too many embryos can turn into too many babies – and multiple pregnancies are considered higher risk for both mum and her brood. The number of embryos that will be transferred will be decided between you and the clinic, using guidelines followed in both NHS and private treatment. For safety's sake (as well as a higher rate of success) a single embryo is considered the ideal, with a maximum of 2 transferred under most circumstances. In exceptional circumstances, or if you are over 40, you may be allowed 3 embryos.

rendezvous, the egg (or eggs) and sperm are combined right after retrieval and then placed soon after laparoscopically (through a small incision in your abdomen) into your fallopian tube. The hope is that sperm and egg will fertilize (usually within hours) and turn into an embryo, which will then make its way down to your uterus for implantation.

Because fertilization (hopefully) happens inside your body instead of inside a lab, the success rate with GIFT is relatively high. Experts speculate that the journey through the fallopian tube nourishes the new embryo, giving it a better chance of being healthy and able to implant in the uterus. Another reason for the increased success rate could be because the embryo arrives in the uterus at the "right" time for implantation (as opposed to IVF, in which the embryo arrives in the uterus when your doctor places it there – and that might not be exactly the time frame nature had in mind). Recovery from a GIFT procedure is the same as IVF done through the laparoscope (a few hours of rest and then taking it easy for a few days).

Zygote Intrafallopian Transfer (ZIFT)

With zygote intrafallopian transfer (ZIFT), the method is similar to GIFT but the eggs are fertilized in the laboratory before being placed (often within hours after fertilization) laparoscopically into your fallopian tube. Why would someone have a ZIFT procedure instead of a GIFT procedure? The advantage to ZIFT is that it's clear fertilization has taken place. With GIFT, the hope that fertilization occurs is there, but there's no way to know right away if egg and sperm are actually getting together to make a zygote (an early embryo). In effect, ZIFT gives a pregnancy a running start. ZIFT, like GIFT, is used very infrequently.

Egg Donation

Time was, a woman who wanted to experience pregnancy and childbirth had no choice but to use her own eggs, conceiving either naturally or with

Can CAM Lend a Hand?

There's definitely no shortage of high-tech techniques – from surgery to medications to IVF and more – that can help couples who are having trouble conceiving get pregnant. But can complementary and alternative medicine (CAM) techniques lend a reproductive hand as well?

The answer could be yes. Though the research is conflicting, some studies show that women receiving acupuncture treatment while undergoing IVF had higher rates of pregnancy (65 percent higher, in fact) than women who didn't use acupuncture. Still other research shows that women who are hypnotized before IVF embryo transfer are more likely to become pregnant than those who aren't. There's also research showing that electro-acupuncture (the application of a pulsating electrical current to acupuncture needles, further stimulating the acupoints) may help induce ovulation in women with PCOS. Whether the benefits come from physiological factors or from a mind-body connection is unclear, but either way, it's hard to argue with the potential of even slightly greater success – especially when it comes at a relatively low price, which CAM therapies typically do (at least, as compared to the fertility treatments they complement).

As more studies are done, low-tech alternative therapies may just become a frequent (or even routine) companion to high-tech fertility treatments. Talk to your doctor about how CAM might be integrated into your conception campaign. Also check on cost before you book your CAM therapies – some can come with a hefty price tag.

the help of ART. Which meant that women without viable eggs (because of age or due to ovarian failure or a genetic disorder, for example) were out of luck in the fertility department. The same went for women who were known carriers of serious diseases that they didn't want to pass on to their offspring. But that all changed with egg donation, technology that gives hope to women who so desperately want a baby of their own. With this ART procedure, an egg (or eggs) from a donor (either fresh or frozen, though fresh are used much more often and with greater success) are mixed with sperm provided by the hopeful father, to produce an embryo. The embryo (or embryos if more than one is being implanted at a time) is then placed in the uterus of the hopeful mum, where it will (hopefully) grow into a healthy pregnancy. Today more than 2,000 babies resulting from donor eggs are born each year with nearly 50 percent of fresh egg donations and 14 percent of frozen egg donations resulting in a live birth.

The first step if you're considering egg donation is to find an egg donor. A close friend or relative may want to be your egg donor (and if she's a relative such as a sister, your baby will contain genes resembling yours). Or you might decide to choose an egg from a donor you don't know through your fertility doctor or through agencies that match donors with recipients (potential donors are screened for genetic disorders, psychological conditions, STDs, and general health, but you will also

ICSI-GIFT: Alphabet Soup Fertility

Some fertility clinics combine ART procedures to try to up the odds of a successful pregnancy even more, combining ICSI (in which a sperm is placed directly inside an egg) with GIFT (in which the egg and sperm or, in this case, the ICSI egg is placed directly into the fallopian tube). The advantage to this approach: it's all done at the same time, from egg retrieval to ICSI to egg-sperm combo transferring – and it allows the embryo to complete fertilization and turn into an embryo in the most natural way (in the fallopian tube). Ask your RE if this type of procedure is available to you.

be able to screen for other genetic factors that matter to you, such as height, hair colour, special talents, and so on). You'll also likely need to involve a lawyer, since there are certain legal issues surrounding egg donation, as well as to factor in any costs involved.

Once you've chosen an egg donor, it's time to get ready for a pregnancy – one that involves, at least at this point, three people. Both you and your donor will have to undergo hormonal treatments to coordinate your cycles (though if the eggs or embryos will be frozen for future use, synchronizing your cycles isn't necessary) and to prepare each of you for your individual job responsibility. Your donor will take fertility drugs (similar to the cocktail of drugs anyone undergoing IVF would use) to stimulate her ovaries to produce multiple eggs – and you'll use fertility drugs to build up your uterine lining so it'll be ready for implantation. When your donor's eggs are mature, they will be retrieved, mixed with your partner's sperm in a Petri dish, and the ensuing embryos will be transferred to your uterus within 2 to 3 days (assuming you coordinated your cycles) just like in a regular IVF cycle. If the embryos are to be frozen, transferring to your uterus can be done at any time.

Sperm Donation

Thanks to advances in sperm-enhancing fertility treatments, the need for donor sperm has decreased somewhat. Still, in many situations sperm donation might be considered. Couples in which the male partner

The Pro-Pregnancy Hormone

Though fertility drugs and IVF may help you get pregnant, the hormone progesterone (known as the pro-pregnancy hormone) keeps you pregnant – preventing miscarriage and helping ensure your pregnancy (and that newly conceived baby) thrives. In women whose natural progesterone levels are low, taking progesterone after conception or an IVF procedure (in injection, vaginal gel, or tablet form) may help keep the pregnancy you've worked so hard to produce going strong. Your doctor or RE can let you know if taking prescribed progesterone is right for your fertility scenario.

Two (or More) for the Price of One?

If anyone deserves a pot of baby gold at the end of the fertility rainbow, it's a couple who's tried long and hard to conceive. But what are your chances of ending up with 2 pots – or maybe 3, or even 4 or more – after having fertility treatments? Actually, pretty good. Though the odds that your pregnancy will be a multiple one are lower than they used to be – thanks to more precise medication dosages and fewer embryo transfers – you still have approximately a 15 percent chance of having twins and a less than 5 percent chance of having triplets (or more) if you're using fertility medications and undergo IUI. There's a nearly 40 percent chance of twins and a 5 percent chance of triplets (or more) if you're undergoing IVF. In fact, around 98 percent of multiple pregnancies these days are the result of fertility treatments.

has an extremely low sperm count, no sperm, sperm of low quality, or sperm that carry a genetic defect might turn to sperm donation. Lesbian couples or single women can also turn to donor sperm to achieve a pregnancy.

Finding a sperm donor is easier – and less expensive – than an egg donor for one simple reason: The sperm donation process is so much simpler than the egg donation process. Sperm banks screen donors for diseases (including STDs), get a family and medical history, and test for some genetic disorders. They'll also allow you, if you wish, to peruse profiles of prospective donors (some offer more detailed profiles than others, though usually such services come at a higher cost). These profiles can provide a snapshot (sometimes literally) of the man behind the sperm – everything from height, hair colour, IQ, education, hobbies, and so on – so you can do some screening of your own. If you'd rather, you can also choose the donor randomly, without knowing any details about him. One pertinent bit of information you'd probably want to know: how many times a particular man has become a biological father through donation. You can also choose to use sperm from someone you know (though he'll have to undergo a screening process as well).

Once a sperm donor is chosen, his frozen sperm will be thawed and you'll either be inseminated with the sperm via IUI or you'll undergo an IVF cycle to mix your egg with the donor sperm in the lab.

Surrogacy

When a woman wants a baby but can't carry a pregnancy, she and her partner can turn to a surrogate – another woman who can carry the pregnancy for them. There are two types of surrogacy: Gestational surrogacy is when a woman (called the gestational carrier) carries a baby that is not biologically related to her. This might be an option if you have viable eggs, want a biological child, but can't carry a baby yourself (because you can't sustain a pregnancy, don't have a uterus, have a medical condition that makes pregnancy dangerous or impossible, or for another reason). The embryo formed in vitro with your eggs (which are retrieved as they would be for IVF) and your partner's sperm is then transferred to the gestational carrier's uterus, where it grows until the baby is ready to be born.

In traditional surrogacy, the surrogate's own egg is inseminated with the sperm from the male partner of an infertile couple. Traditional surrogacy might be an option if you don't have any viable eggs, can't carry a pregnancy, and still want a baby that's biologically related to your partner. It can also be used to make a gay couple parents.

A surrogate can, theoretically, be any woman who volunteers to carry your baby for you (and is physically, practically, and emotionally equipped to do that). But since it is illegal in the UK to advertise surrogacy or have money change hands in the process – even as reimbursement for legitimate expenses – it's likely that your surrogate options would be limited to very close friends or family members.

By law, the woman who carries a pregnancy and gives birth to a child is considered the mother, and her husband (if she is married), the father. If you do choose surrogacy, you and your partner will have to legally adopt the child in order to gain custody.

Pregnancy Tests and ART

Wondering if the fertility medications you're taking can mess up the results on that pregnancy test you're dying to use? Some of them can. If you've received an injection of hCG (or any fertility medication that contains hCG; ask your doctor for the details of your hormone cocktail), testing too early can give you a false positive (because pregnancy tests screen for the presence of hCG normally produced by the baby). You'll need to wait 7 to 14 days after your last injection of hCG to be sure all the hormones (from the shot) are out of your system. If you're taking other fertility medications (either oral like Clomid or via injection), you don't have to worry about them interfering with an HPT.

Beginning Again After a Loss

NO MATTER HOW LONG YOU'VE been trying to conceive, the excitement of a positive pregnancy test is overwhelming. But when the pregnancy ends abruptly in loss, the heartbreak can be overwhelming, too. The blow can be harder still if this is not your first miscarriage, or even your second, or if your path to conception was a long and bumpy one.

A loss can leave you longing for that baby more than ever, but it can also leave you with far more questions than answers as you consider your future fertility – and wonder how you can best improve your odds of carrying a next pregnancy to term. Why did I lose the pregnancy? Are there any treatments that can help prevent a repeat miscarriage? And when can I start trying to conceive again? Whether you've suffered one miscarriage or several, this chapter may help provide you with the answers and reassurance that you're looking for – so you can look forward to a new beginning.

Wondering About a Repeat

It's only natural to wonder – or worry – about having a repeat miscarriage after you've already suffered one loss, or more. Fortunately, in the vast majority of cases, a miscarriage is followed by a healthy pregnancy. Knowing that this happy ending is most likely around the corner for you can make turning that corner much easier.

Chance of a Repeat Miscarriage

"I had a miscarriage last year, and I've finally got up the nerve to TTC again. Do I have a higher chance of having another miscarriage?"

Will It Happen Again?

If you've had a miscarriage, you're likely wondering – understandably – what the chances are that you'll have another. In most cases, you'll be relieved to see, they are probably a lot lower than you'd think (assuming you don't have any other risk factors) – and the chances of your next pregnancy having the happiest ending possible are excellent:

■ If you had a miscarriage during your first pregnancy, your chances of another miscarriage are pretty much the same as they are for someone who hasn't miscarried before (less than 15 percent – which means your chances of a healthy pregnancy next time are over 85 percent).

■ If you've had 2 miscarriages, there is about a 28 percent chance your next pregnancy will end in miscarriage – and a 75 percent chance that you'll carry the next baby to term. The chance of loss is even lower if you've had 1 or more live births.

■ If you've had 3 or more miscarriages, there is about a 43 percent chance you'll miscarry again, and a 65 percent chance that you won't.

All mums-to-be worry about miscarriage at some point in their early pregnancies (some worry pretty much nonstop) – and as someone who's already suffered a pregnancy loss, it's only natural that your stress is stepped up. But happily, it doesn't have to be. Having had one miscarriage does not increase your risk of having another – and, in fact, you have the same excellent chances as someone who's trying for the first time that your next pregnancy will bestow on you the baby you've been hoping for. It's even possible that you can up your odds for a healthy pregnancy by reducing any miscarriage risks that apply to you (see page 181). So relax and enjoy your baby-making activities.

Testing After Miscarriage

"I just had my second miscarriage in a row. Should I get tested to figure out why this is happening?"

While a single loss isn't usually worth investigating (because most of these are random, onetime events, most practitioners won't work up a woman who has had one miscarriage), trying to get to the bottom of recurrent losses definitely makes sense before you try to conceive again. About 75 percent of the time that explanation can be found through testing, which usually involves simple blood tests. Once the cause or causes are uncovered, you can talk to your practitioner about treatment options – as well as how to best care for your next pregnancy (see page 181 for more).

Sometimes no definitive cause turns up. Even then, reducing risk as much as possible can lower the chances of a reoccurrence. No room for improvement? Just remember that the chances that you'll achieve pregnancy success next time around are very good, even if nothing in your preconception profile changes.

Looking to the Future

Just because a pregnancy doesn't take place in your body doesn't mean its loss doesn't hurt you deep inside. And just like your partner, you may approach another baby-making campaign with mixed emotions. On the one hand, you're more anxious than ever to produce that healthy baby (not to mention, hold him or her in your arms). On the other hand, you're worried that another try might lead to another pregnancy failure. If you and your partner have had multiple miscarriages (especially if no cause has been attributed to them, making a targeted treatment trickier), hope may be hard to come by, too, because your hopes were dashed in the past.

But the truth is, there is a lot of hope that your baby dreams will come true. Even when miscarriages have been unexplained and there's no pinpointed cause to treat easily, a couple who has had 2 miscarriages before has a 72 percent chance of carrying the next pregnancy to term. For a couple who has had 3, the rate of success – without any kind of medical intervention – is still 40 to 45 percent. In many cases, the right kind of treatment can significantly reduce or even eliminate the risk of miscarriage in subsequent pregnancies.

Realistically, even the most optimistic statistics may not help you stress less about another miscarriage. So think positive (the more positive you stay, the more positive your partner will stay), but also try venting any lingering fears. Talk to each other, but also to friends who've experienced a pregnancy loss in the past (if you don't know any, look online for message boards devoted to dads). Making positive lifestyle changes, if there's any room for improvement (for instance, cutting back on alcohol, quitting smoking, losing weight, or eating better), can also help, by making you feel like you're contributing to the success of your next pregnancy. And as always, mood-lifting strategies (such as getting regular exercise and learning to relax) can help you see past the past – and keep your eye on the future, a future that will hopefully include that beautiful baby very soon.

Ectopic Pregnancy Repeat

"I had an ectopic pregnancy 3 months ago – does that put me at risk for a repeat?"

Your baby future is likely very bright. The vast majority of women who experience one ectopic (or tubal) pregnancy go on to have a completely normal pregnancy on their very next try. If you've had one ectopic, the repeat risk in your next pregnancy is somewhere between 9 and 12 percent (with the estimated risk on the lower end if you lost a tube, and the higher end if you have both tubes still intact after your ectopic). If you've already had one successful pregnancy after an ectopic, your chances of having another tubal pregnancy are the same as for the general pregnant population (with no increased risk at all). Women who have repeat ectopics (which are rare) usually have other tubal or underlying fertility issues – which means that if you have no fertility issues, your risk of a repeat is lower still.

As for your fertility, that will depend on how your ectopic was managed (medically or surgically). If both of your tubes were preserved, your fertility should be, too. More than half of all women who've had an ectopic go on to conceive a normal pregnancy within a year.

Think Positive

A miscarriage – as sad an event as it is – is a sign that you're capable of conceiving, and that's a very good sign. Even better, it's also a strong indication that you'll most likely conceive again. And even better still, like the vast majority of women who experience a miscarriage, you will very likely go on to have a normal pregnancy and a healthy baby in the near future. All very good reasons to think positive as you move forward in your efforts to become pregnant again.

It's understandable if you're having a hard time seeing a bright side in your baby future. And you may feel afraid to try again, for fear of losing again. As always, turn to your partner for support (remember, you're in this together), as well as to friends and family who've also suffered pregnancy losses and then went on to have healthy babies. Joining a message board for mums who are TTC after a miscarriage (you'll find one at WhatToExpect.com) or other pregnancy loss can also help boost your morale immeasurably.

Anything that helps you relax – and manage your emotions – can also help you think positive. Yoga, visualization techniques, deep breathing techniques, and acupuncture (among other CAM approaches) can ease anxiety; exercise and eating well can lift your mood and brighten your outlook.

Preventing Pregnancy Loss

If you've had a miscarriage, you're undoubtedly wondering what you can do next time around to prevent it from happening again. For most women, a miscarriage is a onetime event and the chances are excellent that the next pregnancy will end with a healthy baby, without any intervention at all – though it doesn't hurt to increase those odds even more by minimizing, modifying, or eliminating any risk factors that apply. If you've had 2 or more miscarriages, trying to uncover the cause and then working to prevent repeats can help put a baby in your future a lot sooner. And luckily, with today's technology and advanced treatments, there are more and more ways to figure out what caused prior miscarriages and how to prevent future ones.

Reducing Risk

"I've had one miscarriage and my doctor says it probably won't happen again. Is there anything I can do now, before I start TTC again, to reduce the risk for next time?"

Your doctor's right – it probably won't happen again. Most single miscarriages are a chance occurrence, and the likelihood that you'll have a second loss is very low – in fact, as low as it is for someone who hasn't miscarried before. Still, it's always smart to maximize your chances for a healthy pregnancy. You're probably very familiar with this pro-pregnancy protocol – and you may already be following it carefully – but it doesn't hurt to check it over to see if you've got any room for improvement in your preconception prep:

- Your weight. Being significantly overweight or underweight can slightly increase the risk of miscarriage, but getting close to your ideal weight before you conceive can eliminate that risk.

- Your diet. A well balanced diet is vital to a healthy pregnancy, so if there's room for improvement in the way you eat, go for it. Deficiencies in certain nutrients (including folic acid and vitamin B_{12}) have been linked to miscarriage risk. A prenatal vitamin (plus a good diet) can get your nutritional reserves up to par if they're not already there, and help reduce the risk of miscarriage.

Could It Be You?

While your health, your diet, and your lifestyle can all have a significant impact on fertility (as well as on the future health of your baby), they don't appear to play a role in miscarriage. Age over 40 in a dad, on the other hand, can slightly increase the risk of miscarriage (chromosomal abnormalities are somewhat more likely in an older man's sperm). But since most repeat miscarriages are related to maternal factors, it's not likely that testing to determine the cause of multiple losses would involve you unless a chromosomal problem is suspected (and then preimplantation genetic diagnosis, or PGD, can be an option; see facing page). So chances are you won't be rolling up your sleeve, just supporting your partner as she undergoes any necessary testing.

- Your caffeine intake. Heavy caffeine intake early in pregnancy slightly increases the risk of miscarriage. Stick to no more than 200 mg of caffeine (about 340 grams of brewed coffee or two shots of espresso) while you're TTC and once you become pregnant.

- A smoking habit. Don't worry about smoking that's in your past – but if you're currently a smoker, quit as soon as possible to cross this risk off your profile. Try as best you can to steer clear of secondhand smoke as well (so if your partner smokes, it's time for him to call it quits, too).

- A drinking habit. As you've most likely heard, alcohol and pregnancy don't mix – and there's growing evidence that too much alcohol can increase the risk for miscarriage. So if you do drink, cut out those cocktails (and beer and wine) once you start TTC.

- Your general health. Untreated chronic conditions (such as diabetes, lupus, high blood pressure), untreated thyroid disorder, and untreated STDs can all increase miscarriage risk. Making sure your body is as healthy as possible before you conceive can help prevent miscarriage, again if there's room for improvement.

- Your stress level. Extremely high stress (not everyday stress, which isn't harmful) has been linked to pregnancy loss. Reducing extreme stress in your life as best you can may help reduce the risk for future miscarriages.

Chromosomal Defect

"I'm 38 and I just had a second miscarriage. My doctor says there were problems with the baby's chromosomes. Will I ever be able to have a healthy baby?"

It's thought that more than half of all miscarriages are caused by a defect in the chromosomal makeup of the embryo or fetus – so your situation is definitely not unusual. It's even less unusual among women in your age group. That's because as you age, so do your eggs. And older eggs – and possibly your partner's older sperm if he's over 40 – are more likely to contain chromosomal abnormalities than younger eggs.

You can't change your age, of course, or the age of your eggs. And knowing that your older egg supply has likely been responsible for the chromosomal problems in your previous pregnancies can be discouraging. After all, won't pregnancy losses keep on happening until the chance healthy egg and sperm meet up? The simple answer is yes – but happily, there is an excellent possibility that this perfect pairing will happen spontaneously with your next conception. That's what happens most of the time in a case like yours.

But what happens if chromosomal problems keep preventing that happy outcome and that healthy embryo? For very few couples (particularly older ones), miscarriages due to chromosomal defects happen again and again. Unfortunately, it's impossible to detect defective chromosomes in an embryo when conception occurs the natural way. But with today's medical technology, physicians are able to screen embryos formed in vitro (in a test tube or Petri dish) for chromosomal abnormalities and choose the healthiest embryos for implantation. This technology, called preimplantation genetic diagnosis (PGD), is basically an embryo biopsy that works in conjunction with in vitro fertilization (IVF). PGD enables your doctor to examine the DNA of one cell of each embryo and identify the healthy embryos. Once it is determined that an embryo is free from identifiable chromosomal abnormalities, it can

Your Age and Your Miscarriage Risk

Miscarriage does become somewhat more likely to happen as you age. That's because older mothers have older eggs, and older eggs have a greater chance of carrying a chromosomal abnormality. Plus, fewer egg follicles means less ovarian hormones are produced, which may make it more difficult for an older mum-to-be to sustain a pregnancy. Still, the increase in risk may not be as high as you'd think. While the odds of a woman under 35 losing a pregnancy is between 11 and 15 percent, a 40-year-old has a 50 percent chance of miscarrying – higher, yes, but still very much in your favour. Though there's nothing you can do about your age, you can definitely maximize your chances of carrying a baby to term by minimizing all the other miscarriage risks that might apply to you (see facing page).

be transferred to your uterus with the hope that it implants and develops into a healthy pregnancy and healthy baby.

Of course, complicated procedures often come with complicated decisions. Before choosing PGD, you and your partner will want to have a conversation with your doctor so that you're clear about the pros and cons of the procedure, as well as the potential risks involved. You'll also need to be comfortable with its implications (there might be embryos that show chromosomal anomalies, and you'll need to think about what will be done with those). It's also important to consider any added cost factor for the procedure – it is available on the NHS but only at a few centres, and strict criteria apply. Also bear in mind that not all chromosomal defects can be detected by PGD. It's also not yet clear whether PGD improves success rates or reduces miscarriage rates. Still, for many couples – especially ones who have been suffering from recurrent pregnancy losses – PGD can tip the healthy-pregnancy scales in their favour.

Keep in mind, too, that other factors may be contributing to your miscarriages. After all, just because the last baby had chromosomal problems, it's impossible to conclude with certainty (unless tests were performed on the other fetus as well) that the same problem led to your previous pregnancy loss. So do make sure you're screened for all other potential risk factors (including hormonal imbalances that are more common in women over 35) to increase your odds of a successful pregnancy next time around, no matter how you decide to conceive.

Hormonal Imbalance

"I have a luteal phase deficiency and I'm wondering if that has anything to do with the miscarriage I just had."

It takes an intricate balance of hormones to deliver a pregnancy safely from conception to delivery. Most of the time, nature takes its hormonal course without incident, but sometimes an imbalance can result in a pregnancy loss. The most common hormonal imbalances associated with miscarriage are:

Luteal phase deficiency. When a woman has a luteal phase (the second half of a cycle) shorter than 10 to 12 days, her progesterone levels remain too low to sustain a pregnancy because there's not enough time in the cycle for the levels to build. This progesterone shortage can lead to an inadequately prepared uterus (there's not enough time for the endometrium to thicken sufficiently). A uterus without a thick lining can make it difficult for an embryo to implant or can result in an early miscarriage. A blood test and possibly a biopsy of your uterine wall can help confirm whether a luteal phase deficiency (LPD) was the cause of your miscarriage. If an LPD is found to be responsible, the right supplementation can reduce the risk of a repeat loss in future pregnancies. Supplemental natural progesterone taken as a vaginal suppository or as an oral tablet – and perhaps vitamin B_6 supplementation as well – prior to conception may help remedy an LPD. In addition, continuing progesterone supplementation through the early stages of pregnancy may help sustain the pregnancy and avoid miscarriage.

Hyperprolactinaemia. Higher-than-normal levels of prolactin (the hormone responsible for breast milk production) have been linked to an increased risk for miscarriage. Signs of hyperprolactinaemia can be a milky discharge from your nipples or anovulation (when you have a period but don't ovulate). Blood tests can reveal if you have excess prolactin. Luckily, once diagnosed, this imbalance can be easily treated with medication that decreases the levels of prolactin and increases the chances that the next pregnancy won't end in miscarriage.

Thyroid condition. Thyroid, another important hormone, though not officially a member of the reproductive hormone team, can directly impact reproduction. Abnormal levels of thyroid hormone can not only reduce fertility, but they can make it less likely that a pregnancy will be sustained. Thyroid conditions, which affect about 15 percent of women of childbearing age, are easily detected through a blood test. Treating hyperthyroidism (too much thyroid hormone) and hypothyroidism (too little thyroid hormone) with medication can easily and dramatically reduce the risk for miscarriage in future pregnancies.

Polycystic ovarian syndrome (PCOS). Women with untreated PCOS are at greater risk of having irregular ovulation and periods because of higher-than-normal levels of testosterone and LH. In some cases, these abnormal hormone levels also increase the risk of miscarriage. Some women with untreated PCOS also have insulin resistance (insulin is a hormone, too), and it is thought that this type of hormonal imbalance can prevent the endometrial lining from maturing properly, making it harder for an embryo to implant properly.

Immune System Malfunction

"Is it true that some miscarriages are caused by the mum's body attacking the baby? Is there anything that can be done to prevent that from happening?"

As implausible as it sounds, what you've heard is true. A very small percentage of miscarriages are thought to be triggered by antibodies in the mother's body. These autoantibodies increase the risk of blood clots, affecting the blood flow to the developing fetus, and causing a miscarriage, usually after 10 weeks.

Autoimmune problems in general account for just 2 percent of recurrent miscarriages. But if you have had multiple miscarriages, blood tests can reveal if you're producing autoantibodies (called antiphospholipid antibodies). Once an immune system malfunction is confirmed, your practitioner may recommend one baby aspirin per day (about one-quarter of an adult aspirin)

throughout your pregnancy and/or heparin (a stronger anticoagulant) injections given during the first half of your pregnancy, to help stop the formation of these fatal-to-the-fetus blood clots.

Anatomical Problems of the Uterus

"My doctor mentioned that I have an unusually shaped uterus. Could that be the cause of my miscarriage? Will that mean I'll have another one?"

Possibly, but not necessarily. While experts believe that 15 percent of all miscarriages result from uterine malformations and other anatomical problems in the uterus and cervix, less than 5 percent of women with a uterine malformation have one that is bad enough to cause a miscarriage. That's because only certain uterine shapes (such as a septate uterus, in which a wall of tissue separates the two sides of the uterus) interfere with the healthy implantation of an embryo or make women more prone to miscarriage. Other anatomical problems in the uterus, such as fibroids, may also interfere with implantation and/or the proper growth of a fetus. Tests such as hysterosalpingogram (HSG; an assessment of the uterus and fallopian tubes using X-ray imaging and dye), hysteroscopy (visualization of the uterus using a camera), sonohystogram (visualization using ultrasound), or an MRI can be used to diagnose a uterine problem.

If it turns out that the unusual shape of your uterus is serious enough to have caused your pregnancy loss and may threaten any future conceptions, surgery before you become pregnant again can be a quick and effective fix. If the issue is fibroids, those can be removed.

If it turns out that the shape of your uterus was not likely the cause of your

Preventing a Repeat with CAM

The list of what complementary and alternative medicine (CAM) can or may be able to do grows longer and longer, as more and more of these alternative therapies are being integrated into more and more traditional treatments. Though there aren't any studies to back it up yet, many women and their practitioners maintain that helping prevent recurrent miscarriages makes the list, too. It's believed that the stress reduction qualities of CAM therapies such as meditation, yoga, tai chi, and acupuncture may explain why they seem to be effective in some cases. Acupuncture may also help promote circulation to the uterus, ensuring a healthy uterine lining and increasing the chances it can sustain a healthy pregnancy.

What about herbal remedies to prevent pregnancy loss? Herbalists say that herbs such as wild yam, partridge berry, red raspberry leaf, black cohosh, and others can help (though red raspberry leaf taken in large amounts can actually trigger contractions). Each herbal practitioner has his or her own cocktail of favourite herbs that are purported to prevent miscarriage, but because herbal treatments do not undergo testing for safety and efficacy, and because there are few or no studies to prove whether they work, herbs are best approached with care. If you do decide to explore the herbal avenue, be sure you do so under the supervision of a licensed practitioner and with the knowledge and go-ahead of your traditional medical team.

---

miscarriage, chances are it was a random event that won't repeat – in which case, your risk of miscarrying a second time is just as low as it is for the general pregnant population.

Infections

"I've heard that infections can cause pregnancy loss. Is it possible the cold I had right when I conceived caused my miscarriage?"

It takes a lot more than a cold to trigger a pregnancy loss. Though there is a small link between infection and miscarriage, it applies to far more serious

(and less common) infections, such as mumps, measles, herpes, CMV, listeria, STDs (sexually transmitted diseases), and a host of others you've probably never even heard of. It does not apply to colds (even bad ones) or the flu, so it couldn't have been responsible for your miscarriage.

So don't worry about a bout with the sniffles when you're next pregnant. But keep in mind that it's always smart to avoid infections when you're expecting (by getting plenty of rest and washing your hands often), and to have any infection that you do come down with treated promptly so it doesn't impact your general health or your pregnancy.

Trying Again

If you're like most hopeful parents-to-be, getting pregnant again is the best possible therapy after a pregnancy loss – and it's something you're likely aching to do as soon as you can. But it's also likely you'll approach trying to conceive again – like most hopeful parents who have suffered a miscarriage – with tempered enthusiasm. After all, you now know that a positive pregnancy test doesn't necessarily come with the promise of a baby 9 months later. The loss of innocence that follows a pregnancy loss – and the trepidation it can bring when you contemplate conceiving again – is understandable, and so common. Just try to remind yourself – and it's true! – that the vast majority of women who have had a miscarriage, or even multiple losses, go on to have healthy pregnancies. Chances are you'll be on your way to starting – or adding to – your family again, just a little later than you originally thought.

When to Try Again

"I just had a miscarriage and I'm wondering when I can start trying to conceive again. I want to so badly."

There's no definitive answer to the question of when you can try to conceive again after a miscarriage, simply because there are no definitive rules. Even guidelines from different practitioners differ – and the same practitioner may recommend a different waiting period to two different women. Many practitioners give the go-head to start trying again as soon as you feel physically and emotionally up to it, whether your miscarriage was natural or you had a D & C after a miscarriage. In fact, some actually encourage a sooner-than-later approach. That's because reproductive hormones may be at high levels following a miscarriage, so fertility could be at its peak for the 3 months after a loss – meaning that you're possibly even more likely to conceive during this time. More encouraging news if you're hoping to get an early start: There does not seem to be an increase in miscarriage rate for women who've conceived immediately after a pregnancy loss.

That said, some practitioners suggest waiting 2 to 3 months before trying to conceive again to allow your cycles to regulate, to give you time to beef up your nutritional reserve (if you hadn't been taking prenatal vitamins before or if your iron stores were depleted due to heavy bleeding), or to give your body time to heal (if the miscarriage was a later one). Still other practitioners recommend waiting until you have your first normal period before actively trying for a baby. Their reasoning: so that the next pregnancy will be easier to date (though that's usually less of an issue

Resuming Sex

Even if you're not ready to start trying for a baby right after a miscarriage, it's perfectly fine to start making love again (if you're up to it emotionally) once the bleeding from the miscarriage (and/or a D & C) stops. Do keep in mind that if you are having sex without birth control, there's a chance you can get pregnant almost immediately – and that might be exactly what you're hoping for.

Endings and Beginnings

Contemplating beginning a pregnancy when one has just ended can leave your feelings all over the emotional map. Of course, you desperately want a baby – and a healthy pregnancy that puts that baby in your arms – as soon as possible. But at the same time, trying for another may make you feel almost disloyal to the baby you've lost, even if that loss came very early in the pregnancy.

How to reconcile a fresh beginning with that painful ending? It may help to keep in mind that you're not replacing one pregnancy with another, or one baby with another. You don't have to stop grieving for your lost pregnancy to start trying to conceive another – and, in fact, you can continue remembering the baby you lost for as long as you need to or want to (by commemorating the day of the loss each year, planting a tree in your garden, honouring your baby's memory by giving to others).

Of course, also keep in mind that you may not have any feelings of ambivalence when it comes to trying again – in fact, you may be nothing but excited to try again – and that's just as normal and understandable. Your reaction is what's right for you.

---

these days because early ultrasound can accurately pinpoint fetal age) and to ensure that all the hCG from the previous pregnancy has left your system completely and your hormone levels are back to normal. For most women, that first period will arrive pretty quickly, usually within 4 to 6 weeks after the miscarriage. Waiting until your cycle has resumed will also allow you to time your baby-making efforts effectively.

Finally, when you'll be given the green light for TTC may also depend on whether or not tests need to be run to rule out conditions that may have caused the miscarriage, or if you have a chronic condition that needs to be better controlled. Either way, taking that extra time – and those extra precautions (if necessary and recommended by your practitioner) – can help ensure that any future conception will turn into a healthy pregnancy.

If your practitioner does give you the immediate go-ahead, go right ahead and begin your baby-making efforts. If he or she recommends waiting, use reliable contraception, preferably of the barrier type – condom, diaphragm – until the waiting time is up. Take advantage of this waiting period – spend it improving your diet and your health habits (if there's any room for improvement) and generally getting your body into tip-top baby-making shape. That way, you'll feel that you're at least doing something constructive while you wait (plus, it'll give you something else to focus on besides the waiting). If your practitioner recommends waiting, but you're not sure why, ask – and if you're super-anxious to start trying again right away, see if there's any wiggle room in that recommendation.

Ready … or Not

"I just had a miscarriage and though my doctor told me I could start TTC again, I'm not sure I'm ready."

For some couples, resuming TTC efforts as soon as possible after a pregnancy loss is just what the doctor ordered. For them, tracking cervical mucus changes, charting BBT, and actively trying for a baby again can help take their focus off their loss and shift it to something positive. It can also help a woman who's suffered a pregnancy loss recover some of the control over her body that the miscarriage (an experience completely out of her control) took from her. For others, however, starting to TTC quickly may not feel right – whether because they're fearful of another miscarriage or because they feel they need more time to grieve. Whichever category you fall into, remember that you need to do what feels right for you. Don't let yourself feel pressured by anyone (your practitioner, your best friend, your mother-in-law) to pick up where you left off and start trying again right away. Maybe you are ready, maybe you're not – but only you and your partner can make that decision.

Just make sure that you do come to that decision together. Though it's your body that has suffered the physical effects of the pregnancy loss, both of you have paid the emotional price. So talk about it. It may help, too, to talk to others who know exactly what you're going through because they're going through it, too – but who are objective in their feedback. In addition to helping you make (or feel better about) your decision, that support can help you heal. You'll likely find such support on TTC or loss message boards, if you don't have friends or family who can personally relate, or if you'd just like all the support you can get.

If you're still on the fence about whether now's the right time (and keeping in mind that there's no time that's right for everyone), you may want to take into account the physical facts. Since women may be more fertile in the 3 months following a miscarriage, beginning again sooner may bring you success

sooner (though it's definitely not a guarantee of success). But don't discount – or second-guess – your emotions, either. If you feel you need to take a break, and take a breath, before you begin to TTC again, then that's absolutely what you should do. Listen to – and follow – your heart, and you'll make the decision that's right for you.

A Return to a Normal Cycle

"When will I start ovulating and get my period again after my miscarriage?"

Your menstrual cycle can't get up and running until your body realizes you're no longer pregnant – and for that to happen, all of the hCG has to be out of your system. For the hCG to get out of your system, the developing placenta has to fully detach from the uterine wall (or be removed in a D & C). Once the hCG is completely gone (it takes about 10 days after the placenta detaches for

Keeping Track Again

Since it's hard to know when you've begun ovulating again after a miscarriage (ovulation may begin before your first period or not until you've had one or two), you may be eager to resume charting. Probably best not to be too eager. If you begin charting immediately after a miscarriage and before you get your first period, you may find those readings all over the place – and largely unreliable. That's normal and to be expected. For better results, wait until after your first normal period and then start your charting anew.

Your Flow Returns

Wondering what your periods will be like after you miscarry? Chances are they'll be pretty much the way they were before. So if you were a heavy bleeder pre-pregnancy loss, you should expect the same now. And if your periods were light and quick – they'll resume that way, too. Cycle length also usually returns to the status quo after a miscarriage, though the first couple of cycles may be a little longer than usual.

hCG to hit zero), you can expect your period to return within 4 to 6 weeks (if your cycles were regular before conceiving), with ovulation occurring 2 to 4 weeks after your hCG reaches zero.

But don't start counting those weeks from the first day you noticed spotting or bleeding. It could take a week or two (or even longer) from the beginning of the miscarriage until the placenta pulls away and that important hormonal shift takes place (you won't notice these changes, you'll only be aware of continuous bleeding). Which means that if you haven't got your period again after 6 weeks from the first day you noticed miscarriage bleeding, there's no need to worry. Wait another week or two before putting in a call to your practitioner. Your period might be just around the corner.

Something else to keep in mind: If your miscarriage occurred late in the first trimester or in the second trimester, you had a lot of hCG in your system (hCG rises as your pregnancy progresses) – and that means it'll take longer to hit that zero mark and, consequently, your period may take a little longer to resume.

Another reason why your period may be late to return: Some women retain tiny fragments of placental tissue after a miscarriage (and more rarely, after a D & C). If that's the case with you, you may have your bleeding taper off only to resume a few days (or even a week or two) later. This bleeding isn't a period yet – it's the continuation of your pregnancy loss. And that means you can't expect to see a true period until at least 4 weeks after the miscarriage has truly completed (in other words, until 4 weeks after all the placental tissue has pulled away from the uterine wall). Though this scenario is normal (if uncommon), do put in a call to your practitioner just for peace of mind. If your hCG levels are at zero but you still continue spotting, your doctor may give you a shot of Provera or some other form of progesterone to trick your body into thinking it's time for a period so your cycles can get back to normal. Of course, if at any time the bleeding becomes very heavy again, call your practitioner as soon as you can.

And though the return of your period may indicate that you've begun ovulating, it's not a sure bet. That's because there may be one (or more) anovulatory cycles (in which you get your period without ovulating) after a miscarriage. To figure out whether you're back to ovulation business as usual, you'll need to start up your cycle tracking again.

Lingering Pregnancy Symptoms

"I had a miscarriage and started TTC again right after. I'm still feeling pregnancy symptoms (tender breasts, bloating) and I'm wondering if that means I'm pregnant again or if they're just residual symptoms from the pregnancy that I lost."

That's a tough call – in fact, it may be an impossible one to make at this point. The problem is, there are several explanations for your symptoms. One is that you're experiencing PMS. As you probably discovered when you were TTC last time, PMS symptoms can be very difficult to distinguish from early pregnancy symptoms (especially those tender breasts and that bloating) and it might be tricky to figure out if those symptoms might be signalling the return of Aunt Flo or a new pregnancy – especially if you haven't had a normal period since you miscarried. Also possible: Your body isn't quite ready for the return of your period but is reacting to hormonal fluctuations – which can be substantial after a pregnancy loss.

Another less likely explanation is that what you're feeling are residual pregnancy symptoms – but for that to be the case, you'd still have to have residual hCG in your system. This is possible if your miscarriage was very recent (the hCG is usually out of your system about 10 days after a miscarriage or D & C is complete) or took place later in the first trimester or in the second (in which case the hCG levels might take a little longer than that to hit zero). Until the hCG is completely gone, you can't ovulate, you can't get your period, and you can't get pregnant. You can, however, possibly have a positive pregnancy test – which would further confuse the picture.

Still another explanation – and this is likely the one you're hoping for – is that you might be pregnant again. It is possible to ovulate and conceive before you've had that first post-loss period, though diagnosing that pregnancy might be tricky initially (a home pregnancy test, again, might be responding to residual hCG in your system, rather than newly generated pregnancy hormone).

Sometimes, pregnancy symptoms after a loss can be triggered by emotional causes – you want to be pregnant still (or again), and so your psyche is clinging to the symptoms (which can feel very real even if they're not physically plausible).

Check in with your doctor if you're unsure of what to think – or if you'd like confirmation of whether or not you're pregnant.

PART 4

Keeping Track

CHAPTER 12

Your Fertility Planner

O F COURSE YOU CAN GET PREG-
nant the old-fashioned way –
stop using birth control, have
sex whenever, wherever, in whatever
position, and wait for that missed
period. Or the even more old-fashioned
way – dispense with the birth control
altogether, and take an "oops" approach
to conception. But there's definitely an
upside to planning your conception –
actually many upsides. Taking charge
of your fertility planning gives you the
opportunity to get your body, your
partner's body, and your life in tip-top
baby-making shape before your conception campaign begins – and gives you a
chance to stack the cards in favour of a
speedier conception, a safer and more
comfortable pregnancy, and a healthier
baby. Plus, it gives you an opportunity
to put that multitasking control freak in
you (yes, you) to work on one of life's
most satisfying projects: baby making.
Let the planning begin.

Countdown to Conception

You can never be fully prepared for
becoming a parent, or even for becoming pregnant. But when time is on your
side (you're just starting to think about
taking the baby plunge), it makes sense to
put those pre-baby-making months to the
most productive possible use.

The following schedule is a general
guide to conception prep (there may be
other items you'll have to add to your
specific plan). Don't stress too much
about the exact time frame – more
important right now is getting most
(if not all) of the items on the agenda
crossed off your to-do list before you get
cracking on conception.

Another consideration as you count
down to conception – just how much to-
doing you've got to get done (for instance,
if you have a hefty number of kilograms to
lose, you'll want to get an earlier start on
weight loss; if you know that you'll never
be able to quit cigarettes in 3 months,
make 6 months your goal). Yet another
consideration: your own time frame for
getting pregnant. If you want to get busier
sooner rather than later, skip right to the
3-month plan.

Six to Twelve Months Out

FOR HER:

☐ Evaluate your weight and BMI. If you have a lot to lose, start a healthy balanced weight-loss programme now. If you're significantly underweight, start eating with an eye on moving those numbers up (and if you have an eating disorder, get treatment now).

☐ Start taking a daily prenatal vitamin, if you want. It's not considered a must-do until 3 months out, but it's never too early to start catching up on any nutritional deficits.

Plus, some research indicates that taking prenatals for a year before conception may reduce the risk for preterm delivery.

☐ If you have substantial problems with your gums and/or teeth, or you suspect you might, get busy having any necessary dental work done.

☐ If you have any chronic medical conditions, take steps to get them under control.

NOTES: _____
_____
_____
_____
_____
_____
_____

FOR HIM:

☐ Evaluate your BMI. If you have a lot of weight to lose, start a healthy balanced weight-loss programme now.

☐ If you have any chronic medical conditions, take steps to get them under control.

NOTES: _____
_____
_____
_____
_____
_____
_____

Three Months Out

FOR HER:

☐ Evaluate your weight and BMI. If it needs a little adjusting (up or down), start a healthy balanced weight-loss (or -gain) programme now.

☐ Take a look at your eating habits and if they're not up to prepregnancy par, ease into a healthy eating plan with baby making in mind.

☐ Start taking a daily prenatal vitamin, if you haven't already.

☐ Cut out smoking. If quitting cold turkey will be too tough, use the next 3 months to cut back slowly until you're nicotine free.

☐ Begin weaning yourself off prescription and over-the-counter medications (under your doctor's guidance) that are not conception compatible and substituting those that are.

☐ Ditch hormonal birth control (the Pill, patch, ring) and use only barrier methods for now (condom, diaphragm, spermicides).

☐ Stop using recreational drugs. If you need help quitting, seek it now.

NOTES: _____

_____

_____

_____

_____

_____

_____

_____

_____

_____

_____

_____

_____

_____

_____

_____

_____

FOR HIM:

☐ Evaluate your weight and BMI. If you could drop a few kilos, now's the time to start a healthy balanced weight-loss programme. If you're too thin, consider beefing up a bit.

☐ Take a look at your eating habits. If there's room for improvement, now's a great time to start eating with fertility optimizing in mind.

☐ Take a multivitamin to make sure your body is well stocked for optimal sperm production.

☐ Cut out smoking. If quitting cold turkey will be too tough, use the next 3 months to cut back slowly until you're nicotine free.

☐ Take stock of your medicine cabinet. With your doctor's help, begin substituting medications that are compatible with baby making for those that aren't.

☐ Stop using recreational drugs. If you need help quitting, seek it now.

NOTES: _____
_____
_____
_____
_____
_____
_____
_____
_____
_____
_____
_____
_____
_____
_____
_____
_____
_____
_____
_____
_____

Two Months Out

FOR HER:

☐ See your doctor and/or midwife for a top-to-bottom checkup to make sure all systems are ready for baby making.

☐ Get a dental checkup and cleaning, if you haven't recently.

☐ Begin (or continue) a moderate exercise programme (aim for 30 minutes each day).

☐ Start to limit the amount of caffeine you get each day (goal: no more than 200 mg, or 2 cups, a day).

☐ Stop dieting for weight loss and continue eating balanced healthy foods that will maintain your loss.

☐ Take a good look at your environment at work. If any occupational hazards might be a problem when trying to conceive (or during pregnancy), find ways to limit your exposure.

☐ Begin charting your basal body temperature (BBT) and your cervical mucus (CM) changes. Mark down any other cycle changes and ovulation signs you notice so you'll be able to pinpoint ovulation.

NOTES: _____

_____

_____

_____

_____

FOR HIM:

☐ See your doctor for a full-body checkup. Be sure to let him or her know you're about to start trying for a family and ask if any special tests or exams might be important now.

☐ Evaluate your work environment. If you're exposed to any hazards that may harm your fertility or the health of your sperm, find ways to limit exposure for now.

☐ Keep cool by staying out of hot tubs, hot baths, and saunas. Treat your laptop as a desktop and keep your mobile phone out of your trouser pocket.

NOTES: _____

_____

_____

_____

One Month Out

FOR HER:

☐ Start reducing your alcohol intake with the aim of cutting it out altogether once you start trying to conceive.

☐ Make sure your finances are in order, including your insurance policies and will.

☐ Learn ways to relax and try to avoid stressful situations starting now (as best you can).

☐ Continue tracking your BBT, your CM changes, and other ovulation signs.

☐ Don't forget that daily vitamin.

☐ Think happy baby thoughts!

NOTES: _____

_____

_____

_____

_____

FOR HIM:

☐ Cut back on alcohol for now to keep your sperm production high and in good baby-making shape.

☐ Cut back on overly strenuous exercise routines (especially heavy-duty bicycling).

☐ Make sure your finances are in order, including your insurance policies and will.

☐ Learn ways to relax and try to avoid stressful situations starting now (as best you can).

NOTES: _____

_____

_____

_____

GO! Now that you're ready to go, make sure to have sex around ovulation each month, keeping in mind that it could take as long as a year of trying before the right sperm and egg get together.

Food Diary

Keep track of your meals and snacks for one week so you can get a clear picture of

	Day 1	Day 2	Day 3
Breakfast			
Lunch			
Dinner			
Snacks			
Protein Foods			
Calcium Foods			
Vegetables			
Fruits			
Whole Grains			
Refined Grains			
Iron-Rich Foods			
High-Fat Foods			
Junk Foods			
Caffeinated Beverages			
Water and Other Fluids			
Calories (approximate)			

how you eat and whether you need to do a little preconception diet tweaking.

Day 4	Day 5	Day 6	Day 7

Health History

When you go for your preconception checkup (which you definitely should), your practitioner will ask you lots of questions about your medical and gynaecological health, and will also do some digging into your lifestyle (and your partner's health and lifestyle, too). To be sure you're armed with all the info you'll be asked for, do your homework before the appointment and bring the answers to these routine questions with you.

Your General Health

Age _____   Weight _____   BMI _____   Blood type_____

Chronic conditions

_____

_____

_____

Medications you take regularly (prescription and over-the-counter)

_____

_____

_____

Allergies (including food allergies)

_____

_____

_____

Previous surgeries

_____

_____

_____

Have you had or been vaccinated for:

Measles _____   Mumps _____   Rubella _____   Chicken Pox _____

Date of your last Td or Tdap booster _____

Do you have a history of depression?

_____

_____

_____

Are you currently being treated for depression? How?

_____

_____

_____

Other general health issues

_____

_____

_____

_____

_____

NOTES: _____

_____

_____

_____

_____

_____

_____

_____

_____

Your Gynaecological History

Date of your last menstrual period _____

Average length of your cycles _____

Date of last Pap smear and results _____

Date(s) of any abnormal Pap smears and treatment you have received _____

_____

_____

Birth control use _____

Do you know if you have fibroids? _____

What symptoms, if any, do you have? _____

_____

_____

Do you know if you have endometriosis? _____

What symptoms do you have? _____

_____

_____

Do you have any other gynaecological conditions? _____

_____

_____

Have you ever had a sexually transmitted disease? _____

_____

_____

NOTES: _____

_____

_____

_____

_____

_____

_____

Your Reproductive History

Have you ever had any fertility issues? _____

Number of previous pregnancies _____ Ages of children _____

Have you ever had a miscarriage? _____

How many? _____ When? _____

How far along was the pregnancy? _____

_____

Have you ever had an ectopic pregnancy? _____ When? _____

_____

Have you ever had an abortion? _____ How many? _____

_____

Have you ever had a stillbirth? _____

_____

Were there any complications during your pregnancies? _____

_____

_____

_____

Were there any delivery complications? _____

_____

_____

_____

Were the deliveries vaginal or via C-section? _____

Did you ever have any postpartum complications? _____

_____

_____

_____

NOTES: _____

_____

_____

_____

Your Lifestyle

Do you smoke? _____ How much? _____

Do you drink alcohol? _____ How much? _____

Do you use any recreational drugs (cocaine, marijuana)?

How much caffeinated coffee, tea, or cola do you drink? _____

_____

How would you describe your eating habits? _____

Typical breakfast: _____

_____

Typical lunch: _____

_____

Typical dinner: _____

_____

Typical snacks: _____

_____

Do you exercise? _____ What type(s) of exercise, and how often?_____

_____

Do you take vitamins or any herbal preparations? _____ If so, what kinds?

_____

_____

Do you use acne medications? _____ If yes, what kind?_____

_____

Are you exposed to any environmental hazards at work or at home?_____

_____

Are you under any excessive emotional stress?_____

_____

NOTES: _____

_____

_____

Your Partner's Health and Lifestyle

Age _____ Height _____ Weight _____ BMI _____ Blood type _____

Chronic conditions _____

Other general health issues _____

Medications he takes regularly _____

Vitamins and supplements he takes regularly _____

Does he smoke? _____ How much? _____

Does he drink alcohol? _____ How much? _____

Does he use recreational drugs? _____

Does he exercise? _____ What type(s) and how often? _____

Is he exposed to environmental hazards at work or at home? _____

NOTES: _____

_____

_____

_____

_____

_____

_____

_____

Your Family History

Your ethnicity _____

Your partner's ethnicity _____

NOTES: _____

_____

_____

_____

_____

_____

_____

_____

Have you, your partner, or anyone in your family or your partner's family had:

	You or Your Family	Your Partner or His Family
Allergies, including food allergies	☐	☐
Autoimmune disorder (rheumatoid arthritis, lupus)	☐	☐
Depression	☐	☐
Diabetes	☐	☐
Heart disease	☐	☐
Hepatitis	☐	☐
Hypertension	☐	☐
Kidney disease	☐	☐
Psychiatric disorders	☐	☐
Seizure disorder	☐	☐
Thyroid disease	☐	☐
Autism	☐	☐
Canavan disease	☐	☐
Chromosomal abnormality	☐	☐
Connective tissue disease	☐	☐

	You or Your Family	Your Partner or His Family
Cystic fibrosis	☐	☐
Down's syndrome	☐	☐
Haemophilia	☐	☐
Hearing loss	☐	☐
Huntington's disease	☐	☐
Mental retardation	☐	☐
Muscular dystrophy	☐	☐
Neural tube defects, including spina bifida, meningocele, and anencephaly	☐	☐
Neurological disorders	☐	☐
Phenylketonuria (PKU)	☐	☐
Sickle-cell disease	☐	☐
Tay-Sachs disease	☐	☐
Thalassaemia	☐	☐
Other genetic disorders	☐	☐
Gestational diabetes	☐	☐
Preeclampsia	☐	☐
Other pregnancy complications	☐	☐
Recurrent miscarriages	☐	☐
Stillbirths	☐	☐

Questions You May Have

_____

_____

_____

_____

_____

_____

_____

Additional Questions or Notes

Tracking Your Cycle

Ready to keep an eye on the calendar? Using this month-at-a-glance calendar (or any calendar you choose), fill in the appropriate dates and then circle the first day of each monthly period. After a few months, you'll be able to determine your natural cycle length. Count back 12 to 16 days each month to get an idea of when you likely ovulated during the previous cycle. This will help narrow down when you'll likely be ovulating next cycle, and when you should schedule in sex. Shade those fertile days to keep track.

Month   Example   **January**

Sun	Mon	Tues	Wed	Thurs	Fri	Sat
1	2	3	4	5	6	7
8	9	10	11	12	13	14
15	16	17	18	19	20	21
22	23	24	25	26	27	28
29	30	31				

Month

Sun	Mon	Tues	Wed	Thurs	Fri	Sat

Month

Sun	Mon	Tues	Wed	Thurs	Fri	Sat

Month

Sun	Mon	Tues	Wed	Thurs	Fri	Sat

Month

Sun	Mon	Tues	Wed	Thurs	Fri	Sat

Month

Sun	Mon	Tues	Wed	Thurs	Fri	Sat

Month

Sun	Mon	Tues	Wed	Thurs	Fri	Sat

Month

Sun	Mon	Tues	Wed	Thurs	Fri	Sat

Your Fertility Charts

This all-in-one fertility chart will let you keep track of all your ovulation and fertility signs, enabling you to better pinpoint when ovulation is happening (and when you should start getting busy in bed). Begin a few months before you start TTC so you can get a head start. Here's how to put it all together:

1. Using a digital basal thermometer, take your temperature each morning before you get out of bed and mark each daily reading on the graph. Connect the dots to help pinpoint ovulation.

2. In the row marked "Cervical Mucus Consistency", note the consistency of your CM (dry, sticky, creamy, or slippery) as detailed on page 88 to help identify when you're most fertile.

3. You can mark down whether your cervix is opened or closed in the row marked "Cervical Position".

4. Fill in the appropriate boxes and corresponding dates in the rows marked "Period/Spotting", "Miscellaneous", and "Intercourse".

5. Finally, if you're using any fertility monitors, OPKs, saliva tests, or chloride ion (fertility watch) tests, you can input the results on this chart as well in the appropriate spaces.

6. If you've figured out your ovulation day, circle it.

7. If you're taking a home pregnancy test (HPT) this month, input the results in the appropriate boxes.

8. Record your thoughts and feelings during the charting cycle, and keep track of the time you spend each month relaxing (important when you're in the baby-making mode).

Not a Charter?

Charting is a great way to keep track of your fertility, but it's definitely not a requirement of TTC. If you're just not into charting, or you'd rather play your cycle by ear – or instinct – skip this section. Or just fill in as much – or as little – of each chart as you'd like (just a few rows each month). Don't feel obliged to keep it up, either, if the charting gets old after a while.

Example

Fertility Chart

Month _October ~ November_ Year_____ Last Month's cycle length _28_ This cycle length _29_

Cycle Day	1	2	3	4	5	6	7	8	9	10	11	12	13	14	15
Date	17	18	19	20	21	22	23	24	25	26	27	28	29	30	31
Time Temp Taken	7:00	~~	~~	~~	~~	8:00	9:30	7:00	~~	~~	~~	~~	~~	8:15	~~

Basal Body Waking Temperature (°F)

	99	99	99	99	99	99	99	99	99	99	99	99	99	99	99
	.9	.9	.9	.9	.9	.9	.9	.9	.9	.9	.9	.9	.9	.9	.9
	.8	.8	.8	.8	.8	.8	.8	.8	.8	.8	.8	.8	.8	.8	.8
	.7	.7	.7	.7	.7	.7	.7	.7	.7	.7	.7	.7	.7	.7	.7
	.6	.6	.6	.6	.6	.6	.6	.6	.6	.6	.6	.6	.6	.6	.6
	.5	.5	.5	.5	.5	.5	.5	.5	.5	.5	.5	.5	.5	.5	.5
	.4	.4	.4	.4	.4	.4	.4	.4	.4	.4	.4	.4	.4	.4	.4
	.3	.3	.3	.3	.3	.3	.3	.3	.3	.3	.3	.3	.3	.3	.3
	.2	.2	.2	.2	.2	.2	.2	.2	.2	.2	.2	.2	.2	.2	.2
	.1	.1	.1	.1	.1	.1	.1	.1	.1	.1	.1	.1	.1	.1	.1
	98	98	98	98	98	98	98	98	98	98	98	98	98	98	98
	.9	.9	.9	.9	.9	.9	.9	.9	.9	.9	.9	.9	.9	.9	.9
	.8	.8	.8	.8	.8	.8	.8	.8	.8	.8	.8	.8	.8	.8	.8
	.7	.7	.7	.7	.7	.7	.7	.7	.7	.7	.7	.7	.7	.7	.7
	.6	.6	.6	.6	.6	.6	.6	.6	.6	.6	.6	.6	.6	.6	.6
	.5	.5	.5	.5	.5	.5	.5	.5	.5	.5	.5	.5	.5	.5	.5
	.4	.4	.4	.4	.4	.4	.4	.4	.4	.4	.4	.4	.4	.4	.4
	.3	.3	.3	.3	.3	.3	.3	.3	.3	.3	.3	.3	.3	.3	.3
	.2	.2	.2	.2	.2	.2	.2	.2	.2	.2	.2	.2	.2	.2	.2
	.1	.1	.1	.1	.1	.1	.1	.1	.1	.1	.1	.1	.1	.1	.1
	97	97	97	97	97	97	97	97	97	97	97	97	97	97	97
	.9	.9	.9	.9	.9	.9	.9	.9	.9	.9	.9	.9	.9	.9	.9

Cycle Day	1	2	3	4	5	6	7	8	9	10	11	12	13	14	15
Period/Spotting	P	P	P	P	P										
Cervical Mucus (CM) Consistency*						D	D	D	S	S	C	C	C	E	E
Cervical Position**										C	C	C	O	O	O
OPK/LH Surge											-	-	-	+	
Fertility Monitor										Low	Low	High	High	Peak	Peak
Saliva Test											-	-	-	+	+
Chloride-ion Surge									~	~	-	+	+		
Miscellaneous (travel, illness, stress, medication, change in schedule, late night, etc.)			Ibuprofen		Late Night										
Intercourse					x									x	x
HPT (pregnancy test)															

*Cervical Fluid Consistency: **D:** Dry **E:** Egg white/Slippery **S:** Sticky **C:** Creamy

Thoughts and feelings _____ | **Ways I relaxed this month** _____

16	17	18	19	20	21	22	23	24	25	26	27	28	29	30	31	32	33	34	35
1	2	3	4	5	6	7	8	9	10	11	12	13	14	15	16	17	18	19	20
7:00	~	~	~	8:00	9:30	7:00	~	~	~	~	~	8:15	~	7:00	~	~	9:00	~	
99	99	99	99	99	99	99	99	99	99	99	99	99	99	99	99	99	99	99	99
.9	.9	.9	.9	.9	.9	.9	.9	.9	.9	.9	.9	.9	.9	.9	.9	.9	.9	.9	.9
.8	.8	.8	.8	.8	.8	.8	.8	.8	.8	.8	.8	.8	.8	.8	.8	.8	.8	.8	.8
.7	.7	.7	.7	.7	.7	.7	.7	.7	.7	.7	.7	.7	.7	.7	.7	.7	.7	.7	.7
.6	.6	.6	.6	.6	.6	.6	.6	.6	.6	.6	.6	.6	.6	.6	.6	.6	.6	.6	.6
.5	.5	.5	.5	.5	.5	.5	.5	.5	.5	.5	.5	.5	.5	.5	.5	.5	.5	.5	.5
.4	.4	.4	.4	.4	.4	.4	.4	.4	.4	.4	.4	.4	.4	.4	.4	.4	.4	.4	.4
.3	.3	.3	.3	.3	.3	.3	.3	.3	.3	.3	.3	.3	.3	.3	.3	.3	.3	.3	.3
.2	.2	.2	.2	.2	.2	.2	.2	.2	.2	.2	.2	.2	.2	.2	.2	.2	.2	.2	.2
.1	.1	.1	.1	.1	.1	.1	.1	.1	.1	.1	.1	.1	.1	.1	.1	.1	.1	.1	.1
98	98	98	98	98	98	98	98	98	98	98	98	98	98	98	98	98	98	98	98
.9	.9	.9	.9	.9	.9	.9	.9	.9	.9	.9	.9	.9	.9	.9	.9	.9	.9	.9	.9
.8	.8	.8	.8	.8	.8	.8	.8	.8	.8	.8	.8	.8	.8	.8	.8	.8	.8	.8	.8
.7	.7	.7	.7	.7	.7	.7	.7	.7	.7	.7	.7	.7	.7	.7	.7	.7	.7	.7	.7
.6	.6	.6	.6	.6	.6	.6	.6	.6	.6	.6	.6	.6	.6	.6	.6	.6	.6	.6	.6
.5	.5	.5	.5	.5	.5	.5	.5	.5	.5	.5	.5	.5	.5	.5	.5	.5	.5	.5	.5
.4	.4	.4	.4	.4	.4	.4	.4	.4	.4	.4	.4	.4	.4	.4	.4	.4	.4	.4	.4
.3	.3	.3	.3	.3	.3	.3	.3	.3	.3	.3	.3	.3	.3	.3	.3	.3	.3	.3	.3
.2	.2	.2	.2	.2	.2	.2	.2	.2	.2	.2	.2	.2	.2	.2	.2	.2	.2	.2	.2
.1	.1	.1	.1	.1	.1	.1	.1	.1	.1	.1	.1	.1	.1	.1	.1	.1	.1	.1	.1
97	97	97	97	97	97	97	97	97	97	97	97	97	97	97	97	97	97	97	97
.9	.9	.9	.9	.9	.9	.9	.9	.9	.9	.9	.9	.9	.9	.9	.9	.9	.9	.9	.9
16	17	18	19	20	21	22	23	24	25	26	27	28	29	30	31	32	33	34	35
E	C	C	S	D	D	D													
O	C	C																	
High	Low																		
x	x			x															
																Neg	Neg	Pos	

Stomach bug

**Cervical Position: O: Open/Soft C: Closed/Firm

Fertility Chart

Month_____ Year_____ Last Month's cycle length_____ This cycle length_____

Cycle Day	1	2	3	4	5	6	7	8	9	10	11	12	13	14	15
Date															
Time Temp Taken															
	99	99	99	99	99	99	99	99	99	99	99	99	99	99	99
	.9	.9	.9	.9	.9	.9	.9	.9	.9	.9	.9	.9	.9	.9	.9
	.8	.8	.8	.8	.8	.8	.8	.8	.8	.8	.8	.8	.8	.8	.8
	.7	.7	.7	.7	.7	.7	.7	.7	.7	.7	.7	.7	.7	.7	.7
	.6	.6	.6	.6	.6	.6	.6	.6	.6	.6	.6	.6	.6	.6	.6
	.5	.5	.5	.5	.5	.5	.5	.5	.5	.5	.5	.5	.5	.5	.5
	.4	.4	.4	.4	.4	.4	.4	.4	.4	.4	.4	.4	.4	.4	.4
	.3	.3	.3	.3	.3	.3	.3	.3	.3	.3	.3	.3	.3	.3	.3
Basal Body	.2	.2	.2	.2	.2	.2	.2	.2	.2	.2	.2	.2	.2	.2	.2
Waking	.1	.1	.1	.1	.1	.1	.1	.1	.1	.1	.1	.1	.1	.1	.1
Temperature (°F)	98	98	98	98	98	98	98	98	98	98	98	98	98	98	98
	.9	.9	.9	.9	.9	.9	.9	.9	.9	.9	.9	.9	.9	.9	.9
	.8	.8	.8	.8	.8	.8	.8	.8	.8	.8	.8	.8	.8	.8	.8
	.7	.7	.7	.7	.7	.7	.7	.7	.7	.7	.7	.7	.7	.7	.7
	.6	.6	.6	.6	.6	.6	.6	.6	.6	.6	.6	.6	.6	.6	.6
	.5	.5	.5	.5	.5	.5	.5	.5	.5	.5	.5	.5	.5	.5	.5
	.4	.4	.4	.4	.4	.4	.4	.4	.4	.4	.4	.4	.4	.4	.4
	.3	.3	.3	.3	.3	.3	.3	.3	.3	.3	.3	.3	.3	.3	.3
	.2	.2	.2	.2	.2	.2	.2	.2	.2	.2	.2	.2	.2	.2	.2
	.1	.1	.1	.1	.1	.1	.1	.1	.1	.1	.1	.1	.1	.1	.1
	97	97	97	97	97	97	97	97	97	97	97	97	97	97	97
	.9	.9	.9	.9	.9	.9	.9	.9	.9	.9	.9	.9	.9	.9	.9
Cycle Day	1	2	3	4	5	6	7	8	9	10	11	12	13	14	15
Period/Spotting															
Cervical Mucus (CM) Consistency*															
Cervical Position**															
OPK/LH Surge															
Fertility Monitor															
Saliva Test															
Chloride-ion Surge															
Miscellaneous (travel, illness, stress, medication, change in schedule, late night, etc.)															
Intercourse															
HPT (pregnancy test)															

*Cervical Fluid Consistency: **D:** Dry **E:** Egg white/Slippery **S:** Sticky **C:** Creamy

Thoughts and feelings _____ | **Ways I relaxed this month** _____

16	17	18	19	20	21	22	23	24	25	26	27	28	29	30	31	32	33	34	35
99	99	99	99	99	99	99	99	99	99	99	99	99	99	99	99	99	99	99	99
.9	.9	.9	.9	.9	.9	.9	.9	.9	.9	.9	.9	.9	.9	.9	.9	.9	.9	.9	.9
.8	.8	.8	.8	.8	.8	.8	.8	.8	.8	.8	.8	.8	.8	.8	.8	.8	.8	.8	.8
.7	.7	.7	.7	.7	.7	.7	.7	.7	.7	.7	.7	.7	.7	.7	.7	.7	.7	.7	.7
.6	.6	.6	.6	.6	.6	.6	.6	.6	.6	.6	.6	.6	.6	.6	.6	.6	.6	.6	.6
.5	.5	.5	.5	.5	.5	.5	.5	.5	.5	.5	.5	.5	.5	.5	.5	.5	.5	.5	.5
.4	.4	.4	.4	.4	.4	.4	.4	.4	.4	.4	.4	.4	.4	.4	.4	.4	.4	.4	.4
.3	.3	.3	.3	.3	.3	.3	.3	.3	.3	.3	.3	.3	.3	.3	.3	.3	.3	.3	.3
.2	.2	.2	.2	.2	.2	.2	.2	.2	.2	.2	.2	.2	.2	.2	.2	.2	.2	.2	.2
.1	.1	.1	.1	.1	.1	.1	.1	.1	.1	.1	.1	.1	.1	.1	.1	.1	.1	.1	.1
98	98	98	98	98	98	98	98	98	98	98	98	98	98	98	98	98	98	98	98
.9	.9	.9	.9	.9	.9	.9	.9	.9	.9	.9	.9	.9	.9	.9	.9	.9	.9	.9	.9
.8	.8	.8	.8	.8	.8	.8	.8	.8	.8	.8	.8	.8	.8	.8	.8	.8	.8	.8	.8
.7	.7	.7	.7	.7	.7	.7	.7	.7	.7	.7	.7	.7	.7	.7	.7	.7	.7	.7	.7
.6	.6	.6	.6	.6	.6	.6	.6	.6	.6	.6	.6	.6	.6	.6	.6	.6	.6	.6	.6
.5	.5	.5	.5	.5	.5	.5	.5	.5	.5	.5	.5	.5	.5	.5	.5	.5	.5	.5	.5
.4	.4	.4	.4	.4	.4	.4	.4	.4	.4	.4	.4	.4	.4	.4	.4	.4	.4	.4	.4
.3	.3	.3	.3	.3	.3	.3	.3	.3	.3	.3	.3	.3	.3	.3	.3	.3	.3	.3	.3
.2	.2	.2	.2	.2	.2	.2	.2	.2	.2	.2	.2	.2	.2	.2	.2	.2	.2	.2	.2
.1	.1	.1	.1	.1	.1	.1	.1	.1	.1	.1	.1	.1	.1	.1	.1	.1	.1	.1	.1
97	97	97	97	97	97	97	97	97	97	97	97	97	97	97	97	97	97	97	97
.9	.9	.9	.9	.9	.9	.9	.9	.9	.9	.9	.9	.9	.9	.9	.9	.9	.9	.9	.9
16	**17**	**18**	**19**	**20**	**21**	**22**	**23**	**24**	**25**	**26**	**27**	**28**	**29**	**30**	**31**	**32**	**33**	**34**	**35**

Cervical Position: O: Open/Soft **C: Closed/Firm

Fertility Chart

Month_____ Year_____ Last Month's cycle length_____ This cycle length_____

Cycle Day	1	2	3	4	5	6	7	8	9	10	11	12	13	14	15
Date															
Time Temp Taken															
	99	99	99	99	99	99	99	99	99	99	99	99	99	99	99
	.9	.9	.9	.9	.9	.9	.9	.9	.9	.9	.9	.9	.9	.9	.9
	.8	.8	.8	.8	.8	.8	.8	.8	.8	.8	.8	.8	.8	.8	.8
	.7	.7	.7	.7	.7	.7	.7	.7	.7	.7	.7	.7	.7	.7	.7
	.6	.6	.6	.6	.6	.6	.6	.6	.6	.6	.6	.6	.6	.6	.6
	.5	.5	.5	.5	.5	.5	.5	.5	.5	.5	.5	.5	.5	.5	.5
	.4	.4	.4	.4	.4	.4	.4	.4	.4	.4	.4	.4	.4	.4	.4
	.3	.3	.3	.3	.3	.3	.3	.3	.3	.3	.3	.3	.3	.3	.3
Basal Body	.2	.2	.2	.2	.2	.2	.2	.2	.2	.2	.2	.2	.2	.2	.2
Waking	.1	.1	.1	.1	.1	.1	.1	.1	.1	.1	.1	.1	.1	.1	.1
Temperature (°F)	98	98	98	98	98	98	98	98	98	98	98	98	98	98	98
	.9	.9	.9	.9	.9	.9	.9	.9	.9	.9	.9	.9	.9	.9	.9
	.8	.8	.8	.8	.8	.8	.8	.8	.8	.8	.8	.8	.8	.8	.8
	.7	.7	.7	.7	.7	.7	.7	.7	.7	.7	.7	.7	.7	.7	.7
	.6	.6	.6	.6	.6	.6	.6	.6	.6	.6	.6	.6	.6	.6	.6
	.5	.5	.5	.5	.5	.5	.5	.5	.5	.5	.5	.5	.5	.5	.5
	.4	.4	.4	.4	.4	.4	.4	.4	.4	.4	.4	.4	.4	.4	.4
	.3	.3	.3	.3	.3	.3	.3	.3	.3	.3	.3	.3	.3	.3	.3
	.2	.2	.2	.2	.2	.2	.2	.2	.2	.2	.2	.2	.2	.2	.2
	.1	.1	.1	.1	.1	.1	.1	.1	.1	.1	.1	.1	.1	.1	.1
	97	97	97	97	97	97	97	97	97	97	97	97	97	97	97
	.9	.9	.9	.9	.9	.9	.9	.9	.9	.9	.9	.9	.9	.9	.9
Cycle Day	1	2	3	4	5	6	7	8	9	10	11	12	13	14	15
Period/Spotting															
Cervical Mucus (CM) Consistency*															
Cervical Position**															
OPK/LH Surge															
Fertility Monitor															
Saliva Test															
Chloride-ion Surge															
Miscellaneous (travel, illness, stress, medication, change in schedule, late night, etc.)															
Intercourse															
HPT (pregnancy test)															

*Cervical Fluid Consistency: **D:** Dry **E:** Egg white/Slippery **S:** Sticky **C:** Creamy

Thoughts and feelings _____ | **Ways I relaxed this month** _____

16	17	18	19	20	21	22	23	24	25	26	27	28	29	30	31	32	33	34	35
99	99	99	99	99	99	99	99	99	99	99	99	99	99	99	99	99	99	99	99
.9	.9	.9	.9	.9	.9	.9	.9	.9	.9	.9	.9	.9	.9	.9	.9	.9	.9	.9	.9
.8	.8	.8	.8	.8	.8	.8	.8	.8	.8	.8	.8	.8	.8	.8	.8	.8	.8	.8	.8
.7	.7	.7	.7	.7	.7	.7	.7	.7	.7	.7	.7	.7	.7	.7	.7	.7	.7	.7	.7
.6	.6	.6	.6	.6	.6	.6	.6	.6	.6	.6	.6	.6	.6	.6	.6	.6	.6	.6	.6
.5	.5	.5	.5	.5	.5	.5	.5	.5	.5	.5	.5	.5	.5	.5	.5	.5	.5	.5	.5
.4	.4	.4	.4	.4	.4	.4	.4	.4	.4	.4	.4	.4	.4	.4	.4	.4	.4	.4	.4
.3	.3	.3	.3	.3	.3	.3	.3	.3	.3	.3	.3	.3	.3	.3	.3	.3	.3	.3	.3
.2	.2	.2	.2	.2	.2	.2	.2	.2	.2	.2	.2	.2	.2	.2	.2	.2	.2	.2	.2
.1	.1	.1	.1	.1	.1	.1	.1	.1	.1	.1	.1	.1	.1	.1	.1	.1	.1	.1	.1
98	98	98	98	98	98	98	98	98	98	98	98	98	98	98	98	98	98	98	98
.9	.9	.9	.9	.9	.9	.9	.9	.9	.9	.9	.9	.9	.9	.9	.9	.9	.9	.9	.9
.8	.8	.8	.8	.8	.8	.8	.8	.8	.8	.8	.8	.8	.8	.8	.8	.8	.8	.8	.8
.7	.7	.7	.7	.7	.7	.7	.7	.7	.7	.7	.7	.7	.7	.7	.7	.7	.7	.7	.7
.6	.6	.6	.6	.6	.6	.6	.6	.6	.6	.6	.6	.6	.6	.6	.6	.6	.6	.6	.6
.5	.5	.5	.5	.5	.5	.5	.5	.5	.5	.5	.5	.5	.5	.5	.5	.5	.5	.5	.5
.4	.4	.4	.4	.4	.4	.4	.4	.4	.4	.4	.4	.4	.4	.4	.4	.4	.4	.4	.4
.3	.3	.3	.3	.3	.3	.3	.3	.3	.3	.3	.3	.3	.3	.3	.3	.3	.3	.3	.3
.2	.2	.2	.2	.2	.2	.2	.2	.2	.2	.2	.2	.2	.2	.2	.2	.2	.2	.2	.2
.1	.1	.1	.1	.1	.1	.1	.1	.1	.1	.1	.1	.1	.1	.1	.1	.1	.1	.1	.1
97	97	97	97	97	97	97	97	97	97	97	97	97	97	97	97	97	97	97	97
.9	.9	.9	.9	.9	.9	.9	.9	.9	.9	.9	.9	.9	.9	.9	.9	.9	.9	.9	.9
16	17	18	19	20	21	22	23	24	25	26	27	28	29	30	31	32	33	34	35

Cervical Position: O: Open/Soft **C: Closed/Firm

Fertility Chart

Month_____ Year_____ Last Month's cycle length_____ This cycle length_____

Cycle Day	1	2	3	4	5	6	7	8	9	10	11	12	13	14	15
Date															
Time Temp Taken															
Basal Body Waking Temperature (°F)	99	99	99	99	99	99	99	99	99	99	99	99	99	99	99
	.9	.9	.9	.9	.9	.9	.9	.9	.9	.9	.9	.9	.9	.9	.9
	.8	.8	.8	.8	.8	.8	.8	.8	.8	.8	.8	.8	.8	.8	.8
	.7	.7	.7	.7	.7	.7	.7	.7	.7	.7	.7	.7	.7	.7	.7
	.6	.6	.6	.6	.6	.6	.6	.6	.6	.6	.6	.6	.6	.6	.6
	.5	.5	.5	.5	.5	.5	.5	.5	.5	.5	.5	.5	.5	.5	.5
	.4	.4	.4	.4	.4	.4	.4	.4	.4	.4	.4	.4	.4	.4	.4
	.3	.3	.3	.3	.3	.3	.3	.3	.3	.3	.3	.3	.3	.3	.3
	.2	.2	.2	.2	.2	.2	.2	.2	.2	.2	.2	.2	.2	.2	.2
	.1	.1	.1	.1	.1	.1	.1	.1	.1	.1	.1	.1	.1	.1	.1
	98	98	98	98	98	98	98	98	98	98	98	98	98	98	98
	.9	.9	.9	.9	.9	.9	.9	.9	.9	.9	.9	.9	.9	.9	.9
	.8	.8	.8	.8	.8	.8	.8	.8	.8	.8	.8	.8	.8	.8	.8
	.7	.7	.7	.7	.7	.7	.7	.7	.7	.7	.7	.7	.7	.7	.7
	.6	.6	.6	.6	.6	.6	.6	.6	.6	.6	.6	.6	.6	.6	.6
	.5	.5	.5	.5	.5	.5	.5	.5	.5	.5	.5	.5	.5	.5	.5
	.4	.4	.4	.4	.4	.4	.4	.4	.4	.4	.4	.4	.4	.4	.4
	.3	.3	.3	.3	.3	.3	.3	.3	.3	.3	.3	.3	.3	.3	.3
	.2	.2	.2	.2	.2	.2	.2	.2	.2	.2	.2	.2	.2	.2	.2
	.1	.1	.1	.1	.1	.1	.1	.1	.1	.1	.1	.1	.1	.1	.1
	97	97	97	97	97	97	97	97	97	97	97	97	97	97	97
	.9	.9	.9	.9	.9	.9	.9	.9	.9	.9	.9	.9	.9	.9	.9

Cycle Day	1	2	3	4	5	6	7	8	9	10	11	12	13	14	15
Period/Spotting															
Cervical Mucus (CM) Consistency*															
Cervical Position**															
OPK/LH Surge															
Fertility Monitor															
Saliva Test															
Chloride-ion Surge															
Miscellaneous (travel, illness, stress, medication, change in schedule, late night, etc.)															
Intercourse															
HPT (pregnancy test)															

*Cervical Fluid Consistency: **D:** Dry **E:** Egg white/Slippery **S:** Sticky **C:** Creamy

Thoughts and feelings _____ | **Ways I relaxed this month** _____

16	17	18	19	20	21	22	23	24	25	26	27	28	29	30	31	32	33	34	35
99	99	99	99	99	99	99	99	99	99	99	99	99	99	99	99	99	99	99	99
.9	.9	.9	.9	.9	.9	.9	.9	.9	.9	.9	.9	.9	.9	.9	.9	.9	.9	.9	.9
.8	.8	.8	.8	.8	.8	.8	.8	.8	.8	.8	.8	.8	.8	.8	.8	.8	.8	.8	.8
.7	.7	.7	.7	.7	.7	.7	.7	.7	.7	.7	.7	.7	.7	.7	.7	.7	.7	.7	.7
.6	.6	.6	.6	.6	.6	.6	.6	.6	.6	.6	.6	.6	.6	.6	.6	.6	.6	.6	.6
.5	.5	.5	.5	.5	.5	.5	.5	.5	.5	.5	.5	.5	.5	.5	.5	.5	.5	.5	.5
.4	.4	.4	.4	.4	.4	.4	.4	.4	.4	.4	.4	.4	.4	.4	.4	.4	.4	.4	.4
.3	.3	.3	.3	.3	.3	.3	.3	.3	.3	.3	.3	.3	.3	.3	.3	.3	.3	.3	.3
.2	.2	.2	.2	.2	.2	.2	.2	.2	.2	.2	.2	.2	.2	.2	.2	.2	.2	.2	.2
.1	.1	.1	.1	.1	.1	.1	.1	.1	.1	.1	.1	.1	.1	.1	.1	.1	.1	.1	.1
98	98	98	98	98	98	98	98	98	98	98	98	98	98	98	98	98	98	98	98
.9	.9	.9	.9	.9	.9	.9	.9	.9	.9	.9	.9	.9	.9	.9	.9	.9	.9	.9	.9
.8	.8	.8	.8	.8	.8	.8	.8	.8	.8	.8	.8	.8	.8	.8	.8	.8	.8	.8	.8
.7	.7	.7	.7	.7	.7	.7	.7	.7	.7	.7	.7	.7	.7	.7	.7	.7	.7	.7	.7
.6	.6	.6	.6	.6	.6	.6	.6	.6	.6	.6	.6	.6	.6	.6	.6	.6	.6	.6	.6
.5	.5	.5	.5	.5	.5	.5	.5	.5	.5	.5	.5	.5	.5	.5	.5	.5	.5	.5	.5
.4	.4	.4	.4	.4	.4	.4	.4	.4	.4	.4	.4	.4	.4	.4	.4	.4	.4	.4	.4
.3	.3	.3	.3	.3	.3	.3	.3	.3	.3	.3	.3	.3	.3	.3	.3	.3	.3	.3	.3
.2	.2	.2	.2	.2	.2	.2	.2	.2	.2	.2	.2	.2	.2	.2	.2	.2	.2	.2	.2
.1	.1	.1	.1	.1	.1	.1	.1	.1	.1	.1	.1	.1	.1	.1	.1	.1	.1	.1	.1
97	97	97	97	97	97	97	97	97	97	97	97	97	97	97	97	97	97	97	97
.9	.9	.9	.9	.9	.9	.9	.9	.9	.9	.9	.9	.9	.9	.9	.9	.9	.9	.9	.9
16	17	18	19	20	21	22	23	24	25	26	27	28	29	30	31	32	33	34	35

Cervical Position: O: Open/Soft **C:** Closed/Firm

Fertility Chart

Month_____ Year_____ Last Month's cycle length_____ This cycle length_____

Cycle Day	1	2	3	4	5	6	7	8	9	10	11	12	13	14	15
Date															
Time Temp Taken															
	99	99	99	99	99	99	99	99	99	99	99	99	99	99	99
	.9	.9	.9	.9	.9	.9	.9	.9	.9	.9	.9	.9	.9	.9	.9
	.8	.8	.8	.8	.8	.8	.8	.8	.8	.8	.8	.8	.8	.8	.8
	.7	.7	.7	.7	.7	.7	.7	.7	.7	.7	.7	.7	.7	.7	.7
	.6	.6	.6	.6	.6	.6	.6	.6	.6	.6	.6	.6	.6	.6	.6
	.5	.5	.5	.5	.5	.5	.5	.5	.5	.5	.5	.5	.5	.5	.5
	.4	.4	.4	.4	.4	.4	.4	.4	.4	.4	.4	.4	.4	.4	.4
	.3	.3	.3	.3	.3	.3	.3	.3	.3	.3	.3	.3	.3	.3	.3
Basal Body	.2	.2	.2	.2	.2	.2	.2	.2	.2	.2	.2	.2	.2	.2	.2
Waking	.1	.1	.1	.1	.1	.1	.1	.1	.1	.1	.1	.1	.1	.1	.1
Temperature (°F)	98	98	98	98	98	98	98	98	98	98	98	98	98	98	98
	.9	.9	.9	.9	.9	.9	.9	.9	.9	.9	.9	.9	.9	.9	.9
	.8	.8	.8	.8	.8	.8	.8	.8	.8	.8	.8	.8	.8	.8	.8
	.7	.7	.7	.7	.7	.7	.7	.7	.7	.7	.7	.7	.7	.7	.7
	.6	.6	.6	.6	.6	.6	.6	.6	.6	.6	.6	.6	.6	.6	.6
	.5	.5	.5	.5	.5	.5	.5	.5	.5	.5	.5	.5	.5	.5	.5
	.4	.4	.4	.4	.4	.4	.4	.4	.4	.4	.4	.4	.4	.4	.4
	.3	.3	.3	.3	.3	.3	.3	.3	.3	.3	.3	.3	.3	.3	.3
	.2	.2	.2	.2	.2	.2	.2	.2	.2	.2	.2	.2	.2	.2	.2
	.1	.1	.1	.1	.1	.1	.1	.1	.1	.1	.1	.1	.1	.1	.1
	97	97	97	97	97	97	97	97	97	97	97	97	97	97	97
	.9	.9	.9	.9	.9	.9	.9	.9	.9	.9	.9	.9	.9	.9	.9
Cycle Day	1	2	3	4	5	6	7	8	9	10	11	12	13	14	15
Period/Spotting															
Cervical Mucus (CM) Consistency*															
Cervical Position**															
OPK/LH Surge															
Fertility Monitor															
Saliva Test															
Chloride-ion Surge															
Miscellaneous (travel, illness, stress, medication, change in schedule, late night, etc.)															
Intercourse															
HPT (pregnancy test)															

*Cervical Fluid Consistency: **D:** Dry **E:** Egg white/Slippery **S:** Sticky **C:** Creamy

Thoughts and feelings _____ | **Ways I relaxed this month** _____

16	17	18	19	20	21	22	23	24	25	26	27	28	29	30	31	32	33	34	35
99	99	99	99	99	99	99	99	99	99	99	99	99	99	99	99	99	99	99	99
.9	.9	.9	.9	.9	.9	.9	.9	.9	.9	.9	.9	.9	.9	.9	.9	.9	.9	.9	.9
.8	.8	.8	.8	.8	.8	.8	.8	.8	.8	.8	.8	.8	.8	.8	.8	.8	.8	.8	.8
.7	.7	.7	.7	.7	.7	.7	.7	.7	.7	.7	.7	.7	.7	.7	.7	.7	.7	.7	.7
.6	.6	.6	.6	.6	.6	.6	.6	.6	.6	.6	.6	.6	.6	.6	.6	.6	.6	.6	.6
.5	.5	.5	.5	.5	.5	.5	.5	.5	.5	.5	.5	.5	.5	.5	.5	.5	.5	.5	.5
.4	.4	.4	.4	.4	.4	.4	.4	.4	.4	.4	.4	.4	.4	.4	.4	.4	.4	.4	.4
.3	.3	.3	.3	.3	.3	.3	.3	.3	.3	.3	.3	.3	.3	.3	.3	.3	.3	.3	.3
.2	.2	.2	.2	.2	.2	.2	.2	.2	.2	.2	.2	.2	.2	.2	.2	.2	.2	.2	.2
.1	.1	.1	.1	.1	.1	.1	.1	.1	.1	.1	.1	.1	.1	.1	.1	.1	.1	.1	.1
98	98	98	98	98	98	98	98	98	98	98	98	98	98	98	98	98	98	98	98
.9	.9	.9	.9	.9	.9	.9	.9	.9	.9	.9	.9	.9	.9	.9	.9	.9	.9	.9	.9
.8	.8	.8	.8	.8	.8	.8	.8	.8	.8	.8	.8	.8	.8	.8	.8	.8	.8	.8	.8
.7	.7	.7	.7	.7	.7	.7	.7	.7	.7	.7	.7	.7	.7	.7	.7	.7	.7	.7	.7
.6	.6	.6	.6	.6	.6	.6	.6	.6	.6	.6	.6	.6	.6	.6	.6	.6	.6	.6	.6
.5	.5	.5	.5	.5	.5	.5	.5	.5	.5	.5	.5	.5	.5	.5	.5	.5	.5	.5	.5
.4	.4	.4	.4	.4	.4	.4	.4	.4	.4	.4	.4	.4	.4	.4	.4	.4	.4	.4	.4
.3	.3	.3	.3	.3	.3	.3	.3	.3	.3	.3	.3	.3	.3	.3	.3	.3	.3	.3	.3
.2	.2	.2	.2	.2	.2	.2	.2	.2	.2	.2	.2	.2	.2	.2	.2	.2	.2	.2	.2
.1	.1	.1	.1	.1	.1	.1	.1	.1	.1	.1	.1	.1	.1	.1	.1	.1	.1	.1	.1
97	97	97	97	97	97	97	97	97	97	97	97	97	97	97	97	97	97	97	97
.9	.9	.9	.9	.9	.9	.9	.9	.9	.9	.9	.9	.9	.9	.9	.9	.9	.9	.9	.9
16	**17**	**18**	**19**	**20**	**21**	**22**	**23**	**24**	**25**	**26**	**27**	**28**	**29**	**30**	**31**	**32**	**33**	**34**	**35**

Cervical Position: **O: Open/Soft **C:** Closed/Firm

Fertility Chart

Month_____ Year_____ Last Month's cycle length_____ This cycle length_____

Cycle Day	1	2	3	4	5	6	7	8	9	10	11	12	13	14	15
Date															
Time Temp Taken															
Basal Body Waking Temperature (°F)	99	99	99	99	99	99	99	99	99	99	99	99	99	99	99
	.9	.9	.9	.9	.9	.9	.9	.9	.9	.9	.9	.9	.9	.9	.9
	.8	.8	.8	.8	.8	.8	.8	.8	.8	.8	.8	.8	.8	.8	.8
	.7	.7	.7	.7	.7	.7	.7	.7	.7	.7	.7	.7	.7	.7	.7
	.6	.6	.6	.6	.6	.6	.6	.6	.6	.6	.6	.6	.6	.6	.6
	.5	.5	.5	.5	.5	.5	.5	.5	.5	.5	.5	.5	.5	.5	.5
	.4	.4	.4	.4	.4	.4	.4	.4	.4	.4	.4	.4	.4	.4	.4
	.3	.3	.3	.3	.3	.3	.3	.3	.3	.3	.3	.3	.3	.3	.3
	.2	.2	.2	.2	.2	.2	.2	.2	.2	.2	.2	.2	.2	.2	.2
	.1	.1	.1	.1	.1	.1	.1	.1	.1	.1	.1	.1	.1	.1	.1
	98	98	98	98	98	98	98	98	98	98	98	98	98	98	98
	.9	.9	.9	.9	.9	.9	.9	.9	.9	.9	.9	.9	.9	.9	.9
	.8	.8	.8	.8	.8	.8	.8	.8	.8	.8	.8	.8	.8	.8	.8
	.7	.7	.7	.7	.7	.7	.7	.7	.7	.7	.7	.7	.7	.7	.7
	.6	.6	.6	.6	.6	.6	.6	.6	.6	.6	.6	.6	.6	.6	.6
	.5	.5	.5	.5	.5	.5	.5	.5	.5	.5	.5	.5	.5	.5	.5
	.4	.4	.4	.4	.4	.4	.4	.4	.4	.4	.4	.4	.4	.4	.4
	.3	.3	.3	.3	.3	.3	.3	.3	.3	.3	.3	.3	.3	.3	.3
	.2	.2	.2	.2	.2	.2	.2	.2	.2	.2	.2	.2	.2	.2	.2
	.1	.1	.1	.1	.1	.1	.1	.1	.1	.1	.1	.1	.1	.1	.1
	97	97	97	97	97	97	97	97	97	97	97	97	97	97	97
	.9	.9	.9	.9	.9	.9	.9	.9	.9	.9	.9	.9	.9	.9	.9
Cycle Day	1	2	3	4	5	6	7	8	9	10	11	12	13	14	15
Period/Spotting															
Cervical Mucus (CM) Consistency*															
Cervical Position**															
OPK/LH Surge															
Fertility Monitor															
Saliva Test															
Chloride-ion Surge															
Miscellaneous (travel, illness, stress, medication, change in schedule, late night, etc.)															
Intercourse															
HPT (pregnancy test)															

*Cervical Fluid Consistency: **D:** Dry **E:** Egg white/Slippery **S:** Sticky **C:** Creamy

Thoughts and feelings _____ | **Ways I relaxed this month** _____

16	17	18	19	20	21	22	23	24	25	26	27	28	29	30	31	32	33	34	35
99	99	99	99	99	99	99	99	99	99	99	99	99	99	99	99	99	99	99	99
.9	.9	.9	.9	.9	.9	.9	.9	.9	.9	.9	.9	.9	.9	.9	.9	.9	.9	.9	.9
.8	.8	.8	.8	.8	.8	.8	.8	.8	.8	.8	.8	.8	.8	.8	.8	.8	.8	.8	.8
.7	.7	.7	.7	.7	.7	.7	.7	.7	.7	.7	.7	.7	.7	.7	.7	.7	.7	.7	.7
.6	.6	.6	.6	.6	.6	.6	.6	.6	.6	.6	.6	.6	.6	.6	.6	.6	.6	.6	.6
.5	.5	.5	.5	.5	.5	.5	.5	.5	.5	.5	.5	.5	.5	.5	.5	.5	.5	.5	.5
.4	.4	.4	.4	.4	.4	.4	.4	.4	.4	.4	.4	.4	.4	.4	.4	.4	.4	.4	.4
.3	.3	.3	.3	.3	.3	.3	.3	.3	.3	.3	.3	.3	.3	.3	.3	.3	.3	.3	.3
.2	.2	.2	.2	.2	.2	.2	.2	.2	.2	.2	.2	.2	.2	.2	.2	.2	.2	.2	.2
.1	.1	.1	.1	.1	.1	.1	.1	.1	.1	.1	.1	.1	.1	.1	.1	.1	.1	.1	.1
98	98	98	98	98	98	98	98	98	98	98	98	98	98	98	98	98	98	98	98
.9	.9	.9	.9	.9	.9	.9	.9	.9	.9	.9	.9	.9	.9	.9	.9	.9	.9	.9	.9
.8	.8	.8	.8	.8	.8	.8	.8	.8	.8	.8	.8	.8	.8	.8	.8	.8	.8	.8	.8
.7	.7	.7	.7	.7	.7	.7	.7	.7	.7	.7	.7	.7	.7	.7	.7	.7	.7	.7	.7
.6	.6	.6	.6	.6	.6	.6	.6	.6	.6	.6	.6	.6	.6	.6	.6	.6	.6	.6	.6
.5	.5	.5	.5	.5	.5	.5	.5	.5	.5	.5	.5	.5	.5	.5	.5	.5	.5	.5	.5
.4	.4	.4	.4	.4	.4	.4	.4	.4	.4	.4	.4	.4	.4	.4	.4	.4	.4	.4	.4
.3	.3	.3	.3	.3	.3	.3	.3	.3	.3	.3	.3	.3	.3	.3	.3	.3	.3	.3	.3
.2	.2	.2	.2	.2	.2	.2	.2	.2	.2	.2	.2	.2	.2	.2	.2	.2	.2	.2	.2
.1	.1	.1	.1	.1	.1	.1	.1	.1	.1	.1	.1	.1	.1	.1	.1	.1	.1	.1	.1
97	97	97	97	97	97	97	97	97	97	97	97	97	97	97	97	97	97	97	97
.9	.9	.9	.9	.9	.9	.9	.9	.9	.9	.9	.9	.9	.9	.9	.9	.9	.9	.9	.9
16	17	18	19	20	21	22	23	24	25	26	27	28	29	30	31	32	33	34	35

Cervical Position: O: Open/Soft **C:** Closed/Firm

Fertility Chart

Month_____ Year_____ Last Month's cycle length_____ This cycle length_____

Cycle Day	1	2	3	4	5	6	7	8	9	10	11	12	13	14	15
Date															
Time Temp Taken															
	99	99	99	99	99	99	99	99	99	99	99	99	99	99	99
	.9	.9	.9	.9	.9	.9	.9	.9	.9	.9	.9	.9	.9	.9	.9
	.8	.8	.8	.8	.8	.8	.8	.8	.8	.8	.8	.8	.8	.8	.8
	.7	.7	.7	.7	.7	.7	.7	.7	.7	.7	.7	.7	.7	.7	.7
	.6	.6	.6	.6	.6	.6	.6	.6	.6	.6	.6	.6	.6	.6	.6
	.5	.5	.5	.5	.5	.5	.5	.5	.5	.5	.5	.5	.5	.5	.5
	.4	.4	.4	.4	.4	.4	.4	.4	.4	.4	.4	.4	.4	.4	.4
	.3	.3	.3	.3	.3	.3	.3	.3	.3	.3	.3	.3	.3	.3	.3
Basal Body	.2	.2	.2	.2	.2	.2	.2	.2	.2	.2	.2	.2	.2	.2	.2
Waking	.1	.1	.1	.1	.1	.1	.1	.1	.1	.1	.1	.1	.1	.1	.1
Temperature (°F)	98	98	98	98	98	98	98	98	98	98	98	98	98	98	98
	.9	.9	.9	.9	.9	.9	.9	.9	.9	.9	.9	.9	.9	.9	.9
	.8	.8	.8	.8	.8	.8	.8	.8	.8	.8	.8	.8	.8	.8	.8
	.7	.7	.7	.7	.7	.7	.7	.7	.7	.7	.7	.7	.7	.7	.7
	.6	.6	.6	.6	.6	.6	.6	.6	.6	.6	.6	.6	.6	.6	.6
	.5	.5	.5	.5	.5	.5	.5	.5	.5	.5	.5	.5	.5	.5	.5
	.4	.4	.4	.4	.4	.4	.4	.4	.4	.4	.4	.4	.4	.4	.4
	.3	.3	.3	.3	.3	.3	.3	.3	.3	.3	.3	.3	.3	.3	.3
	.2	.2	.2	.2	.2	.2	.2	.2	.2	.2	.2	.2	.2	.2	.2
	.1	.1	.1	.1	.1	.1	.1	.1	.1	.1	.1	.1	.1	.1	.1
	97	97	97	97	97	97	97	97	97	97	97	97	97	97	97
	.9	.9	.9	.9	.9	.9	.9	.9	.9	.9	.9	.9	.9	.9	.9
Cycle Day	1	2	3	4	5	6	7	8	9	10	11	12	13	14	15
Period/Spotting															
Cervical Mucus (CM) Consistency*															
Cervical Position**															
OPK/LH Surge															
Fertility Monitor															
Saliva Test															
Chloride-ion Surge															
Miscellaneous (travel, illness, stress, medication, change in schedule, late night, etc.)															
Intercourse															
HPT (pregnancy test)															

*Cervical Fluid Consistency: **D:** Dry **E:** Egg white/Slippery **S:** Sticky **C:** Creamy

Thoughts and feelings _____ | **Ways I relaxed this month** _____

16	17	18	19	20	21	22	23	24	25	26	27	28	29	30	31	32	33	34	35
99	99	99	99	99	99	99	99	99	99	99	99	99	99	99	99	99	99	99	99
.9	.9	.9	.9	.9	.9	.9	.9	.9	.9	.9	.9	.9	.9	.9	.9	.9	.9	.9	.9
.8	.8	.8	.8	.8	.8	.8	.8	.8	.8	.8	.8	.8	.8	.8	.8	.8	.8	.8	.8
.7	.7	.7	.7	.7	.7	.7	.7	.7	.7	.7	.7	.7	.7	.7	.7	.7	.7	.7	.7
.6	.6	.6	.6	.6	.6	.6	.6	.6	.6	.6	.6	.6	.6	.6	.6	.6	.6	.6	.6
.5	.5	.5	.5	.5	.5	.5	.5	.5	.5	.5	.5	.5	.5	.5	.5	.5	.5	.5	.5
.4	.4	.4	.4	.4	.4	.4	.4	.4	.4	.4	.4	.4	.4	.4	.4	.4	.4	.4	.4
.3	.3	.3	.3	.3	.3	.3	.3	.3	.3	.3	.3	.3	.3	.3	.3	.3	.3	.3	.3
.2	.2	.2	.2	.2	.2	.2	.2	.2	.2	.2	.2	.2	.2	.2	.2	.2	.2	.2	.2
.1	.1	.1	.1	.1	.1	.1	.1	.1	.1	.1	.1	.1	.1	.1	.1	.1	.1	.1	.1
98	98	98	98	98	98	98	98	98	98	98	98	98	98	98	98	98	98	98	98
.9	.9	.9	.9	.9	.9	.9	.9	.9	.9	.9	.9	.9	.9	.9	.9	.9	.9	.9	.9
.8	.8	.8	.8	.8	.8	.8	.8	.8	.8	.8	.8	.8	.8	.8	.8	.8	.8	.8	.8
.7	.7	.7	.7	.7	.7	.7	.7	.7	.7	.7	.7	.7	.7	.7	.7	.7	.7	.7	.7
.6	.6	.6	.6	.6	.6	.6	.6	.6	.6	.6	.6	.6	.6	.6	.6	.6	.6	.6	.6
.5	.5	.5	.5	.5	.5	.5	.5	.5	.5	.5	.5	.5	.5	.5	.5	.5	.5	.5	.5
.4	.4	.4	.4	.4	.4	.4	.4	.4	.4	.4	.4	.4	.4	.4	.4	.4	.4	.4	.4
.3	.3	.3	.3	.3	.3	.3	.3	.3	.3	.3	.3	.3	.3	.3	.3	.3	.3	.3	.3
.2	.2	.2	.2	.2	.2	.2	.2	.2	.2	.2	.2	.2	.2	.2	.2	.2	.2	.2	.2
.1	.1	.1	.1	.1	.1	.1	.1	.1	.1	.1	.1	.1	.1	.1	.1	.1	.1	.1	.1
97	97	97	97	97	97	97	97	97	97	97	97	97	97	97	97	97	97	97	97
.9	.9	.9	.9	.9	.9	.9	.9	.9	.9	.9	.9	.9	.9	.9	.9	.9	.9	.9	.9
16	**17**	**18**	**19**	**20**	**21**	**22**	**23**	**24**	**25**	**26**	**27**	**28**	**29**	**30**	**31**	**32**	**33**	**34**	**35**

Cervical Position: O: Open/Soft **C: Closed/Firm

Fertility Chart

Month_____ Year_____ Last Month's cycle length_____ This cycle length_____

Cycle Day	1	2	3	4	5	6	7	8	9	10	11	12	13	14	15
Date															
Time Temp Taken															
	99	99	99	99	99	99	99	99	99	99	99	99	99	99	99
	.9	.9	.9	.9	.9	.9	.9	.9	.9	.9	.9	.9	.9	.9	.9
	.8	.8	.8	.8	.8	.8	.8	.8	.8	.8	.8	.8	.8	.8	.8
	.7	.7	.7	.7	.7	.7	.7	.7	.7	.7	.7	.7	.7	.7	.7
	.6	.6	.6	.6	.6	.6	.6	.6	.6	.6	.6	.6	.6	.6	.6
	.5	.5	.5	.5	.5	.5	.5	.5	.5	.5	.5	.5	.5	.5	.5
	.4	.4	.4	.4	.4	.4	.4	.4	.4	.4	.4	.4	.4	.4	.4
	.3	.3	.3	.3	.3	.3	.3	.3	.3	.3	.3	.3	.3	.3	.3
Basal Body	.2	.2	.2	.2	.2	.2	.2	.2	.2	.2	.2	.2	.2	.2	.2
Waking	.1	.1	.1	.1	.1	.1	.1	.1	.1	.1	.1	.1	.1	.1	.1
Temperature (°F)	98	98	98	98	98	98	98	98	98	98	98	98	98	98	98
	.9	.9	.9	.9	.9	.9	.9	.9	.9	.9	.9	.9	.9	.9	.9
	.8	.8	.8	.8	.8	.8	.8	.8	.8	.8	.8	.8	.8	.8	.8
	.7	.7	.7	.7	.7	.7	.7	.7	.7	.7	.7	.7	.7	.7	.7
	.6	.6	.6	.6	.6	.6	.6	.6	.6	.6	.6	.6	.6	.6	.6
	.5	.5	.5	.5	.5	.5	.5	.5	.5	.5	.5	.5	.5	.5	.5
	.4	.4	.4	.4	.4	.4	.4	.4	.4	.4	.4	.4	.4	.4	.4
	.3	.3	.3	.3	.3	.3	.3	.3	.3	.3	.3	.3	.3	.3	.3
	.2	.2	.2	.2	.2	.2	.2	.2	.2	.2	.2	.2	.2	.2	.2
	.1	.1	.1	.1	.1	.1	.1	.1	.1	.1	.1	.1	.1	.1	.1
	97	97	97	97	97	97	97	97	97	97	97	97	97	97	97
	.9	.9	.9	.9	.9	.9	.9	.9	.9	.9	.9	.9	.9	.9	.9
Cycle Day	1	2	3	4	5	6	7	8	9	10	11	12	13	14	15
Period/Spotting															
Cervical Mucus (CM) Consistency*															
Cervical Position**															
OPK/LH Surge															
Fertility Monitor															
Saliva Test															
Chloride-ion Surge															
Miscellaneous (travel, illness, stress, medication, change in schedule, late night, etc.)															
Intercourse															
HPT (pregnancy test)															

*Cervical Fluid Consistency: **D:** Dry **E:** Egg white/Slippery **S:** Sticky **C:** Creamy

Thoughts and feelings _____ | **Ways I relaxed this month** _____

16	17	18	19	20	21	22	23	24	25	26	27	28	29	30	31	32	33	34	35
99	99	99	99	99	99	99	99	99	99	99	99	99	99	99	99	99	99	99	99
.9	.9	.9	.9	.9	.9	.9	.9	.9	.9	.9	.9	.9	.9	.9	.9	.9	.9	.9	.9
.8	.8	.8	.8	.8	.8	.8	.8	.8	.8	.8	.8	.8	.8	.8	.8	.8	.8	.8	.8
.7	.7	.7	.7	.7	.7	.7	.7	.7	.7	.7	.7	.7	.7	.7	.7	.7	.7	.7	.7
.6	.6	.6	.6	.6	.6	.6	.6	.6	.6	.6	.6	.6	.6	.6	.6	.6	.6	.6	.6
.5	.5	.5	.5	.5	.5	.5	.5	.5	.5	.5	.5	.5	.5	.5	.5	.5	.5	.5	.5
.4	.4	.4	.4	.4	.4	.4	.4	.4	.4	.4	.4	.4	.4	.4	.4	.4	.4	.4	.4
.3	.3	.3	.3	.3	.3	.3	.3	.3	.3	.3	.3	.3	.3	.3	.3	.3	.3	.3	.3
.2	.2	.2	.2	.2	.2	.2	.2	.2	.2	.2	.2	.2	.2	.2	.2	.2	.2	.2	.2
.1	.1	.1	.1	.1	.1	.1	.1	.1	.1	.1	.1	.1	.1	.1	.1	.1	.1	.1	.1
98	98	98	98	98	98	98	98	98	98	98	98	98	98	98	98	98	98	98	98
.9	.9	.9	.9	.9	.9	.9	.9	.9	.9	.9	.9	.9	.9	.9	.9	.9	.9	.9	.9
.8	.8	.8	.8	.8	.8	.8	.8	.8	.8	.8	.8	.8	.8	.8	.8	.8	.8	.8	.8
.7	.7	.7	.7	.7	.7	.7	.7	.7	.7	.7	.7	.7	.7	.7	.7	.7	.7	.7	.7
.6	.6	.6	.6	.6	.6	.6	.6	.6	.6	.6	.6	.6	.6	.6	.6	.6	.6	.6	.6
.5	.5	.5	.5	.5	.5	.5	.5	.5	.5	.5	.5	.5	.5	.5	.5	.5	.5	.5	.5
.4	.4	.4	.4	.4	.4	.4	.4	.4	.4	.4	.4	.4	.4	.4	.4	.4	.4	.4	.4
.3	.3	.3	.3	.3	.3	.3	.3	.3	.3	.3	.3	.3	.3	.3	.3	.3	.3	.3	.3
.2	.2	.2	.2	.2	.2	.2	.2	.2	.2	.2	.2	.2	.2	.2	.2	.2	.2	.2	.2
.1	.1	.1	.1	.1	.1	.1	.1	.1	.1	.1	.1	.1	.1	.1	.1	.1	.1	.1	.1
97	97	97	97	97	97	97	97	97	97	97	97	97	97	97	97	97	97	97	97
.9	.9	.9	.9	.9	.9	.9	.9	.9	.9	.9	.9	.9	.9	.9	.9	.9	.9	.9	.9
16	17	18	19	20	21	22	23	24	25	26	27	28	29	30	31	32	33	34	35

Cervical Position: O: Open/Soft **C:** Closed/Firm

Fertility Chart

Month_____ Year_____ Last Month's cycle length_____ This cycle length_____

Cycle Day	1	2	3	4	5	6	7	8	9	10	11	12	13	14	15
Date															
Time Temp Taken															
	99	99	99	99	99	99	99	99	99	99	99	99	99	99	99
	.9	.9	.9	.9	.9	.9	.9	.9	.9	.9	.9	.9	.9	.9	.9
	.8	.8	.8	.8	.8	.8	.8	.8	.8	.8	.8	.8	.8	.8	.8
	.7	.7	.7	.7	.7	.7	.7	.7	.7	.7	.7	.7	.7	.7	.7
	.6	.6	.6	.6	.6	.6	.6	.6	.6	.6	.6	.6	.6	.6	.6
	.5	.5	.5	.5	.5	.5	.5	.5	.5	.5	.5	.5	.5	.5	.5
	.4	.4	.4	.4	.4	.4	.4	.4	.4	.4	.4	.4	.4	.4	.4
	.3	.3	.3	.3	.3	.3	.3	.3	.3	.3	.3	.3	.3	.3	.3
Basal Body	.2	.2	.2	.2	.2	.2	.2	.2	.2	.2	.2	.2	.2	.2	.2
Waking	.1	.1	.1	.1	.1	.1	.1	.1	.1	.1	.1	.1	.1	.1	.1
Temperature (°F)	98	98	98	98	98	98	98	98	98	98	98	98	98	98	98
	.9	.9	.9	.9	.9	.9	.9	.9	.9	.9	.9	.9	.9	.9	.9
	.8	.8	.8	.8	.8	.8	.8	.8	.8	.8	.8	.8	.8	.8	.8
	.7	.7	.7	.7	.7	.7	.7	.7	.7	.7	.7	.7	.7	.7	.7
	.6	.6	.6	.6	.6	.6	.6	.6	.6	.6	.6	.6	.6	.6	.6
	.5	.5	.5	.5	.5	.5	.5	.5	.5	.5	.5	.5	.5	.5	.5
	.4	.4	.4	.4	.4	.4	.4	.4	.4	.4	.4	.4	.4	.4	.4
	.3	.3	.3	.3	.3	.3	.3	.3	.3	.3	.3	.3	.3	.3	.3
	.2	.2	.2	.2	.2	.2	.2	.2	.2	.2	.2	.2	.2	.2	.2
	.1	.1	.1	.1	.1	.1	.1	.1	.1	.1	.1	.1	.1	.1	.1
	97	97	97	97	97	97	97	97	97	97	97	97	97	97	97
	.9	.9	.9	.9	.9	.9	.9	.9	.9	.9	.9	.9	.9	.9	.9
Cycle Day	1	2	3	4	5	6	7	8	9	10	11	12	13	14	15
Period/Spotting															
Cervical Mucus (CM) Consistency*															
Cervical Position**															
OPK/LH Surge															
Fertility Monitor															
Saliva Test															
Chloride-ion Surge															
Miscellaneous (travel, illness, stress, medication, change in schedule, late night, etc.)															
Intercourse															
HPT (pregnancy test)															

*Cervical Fluid Consistency: **D:** Dry **E:** Egg white/Slippery **S:** Sticky **C:** Creamy

Thoughts and feelings _____ | **Ways I relaxed this month** _____

16	17	18	19	20	21	22	23	24	25	26	27	28	29	30	31	32	33	34	35
99	99	99	99	99	99	99	99	99	99	99	99	99	99	99	99	99	99	99	99
.9	.9	.9	.9	.9	.9	.9	.9	.9	.9	.9	.9	.9	.9	.9	.9	.9	.9	.9	.9
.8	.8	.8	.8	.8	.8	.8	.8	.8	.8	.8	.8	.8	.8	.8	.8	.8	.8	.8	.8
.7	.7	.7	.7	.7	.7	.7	.7	.7	.7	.7	.7	.7	.7	.7	.7	.7	.7	.7	.7
.6	.6	.6	.6	.6	.6	.6	.6	.6	.6	.6	.6	.6	.6	.6	.6	.6	.6	.6	.6
.5	.5	.5	.5	.5	.5	.5	.5	.5	.5	.5	.5	.5	.5	.5	.5	.5	.5	.5	.5
.4	.4	.4	.4	.4	.4	.4	.4	.4	.4	.4	.4	.4	.4	.4	.4	.4	.4	.4	.4
.3	.3	.3	.3	.3	.3	.3	.3	.3	.3	.3	.3	.3	.3	.3	.3	.3	.3	.3	.3
.2	.2	.2	.2	.2	.2	.2	.2	.2	.2	.2	.2	.2	.2	.2	.2	.2	.2	.2	.2
.1	.1	.1	.1	.1	.1	.1	.1	.1	.1	.1	.1	.1	.1	.1	.1	.1	.1	.1	.1
98	98	98	98	98	98	98	98	98	98	98	98	98	98	98	98	98	98	98	98
.9	.9	.9	.9	.9	.9	.9	.9	.9	.9	.9	.9	.9	.9	.9	.9	.9	.9	.9	.9
.8	.8	.8	.8	.8	.8	.8	.8	.8	.8	.8	.8	.8	.8	.8	.8	.8	.8	.8	.8
.7	.7	.7	.7	.7	.7	.7	.7	.7	.7	.7	.7	.7	.7	.7	.7	.7	.7	.7	.7
.6	.6	.6	.6	.6	.6	.6	.6	.6	.6	.6	.6	.6	.6	.6	.6	.6	.6	.6	.6
.5	.5	.5	.5	.5	.5	.5	.5	.5	.5	.5	.5	.5	.5	.5	.5	.5	.5	.5	.5
.4	.4	.4	.4	.4	.4	.4	.4	.4	.4	.4	.4	.4	.4	.4	.4	.4	.4	.4	.4
.3	.3	.3	.3	.3	.3	.3	.3	.3	.3	.3	.3	.3	.3	.3	.3	.3	.3	.3	.3
.2	.2	.2	.2	.2	.2	.2	.2	.2	.2	.2	.2	.2	.2	.2	.2	.2	.2	.2	.2
.1	.1	.1	.1	.1	.1	.1	.1	.1	.1	.1	.1	.1	.1	.1	.1	.1	.1	.1	.1
97	97	97	97	97	97	97	97	97	97	97	97	97	97	97	97	97	97	97	97
.9	.9	.9	.9	.9	.9	.9	.9	.9	.9	.9	.9	.9	.9	.9	.9	.9	.9	.9	.9
16	17	18	19	20	21	22	23	24	25	26	27	28	29	30	31	32	33	34	35

Cervical Position: O: Open/Soft **C:** Closed/Firm

Fertility Chart

Month_____ Year_____ Last Month's cycle length_____ This cycle length_____

Cycle Day	1	2	3	4	5	6	7	8	9	10	11	12	13	14	15
Date															
Time Temp Taken															
	99	99	99	99	99	99	99	99	99	99	99	99	99	99	99
	.9	.9	.9	.9	.9	.9	.9	.9	.9	.9	.9	.9	.9	.9	.9
	.8	.8	.8	.8	.8	.8	.8	.8	.8	.8	.8	.8	.8	.8	.8
	.7	.7	.7	.7	.7	.7	.7	.7	.7	.7	.7	.7	.7	.7	.7
	.6	.6	.6	.6	.6	.6	.6	.6	.6	.6	.6	.6	.6	.6	.6
	.5	.5	.5	.5	.5	.5	.5	.5	.5	.5	.5	.5	.5	.5	.5
	.4	.4	.4	.4	.4	.4	.4	.4	.4	.4	.4	.4	.4	.4	.4
	.3	.3	.3	.3	.3	.3	.3	.3	.3	.3	.3	.3	.3	.3	.3
Basal Body	.2	.2	.2	.2	.2	.2	.2	.2	.2	.2	.2	.2	.2	.2	.2
Waking	.1	.1	.1	.1	.1	.1	.1	.1	.1	.1	.1	.1	.1	.1	.1
Temperature (°F)	98	98	98	98	98	98	98	98	98	98	98	98	98	98	98
	.9	.9	.9	.9	.9	.9	.9	.9	.9	.9	.9	.9	.9	.9	.9
	.8	.8	.8	.8	.8	.8	.8	.8	.8	.8	.8	.8	.8	.8	.8
	.7	.7	.7	.7	.7	.7	.7	.7	.7	.7	.7	.7	.7	.7	.7
	.6	.6	.6	.6	.6	.6	.6	.6	.6	.6	.6	.6	.6	.6	.6
	.5	.5	.5	.5	.5	.5	.5	.5	.5	.5	.5	.5	.5	.5	.5
	.4	.4	.4	.4	.4	.4	.4	.4	.4	.4	.4	.4	.4	.4	.4
	.3	.3	.3	.3	.3	.3	.3	.3	.3	.3	.3	.3	.3	.3	.3
	.2	.2	.2	.2	.2	.2	.2	.2	.2	.2	.2	.2	.2	.2	.2
	.1	.1	.1	.1	.1	.1	.1	.1	.1	.1	.1	.1	.1	.1	.1
	97	97	97	97	97	97	97	97	97	97	97	97	97	97	97
	.9	.9	.9	.9	.9	.9	.9	.9	.9	.9	.9	.9	.9	.9	.9
Cycle Day	1	2	3	4	5	6	7	8	9	10	11	12	13	14	15
Period/Spotting															
Cervical Mucus (CM) Consistency*															
Cervical Position**															
OPK/LH Surge															
Fertility Monitor															
Saliva Test															
Chloride-ion Surge															
Miscellaneous (travel, illness, stress, medication, change in schedule, late night, etc.)															
Intercourse															
HPT (pregnancy test)															

*Cervical Fluid Consistency: **D:** Dry **E:** Egg white/Slippery **S:** Sticky **C:** Creamy

Thoughts and feelings _____ | **Ways I relaxed this month** _____

16	17	18	19	20	21	22	23	24	25	26	27	28	29	30	31	32	33	34	35
99	99	99	99	99	99	99	99	99	99	99	99	99	99	99	99	99	99	99	99
.9	.9	.9	.9	.9	.9	.9	.9	.9	.9	.9	.9	.9	.9	.9	.9	.9	.9	.9	.9
.8	.8	.8	.8	.8	.8	.8	.8	.8	.8	.8	.8	.8	.8	.8	.8	.8	.8	.8	.8
.7	.7	.7	.7	.7	.7	.7	.7	.7	.7	.7	.7	.7	.7	.7	.7	.7	.7	.7	.7
.6	.6	.6	.6	.6	.6	.6	.6	.6	.6	.6	.6	.6	.6	.6	.6	.6	.6	.6	.6
.5	.5	.5	.5	.5	.5	.5	.5	.5	.5	.5	.5	.5	.5	.5	.5	.5	.5	.5	.5
.4	.4	.4	.4	.4	.4	.4	.4	.4	.4	.4	.4	.4	.4	.4	.4	.4	.4	.4	.4
.3	.3	.3	.3	.3	.3	.3	.3	.3	.3	.3	.3	.3	.3	.3	.3	.3	.3	.3	.3
.2	.2	.2	.2	.2	.2	.2	.2	.2	.2	.2	.2	.2	.2	.2	.2	.2	.2	.2	.2
.1	.1	.1	.1	.1	.1	.1	.1	.1	.1	.1	.1	.1	.1	.1	.1	.1	.1	.1	.1
98	98	98	98	98	98	98	98	98	98	98	98	98	98	98	98	98	98	98	98
.9	.9	.9	.9	.9	.9	.9	.9	.9	.9	.9	.9	.9	.9	.9	.9	.9	.9	.9	.9
.8	.8	.8	.8	.8	.8	.8	.8	.8	.8	.8	.8	.8	.8	.8	.8	.8	.8	.8	.8
.7	.7	.7	.7	.7	.7	.7	.7	.7	.7	.7	.7	.7	.7	.7	.7	.7	.7	.7	.7
.6	.6	.6	.6	.6	.6	.6	.6	.6	.6	.6	.6	.6	.6	.6	.6	.6	.6	.6	.6
.5	.5	.5	.5	.5	.5	.5	.5	.5	.5	.5	.5	.5	.5	.5	.5	.5	.5	.5	.5
.4	.4	.4	.4	.4	.4	.4	.4	.4	.4	.4	.4	.4	.4	.4	.4	.4	.4	.4	.4
.3	.3	.3	.3	.3	.3	.3	.3	.3	.3	.3	.3	.3	.3	.3	.3	.3	.3	.3	.3
.2	.2	.2	.2	.2	.2	.2	.2	.2	.2	.2	.2	.2	.2	.2	.2	.2	.2	.2	.2
.1	.1	.1	.1	.1	.1	.1	.1	.1	.1	.1	.1	.1	.1	.1	.1	.1	.1	.1	.1
97	97	97	97	97	97	97	97	97	97	97	97	97	97	97	97	97	97	97	97
.9	.9	.9	.9	.9	.9	.9	.9	.9	.9	.9	.9	.9	.9	.9	.9	.9	.9	.9	.9
16	**17**	**18**	**19**	**20**	**21**	**22**	**23**	**24**	**25**	**26**	**27**	**28**	**29**	**30**	**31**	**32**	**33**	**34**	**35**

Cervical Position: O: Open/Soft **C: Closed/Firm

Fertility Chart

Month_____ Year_____ Last Month's cycle length_____ This cycle length_____

Cycle Day	1	2	3	4	5	6	7	8	9	10	11	12	13	14	15
Date															
Time Temp Taken															
Basal Body Waking Temperature (°F)	99	99	99	99	99	99	99	99	99	99	99	99	99	99	99
	.9	.9	.9	.9	.9	.9	.9	.9	.9	.9	.9	.9	.9	.9	.9
	.8	.8	.8	.8	.8	.8	.8	.8	.8	.8	.8	.8	.8	.8	.8
	.7	.7	.7	.7	.7	.7	.7	.7	.7	.7	.7	.7	.7	.7	.7
	.6	.6	.6	.6	.6	.6	.6	.6	.6	.6	.6	.6	.6	.6	.6
	.5	.5	.5	.5	.5	.5	.5	.5	.5	.5	.5	.5	.5	.5	.5
	.4	.4	.4	.4	.4	.4	.4	.4	.4	.4	.4	.4	.4	.4	.4
	.3	.3	.3	.3	.3	.3	.3	.3	.3	.3	.3	.3	.3	.3	.3
	.2	.2	.2	.2	.2	.2	.2	.2	.2	.2	.2	.2	.2	.2	.2
	.1	.1	.1	.1	.1	.1	.1	.1	.1	.1	.1	.1	.1	.1	.1
	98	98	98	98	98	98	98	98	98	98	98	98	98	98	98
	.9	.9	.9	.9	.9	.9	.9	.9	.9	.9	.9	.9	.9	.9	.9
	.8	.8	.8	.8	.8	.8	.8	.8	.8	.8	.8	.8	.8	.8	.8
	.7	.7	.7	.7	.7	.7	.7	.7	.7	.7	.7	.7	.7	.7	.7
	.6	.6	.6	.6	.6	.6	.6	.6	.6	.6	.6	.6	.6	.6	.6
	.5	.5	.5	.5	.5	.5	.5	.5	.5	.5	.5	.5	.5	.5	.5
	.4	.4	.4	.4	.4	.4	.4	.4	.4	.4	.4	.4	.4	.4	.4
	.3	.3	.3	.3	.3	.3	.3	.3	.3	.3	.3	.3	.3	.3	.3
	.2	.2	.2	.2	.2	.2	.2	.2	.2	.2	.2	.2	.2	.2	.2
	.1	.1	.1	.1	.1	.1	.1	.1	.1	.1	.1	.1	.1	.1	.1
	97	97	97	97	97	97	97	97	97	97	97	97	97	97	97
	.9	.9	.9	.9	.9	.9	.9	.9	.9	.9	.9	.9	.9	.9	.9
Cycle Day	1	2	3	4	5	6	7	8	9	10	11	12	13	14	15
Period/Spotting															
Cervical Mucus (CM) Consistency*															
Cervical Position**															
OPK/LH Surge															
Fertility Monitor															
Saliva Test															
Chloride-ion Surge															
Miscellaneous (travel, illness, stress, medication, change in schedule, late night, etc.)															
Intercourse															
HPT (pregnancy test)															

*Cervical Fluid Consistency: **D:** Dry **E:** Egg white/Slippery **S:** Sticky **C:** Creamy

Thoughts and feelings _____ | Ways I relaxed this month _____

16	17	18	19	20	21	22	23	24	25	26	27	28	29	30	31	32	33	34	35
99	99	99	99	99	99	99	99	99	99	99	99	99	99	99	99	99	99	99	99
.9	.9	.9	.9	.9	.9	.9	.9	.9	.9	.9	.9	.9	.9	.9	.9	.9	.9	.9	.9
.8	.8	.8	.8	.8	.8	.8	.8	.8	.8	.8	.8	.8	.8	.8	.8	.8	.8	.8	.8
.7	.7	.7	.7	.7	.7	.7	.7	.7	.7	.7	.7	.7	.7	.7	.7	.7	.7	.7	.7
.6	.6	.6	.6	.6	.6	.6	.6	.6	.6	.6	.6	.6	.6	.6	.6	.6	.6	.6	.6
.5	.5	.5	.5	.5	.5	.5	.5	.5	.5	.5	.5	.5	.5	.5	.5	.5	.5	.5	.5
.4	.4	.4	.4	.4	.4	.4	.4	.4	.4	.4	.4	.4	.4	.4	.4	.4	.4	.4	.4
.3	.3	.3	.3	.3	.3	.3	.3	.3	.3	.3	.3	.3	.3	.3	.3	.3	.3	.3	.3
.2	.2	.2	.2	.2	.2	.2	.2	.2	.2	.2	.2	.2	.2	.2	.2	.2	.2	.2	.2
.1	.1	.1	.1	.1	.1	.1	.1	.1	.1	.1	.1	.1	.1	.1	.1	.1	.1	.1	.1
98	98	98	98	98	98	98	98	98	98	98	98	98	98	98	98	98	98	98	98
.9	.9	.9	.9	.9	.9	.9	.9	.9	.9	.9	.9	.9	.9	.9	.9	.9	.9	.9	.9
.8	.8	.8	.8	.8	.8	.8	.8	.8	.8	.8	.8	.8	.8	.8	.8	.8	.8	.8	.8
.7	.7	.7	.7	.7	.7	.7	.7	.7	.7	.7	.7	.7	.7	.7	.7	.7	.7	.7	.7
.6	.6	.6	.6	.6	.6	.6	.6	.6	.6	.6	.6	.6	.6	.6	.6	.6	.6	.6	.6
.5	.5	.5	.5	.5	.5	.5	.5	.5	.5	.5	.5	.5	.5	.5	.5	.5	.5	.5	.5
.4	.4	.4	.4	.4	.4	.4	.4	.4	.4	.4	.4	.4	.4	.4	.4	.4	.4	.4	.4
.3	.3	.3	.3	.3	.3	.3	.3	.3	.3	.3	.3	.3	.3	.3	.3	.3	.3	.3	.3
.2	.2	.2	.2	.2	.2	.2	.2	.2	.2	.2	.2	.2	.2	.2	.2	.2	.2	.2	.2
.1	.1	.1	.1	.1	.1	.1	.1	.1	.1	.1	.1	.1	.1	.1	.1	.1	.1	.1	.1
97	97	97	97	97	97	97	97	97	97	97	97	97	97	97	97	97	97	97	97
.9	.9	.9	.9	.9	.9	.9	.9	.9	.9	.9	.9	.9	.9	.9	.9	.9	.9	.9	.9
16	**17**	**18**	**19**	**20**	**21**	**22**	**23**	**24**	**25**	**26**	**27**	**28**	**29**	**30**	**31**	**32**	**33**	**34**	**35**

Cervical Position: O: Open/Soft **C:** Closed/Firm

Fertility Chart

Month_____ Year_____ Last Month's cycle length_____ This cycle length_____

Cycle Day	1	2	3	4	5	6	7	8	9	10	11	12	13	14	15
Date															
Time Temp Taken															
	99	99	99	99	99	99	99	99	99	99	99	99	99	99	99
	.9	.9	.9	.9	.9	.9	.9	.9	.9	.9	.9	.9	.9	.9	.9
	.8	.8	.8	.8	.8	.8	.8	.8	.8	.8	.8	.8	.8	.8	.8
	.7	.7	.7	.7	.7	.7	.7	.7	.7	.7	.7	.7	.7	.7	.7
	.6	.6	.6	.6	.6	.6	.6	.6	.6	.6	.6	.6	.6	.6	.6
	.5	.5	.5	.5	.5	.5	.5	.5	.5	.5	.5	.5	.5	.5	.5
	.4	.4	.4	.4	.4	.4	.4	.4	.4	.4	.4	.4	.4	.4	.4
	.3	.3	.3	.3	.3	.3	.3	.3	.3	.3	.3	.3	.3	.3	.3
Basal Body	.2	.2	.2	.2	.2	.2	.2	.2	.2	.2	.2	.2	.2	.2	.2
Waking	.1	.1	.1	.1	.1	.1	.1	.1	.1	.1	.1	.1	.1	.1	.1
Temperature (°F)	98	98	98	98	98	98	98	98	98	98	98	98	98	98	98
	.9	.9	.9	.9	.9	.9	.9	.9	.9	.9	.9	.9	.9	.9	.9
	.8	.8	.8	.8	.8	.8	.8	.8	.8	.8	.8	.8	.8	.8	.8
	.7	.7	.7	.7	.7	.7	.7	.7	.7	.7	.7	.7	.7	.7	.7
	.6	.6	.6	.6	.6	.6	.6	.6	.6	.6	.6	.6	.6	.6	.6
	.5	.5	.5	.5	.5	.5	.5	.5	.5	.5	.5	.5	.5	.5	.5
	.4	.4	.4	.4	.4	.4	.4	.4	.4	.4	.4	.4	.4	.4	.4
	.3	.3	.3	.3	.3	.3	.3	.3	.3	.3	.3	.3	.3	.3	.3
	.2	.2	.2	.2	.2	.2	.2	.2	.2	.2	.2	.2	.2	.2	.2
	.1	.1	.1	.1	.1	.1	.1	.1	.1	.1	.1	.1	.1	.1	.1
	97	97	97	97	97	97	97	97	97	97	97	97	97	97	97
	.9	.9	.9	.9	.9	.9	.9	.9	.9	.9	.9	.9	.9	.9	.9
Cycle Day	1	2	3	4	5	6	7	8	9	10	11	12	13	14	15
Period/Spotting															
Cervical Mucus (CM) Consistency*															
Cervical Position**															
OPK/LH Surge															
Fertility Monitor															
Saliva Test															
Chloride-ion Surge															
Miscellaneous (travel, illness, stress, medication, change in schedule, late night, etc.)															
Intercourse															
HPT (pregnancy test)															

*Cervical Fluid Consistency: **D:** Dry **E:** Egg white/Slippery **S:** Sticky **C:** Creamy

Thoughts and feelings _____ | **Ways I relaxed this month** _____

16	17	18	19	20	21	22	23	24	25	26	27	28	29	30	31	32	33	34	35
99	99	99	99	99	99	99	99	99	99	99	99	99	99	99	99	99	99	99	99
.9	.9	.9	.9	.9	.9	.9	.9	.9	.9	.9	.9	.9	.9	.9	.9	.9	.9	.9	.9
.8	.8	.8	.8	.8	.8	.8	.8	.8	.8	.8	.8	.8	.8	.8	.8	.8	.8	.8	.8
.7	.7	.7	.7	.7	.7	.7	.7	.7	.7	.7	.7	.7	.7	.7	.7	.7	.7	.7	.7
.6	.6	.6	.6	.6	.6	.6	.6	.6	.6	.6	.6	.6	.6	.6	.6	.6	.6	.6	.6
.5	.5	.5	.5	.5	.5	.5	.5	.5	.5	.5	.5	.5	.5	.5	.5	.5	.5	.5	.5
.4	.4	.4	.4	.4	.4	.4	.4	.4	.4	.4	.4	.4	.4	.4	.4	.4	.4	.4	.4
.3	.3	.3	.3	.3	.3	.3	.3	.3	.3	.3	.3	.3	.3	.3	.3	.3	.3	.3	.3
.2	.2	.2	.2	.2	.2	.2	.2	.2	.2	.2	.2	.2	.2	.2	.2	.2	.2	.2	.2
.1	.1	.1	.1	.1	.1	.1	.1	.1	.1	.1	.1	.1	.1	.1	.1	.1	.1	.1	.1
98	98	98	98	98	98	98	98	98	98	98	98	98	98	98	98	98	98	98	98
.9	.9	.9	.9	.9	.9	.9	.9	.9	.9	.9	.9	.9	.9	.9	.9	.9	.9	.9	.9
.8	.8	.8	.8	.8	.8	.8	.8	.8	.8	.8	.8	.8	.8	.8	.8	.8	.8	.8	.8
.7	.7	.7	.7	.7	.7	.7	.7	.7	.7	.7	.7	.7	.7	.7	.7	.7	.7	.7	.7
.6	.6	.6	.6	.6	.6	.6	.6	.6	.6	.6	.6	.6	.6	.6	.6	.6	.6	.6	.6
.5	.5	.5	.5	.5	.5	.5	.5	.5	.5	.5	.5	.5	.5	.5	.5	.5	.5	.5	.5
.4	.4	.4	.4	.4	.4	.4	.4	.4	.4	.4	.4	.4	.4	.4	.4	.4	.4	.4	.4
.3	.3	.3	.3	.3	.3	.3	.3	.3	.3	.3	.3	.3	.3	.3	.3	.3	.3	.3	.3
.2	.2	.2	.2	.2	.2	.2	.2	.2	.2	.2	.2	.2	.2	.2	.2	.2	.2	.2	.2
.1	.1	.1	.1	.1	.1	.1	.1	.1	.1	.1	.1	.1	.1	.1	.1	.1	.1	.1	.1
97	97	97	97	97	97	97	97	97	97	97	97	97	97	97	97	97	97	97	97
.9	.9	.9	.9	.9	.9	.9	.9	.9	.9	.9	.9	.9	.9	.9	.9	.9	.9	.9	.9
16	**17**	**18**	**19**	**20**	**21**	**22**	**23**	**24**	**25**	**26**	**27**	**28**	**29**	**30**	**31**	**32**	**33**	**34**	**35**

Cervical Position: O: Open/Soft **C:** Closed/Firm

Fertility Chart

Month_____ Year_____ Last Month's cycle length_____ This cycle length_____

Cycle Day	1	2	3	4	5	6	7	8	9	10	11	12	13	14	15
Date															
Time Temp Taken															
Basal Body Waking Temperature (°F)	99	99	99	99	99	99	99	99	99	99	99	99	99	99	99
	.9	.9	.9	.9	.9	.9	.9	.9	.9	.9	.9	.9	.9	.9	.9
	.8	.8	.8	.8	.8	.8	.8	.8	.8	.8	.8	.8	.8	.8	.8
	.7	.7	.7	.7	.7	.7	.7	.7	.7	.7	.7	.7	.7	.7	.7
	.6	.6	.6	.6	.6	.6	.6	.6	.6	.6	.6	.6	.6	.6	.6
	.5	.5	.5	.5	.5	.5	.5	.5	.5	.5	.5	.5	.5	.5	.5
	.4	.4	.4	.4	.4	.4	.4	.4	.4	.4	.4	.4	.4	.4	.4
	.3	.3	.3	.3	.3	.3	.3	.3	.3	.3	.3	.3	.3	.3	.3
	.2	.2	.2	.2	.2	.2	.2	.2	.2	.2	.2	.2	.2	.2	.2
	.1	.1	.1	.1	.1	.1	.1	.1	.1	.1	.1	.1	.1	.1	.1
	98	98	98	98	98	98	98	98	98	98	98	98	98	98	98
	.9	.9	.9	.9	.9	.9	.9	.9	.9	.9	.9	.9	.9	.9	.9
	.8	.8	.8	.8	.8	.8	.8	.8	.8	.8	.8	.8	.8	.8	.8
	.7	.7	.7	.7	.7	.7	.7	.7	.7	.7	.7	.7	.7	.7	.7
	.6	.6	.6	.6	.6	.6	.6	.6	.6	.6	.6	.6	.6	.6	.6
	.5	.5	.5	.5	.5	.5	.5	.5	.5	.5	.5	.5	.5	.5	.5
	.4	.4	.4	.4	.4	.4	.4	.4	.4	.4	.4	.4	.4	.4	.4
	.3	.3	.3	.3	.3	.3	.3	.3	.3	.3	.3	.3	.3	.3	.3
	.2	.2	.2	.2	.2	.2	.2	.2	.2	.2	.2	.2	.2	.2	.2
	.1	.1	.1	.1	.1	.1	.1	.1	.1	.1	.1	.1	.1	.1	.1
	97	97	97	97	97	97	97	97	97	97	97	97	97	97	97
	.9	.9	.9	.9	.9	.9	.9	.9	.9	.9	.9	.9	.9	.9	.9
Cycle Day	**1**	**2**	**3**	**4**	**5**	**6**	**7**	**8**	**9**	**10**	**11**	**12**	**13**	**14**	**15**
Period/Spotting															
Cervical Mucus (CM) Consistency*															
Cervical Position**															
OPK/LH Surge															
Fertility Monitor															
Saliva Test															
Chloride-ion Surge															
Miscellaneous (travel, illness, stress, medication, change in schedule, late night, etc.)															
Intercourse															
HPT (pregnancy test)															

*Cervical Fluid Consistency: **D:** Dry **E:** Egg white/Slippery **S:** Sticky **C:** Creamy

Thoughts and feelings _____ | **Ways I relaxed this month** _____

16	17	18	19	20	21	22	23	24	25	26	27	28	29	30	31	32	33	34	35
99	99	99	99	99	99	99	99	99	99	99	99	99	99	99	99	99	99	99	99
.9	.9	.9	.9	.9	.9	.9	.9	.9	.9	.9	.9	.9	.9	.9	.9	.9	.9	.9	.9
.8	.8	.8	.8	.8	.8	.8	.8	.8	.8	.8	.8	.8	.8	.8	.8	.8	.8	.8	.8
.7	.7	.7	.7	.7	.7	.7	.7	.7	.7	.7	.7	.7	.7	.7	.7	.7	.7	.7	.7
.6	.6	.6	.6	.6	.6	.6	.6	.6	.6	.6	.6	.6	.6	.6	.6	.6	.6	.6	.6
.5	.5	.5	.5	.5	.5	.5	.5	.5	.5	.5	.5	.5	.5	.5	.5	.5	.5	.5	.5
.4	.4	.4	.4	.4	.4	.4	.4	.4	.4	.4	.4	.4	.4	.4	.4	.4	.4	.4	.4
.3	.3	.3	.3	.3	.3	.3	.3	.3	.3	.3	.3	.3	.3	.3	.3	.3	.3	.3	.3
.2	.2	.2	.2	.2	.2	.2	.2	.2	.2	.2	.2	.2	.2	.2	.2	.2	.2	.2	.2
.1	.1	.1	.1	.1	.1	.1	.1	.1	.1	.1	.1	.1	.1	.1	.1	.1	.1	.1	.1
98	98	98	98	98	98	98	98	98	98	98	98	98	98	98	98	98	98	98	98
.9	.9	.9	.9	.9	.9	.9	.9	.9	.9	.9	.9	.9	.9	.9	.9	.9	.9	.9	.9
.8	.8	.8	.8	.8	.8	.8	.8	.8	.8	.8	.8	.8	.8	.8	.8	.8	.8	.8	.8
.7	.7	.7	.7	.7	.7	.7	.7	.7	.7	.7	.7	.7	.7	.7	.7	.7	.7	.7	.7
.6	.6	.6	.6	.6	.6	.6	.6	.6	.6	.6	.6	.6	.6	.6	.6	.6	.6	.6	.6
.5	.5	.5	.5	.5	.5	.5	.5	.5	.5	.5	.5	.5	.5	.5	.5	.5	.5	.5	.5
.4	.4	.4	.4	.4	.4	.4	.4	.4	.4	.4	.4	.4	.4	.4	.4	.4	.4	.4	.4
.3	.3	.3	.3	.3	.3	.3	.3	.3	.3	.3	.3	.3	.3	.3	.3	.3	.3	.3	.3
.2	.2	.2	.2	.2	.2	.2	.2	.2	.2	.2	.2	.2	.2	.2	.2	.2	.2	.2	.2
.1	.1	.1	.1	.1	.1	.1	.1	.1	.1	.1	.1	.1	.1	.1	.1	.1	.1	.1	.1
97	97	97	97	97	97	97	97	97	97	97	97	97	97	97	97	97	97	97	97
.9	.9	.9	.9	.9	.9	.9	.9	.9	.9	.9	.9	.9	.9	.9	.9	.9	.9	.9	.9
16	17	18	19	20	21	22	23	24	25	26	27	28	29	30	31	32	33	34	35

Cervical Position: O: Open/Soft **C:** Closed/Firm

Fertility Treatment Planner

Do your conception plans need a little push in the right direction from reproductive science? If so, you're probably going to have a lot more doctor appointments, medications, tests, and other treatments to keep track of. Use this fertility treatment planner to stay on top of it all.

Fertility Tests

Test _____

Date/Place _____

_____

Doctor _____

When/Where to call for results _____

_____

Results _____

_____

_____

Follow-up tests needed, if any _____

_____

Test _____

Date/Place _____

_____

Doctor _____

When/Where to call for results _____

_____

Results _____

_____

_____

Follow-up tests needed, if any _____

_____

Test _____

Date/Place _____

_____

Doctor _____

When/Where to call for results _____

_____

Results _____

_____

_____

Follow-up tests needed, if any _____

_____

Test _____

Date/Place _____

_____

Doctor _____

When/Where to call for results _____

_____

Results _____

_____

_____

Follow-up tests needed, if any _____

_____

Test _____

Date/Place _____

_____

Doctor _____

When/Where to call for results _____

_____

Results _____

_____

_____

Follow-up tests needed, if any _____

_____

Fertility Specialist Visits

Date _____

Doctor seen _____

Doctor's recommendations _____

_____

_____

_____

Date _____

Doctor seen _____

Doctor's recommendations _____

_____

_____

Date _____

Doctor seen _____

Doctor's recommendations _____

_____

_____

Date _____

Doctor seen _____

Doctor's recommendations _____

_____

_____

Date _____

Doctor seen _____

Doctor's recommendations _____

_____

_____

Date _____

Doctor seen _____

Doctor's recommendations _____

_____

_____

Date _____

Doctor seen _____

Doctor's recommendations _____

_____

_____

Date _____

Doctor seen _____

Doctor's recommendations _____

_____

_____

Date _____

Doctor seen _____

Doctor's recommendations _____

_____

_____

Date _____

Doctor seen _____

Doctor's recommendations _____

_____

_____

Fertility Medications

Name of medication/injection _____

_____

Amount to take _____ How to take _____

Time of day _____ For this long _____

NOTES: _____

_____

_____

Name of medication/injection _____

_____

Amount to take _____ How to take _____

Time of day _____ For this long _____

NOTES: _____

_____

_____

Name of medication/injection _____

_____

Amount to take _____ How to take _____

Time of day _____ For this long _____

NOTES: _____

_____

_____

Name of medication/injection _____

_____

Amount to take _____ How to take _____

Time of day _____ For this long _____

NOTES: _____

_____

_____

Name of medication/injection _____

Amount to take _____ How to take _____
Time of day _____ For this long _____
NOTES: _____
_____
_____

Name of medication/injection _____

Amount to take _____ How to take _____
Time of day _____ For this long _____
NOTES: _____
_____
_____

Name of medication/injection _____

Amount to take _____ How to take _____
Time of day _____ For this long _____
NOTES: _____
_____
_____

Name of medication/injection _____

Amount to take _____ How to take _____
Time of day _____ For this long _____
NOTES: _____
_____
_____

Fertility Procedures

Procedure _____

Date/Place _____

Doctor _____

Follow-up needed, if any _____

NOTES: _____

_____

_____

Procedure _____

Date/Place _____

Doctor _____

Follow-up needed, if any _____

NOTES: _____

_____

_____

Procedure _____

Date/Place _____

Doctor _____

Follow-up needed, if any _____

NOTES: _____

_____

_____

Procedure _____

Date/Place _____

Doctor _____

Follow-up needed, if any _____

NOTES: _____

_____

_____

Procedure _____

Date/Place _____

Doctor _____

Follow-up needed, if any _____

NOTES: _____

_____

_____

_____

Procedure _____

Date/Place _____

Doctor _____

Follow-up needed, if any _____

NOTES: _____

_____

_____

_____

Procedure _____

Date/Place _____

Doctor _____

Follow-up needed, if any _____

NOTES: _____

_____

_____

_____

Procedure _____

Date/Place _____

Doctor _____

Follow-up needed, if any _____

NOTES: _____

_____

_____

Contacts

General Practitioner (GP)

Name _____

Address _____

Telephone _____

Fax _____

E-mail _____

Gynaecologist (GYN)

Name _____

Address _____

Telephone _____

Fax _____

E-mail _____

Midwife

Name _____

Address _____

Telephone _____

Fax _____

E-mail _____

Reproductive Endocrinologist (RE)

Name _____

Address _____

Telephone _____

Fax _____

E-mail _____

Ultrasound Centre

Name _____

Address _____

Telephone _____

Fax _____

CAM Therapist

Name _____

Address _____

Telephone _____

Fax _____

E-mail _____

CAM Therapist

Name _____

Address _____

Telephone _____

Fax _____

E-mail _____

Therapist

Name _____

Address _____

Telephone _____

Fax _____

E-mail _____

NOTES: _____

_____

_____

_____

Other Specialist

Name _____

Address _____

Telephone _____

Fax _____

E-mail _____

Lab

Name _____

Address _____

Telephone _____

Fax _____

Hours _____

Pharmacy

Name _____

Address _____

Telephone _____

Fax _____

Hours _____

Insurance Company

Name _____

Address _____

Telephone _____

Fax _____

Website _____

NOTES: _____

_____

_____

Other Contacts

Name _____

Address _____

Telephone _____

Fax _____

E-mail _____

Name _____

Address _____

Telephone _____

Fax _____

E-mail _____

Name _____

Address _____

Telephone _____

Fax _____

E-mail _____

Name _____

Address _____

Telephone _____

Fax _____

E-mail _____

NOTES: _____

_____

_____

TTC Glossary

Spend a little time on those TTC message boards, and you'll soon discover that "TTC" is far from the only acronym used by those who are trying to conceive. Here's a short – though still pretty long – list of some of the acronyms you may encounter during your conception adventure. You may well come across others – and if you do, you can jot them down here so you can keep them straight:

2WW .... Two-Week Wait (until you can take a pregnancy test)
AF .... Aunt Flo(w), your period
BBT .... Basal Body Temperature
BD .... Baby Dance, sex
BFN .... Big Fat Negative (pregnancy test result)
BFP .... Big Fat Positive (pregnancy test result)
BMS .... Baby-Making Sex
CD .... Cycle Day
CF .... Cervical Fluid
CL .... Corpus Luteum
CM .... Cervical Mucus
CP .... Cervical Position
CY .... Cycle
DI .... Donor Insemination
DP .... "Dancing" Partner; spouse or significant other
DPO .... Days Past Ovulation
DTD .... Doing The Dance, sex
EW .... Egg White (re: consistency of cervical mucus)
FTTA .... Fertile Thoughts To All
FMU .... First Morning Urine
hCG .... Human Chorionic Gonadotropin (pregnancy hormone)
HPT .... Home Pregnancy Test
IF .... Infertility
IUI .... Intrauterine Insemination
IVF .... In Vitro Fertilization
LH .... Luteinizing Hormone
LMP .... Last Menstrual Period
LP .... Luteal Phase
O .... Ovulation
OPK .... Ovulation Predictor Kit
PCOS .... Polycystic Ovarian Syndrome
PG .... Pregnancy, Pregnant
S/A .... Sperm/Semen Analysis
TTC .... Trying To Conceive

Other TTC Terms

Your TTC Journal

Your feelings may be all over the emotional map while you're on your TTC journey – excited, hopeful, sometimes frustrated, often a little nervous. Whether you've just started out, or you've been on the road-to-baby for a while, use these pages to keep track of everything you're feeling, thinking, stressing about, and dreaming of.

Index

More from *What to Expect*®

What to Expect® When You're Expecting
The pregnancy guide that reassuringly answers the questions of mothers- and father-to-be, from the planning stage through postpartum.

"Like having a personal obstetrician to guide you . . . one who is wise but funny, thorough but practical, experienced but enthusiastic, organized but empathetic."
– Charles J. Lockwood, MD, Chair, Department of Obstetrics, Gynecology, and Reproductive Sciences, Yale University School of Medicine

□□□

What to Expect® the First Year
The reassuring and comprehensive month-by-month guide to child care in the first year.

"It delivers on its promise . . . Better than any current book on infant care."
– Mark D. Widome, MD, MPH, Professor of Pediatrics, The Penn State Children's Hospital

□□□

What to Expect® the Toddler Years
An all-inclusive guide for the parents of toddlers.

"This wonderful guide . . . is essential in every parent's library."
– Marian Wright Edelman, President and Founder of The Children's Defense Fund

□□□

What to Expect® Eating Well When You're Expecting
Everything you need to know to nourish a healthy pregnancy, including 175 delicious recipes.

"The recipes are delicious – and just right for today's mother-to-be."
– Sheila Lukins, Food Editor, *Parade*; co-author, *The New Basics and Silver Palate* cookbooks

□□□

What to Expect® Babysitter and Nanny Handbook
Everything a babysitter needs to know about caring for a child, from newborn to preschooler.

Expecting to Expect?

Join me on WhatToExpect.com!

TTC loves company – and support – and you'll find plenty of both on WhatToExpect.com, the interactive companion to the What to Expect® books. Join me and a whole online community of hopeful mums- (and dads-) to-be who know exactly what you're going through – friends to share the excitement and anticipation, the ups and downs, the twists and turns of the amazing journey from baby prep to baby making, pregnancy to parenthood.

Hope to see you on WhatToExpect.com, and may all your greatest expectations come true!

heidi